T0355218

The Self and its Disorders

The Self and its Disorders

SHAUN GALLAGHER

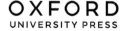
OXFORD
UNIVERSITY PRESS

OXFORD
UNIVERSITY PRESS

Great Clarendon Street, Oxford, OX2 6DP,
United Kingdom

Oxford University Press is a department of the University of Oxford.
It furthers the University's objective of excellence in research, scholarship,
and education by publishing worldwide. Oxford is a registered trade mark of
Oxford University Press in the UK and in certain other countries

Published in the United States of America by Oxford University Press
198 Madison Avenue, New York, NY 10016, United States of America

British Library Cataloguing in Publication Data
Data available

Library of Congress Control Number: 2023939206

ISBN 978-0-19-887306-8

DOI: 10.1093/oso/9780198873068.001.0001

Printed and bound by
CPI Group (UK) Ltd, Croydon, CR0 4YY

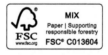

MIX
Paper | Supporting
responsible forestry
FSC® C013604

To my daughter Laura

Contents

Acknowledgments

This book has been helped along by numerous colleagues, including co-authors, conference audiences, and researchers who have commented on some of the material that make up the following chapters. Several of the chapters, in part, draw on some of my published papers, including papers co-authored with Yochai Ataria, Anya Daly, Josef Parnas, Laura Sparaci, Dylan Trigg, and Somogy Varga. Chapter 9 has been fully informed by some work that started (and continues) with a group of researchers at a workshop in 2019 at the Lorentz Center at the University of Leiden (I list those scholars in the first footnote in Section 9.1). I have also benefited from ongoing discussions with Albert Newen. My work was well supported by the Lillian and Morrie Moss Chair of Excellence at the University of Memphis, and a sabbatical in the pandemic year of 2021 allowed me to gather and refine these chapters. Research for Chapter 3 was supported by an Australian Research Council grant, led by Daniel Hutto: Minds in skilled performance (DP170102987), and my position as Professorial Fellow at the University of Wollongong. I also want to thank Antonino Raffone and the Psychology Department at the University of Rome-Sapienza for funding and hosting me as a visiting professor in the spring-summer of 2022, giving me the opportunity to finish my revisions of this book. As always, my wife Elaine has provided essential support, especially during our shared pandemic lock-down and our long therapeutic walks by the sea.

I thank Peter Momtchiloff at Oxford University Press for guiding this project to publication, and two anonymous reviewers who provided critical comments which led to an improved final product. I also need to thank numerous anonymous reviewers for their critical and helpful comments on earlier published papers that form the basis of some sections or chapters. I also thank the various journals for permission to include this material.

Chapter 1 is a revised and updated version of the 2013 paper "A pattern theory of self", *Frontiers in Human Neuroscience* 7(443): 1–7. doi: 10.3389/fnhum.2013.00443

Chapter 3 applies an approach developed in several papers, including:

Gallagher, S. (2022). Integration and causality in enactive approaches to psychiatry. *Frontiers in Psychiatry* 13: 870122. doi: 10.3389/fpsyt.2022.870122

Gallagher, S. and Varga, S. (2020). The meshed architecture of performance as a model of situated cognition. *Frontiers in Psychology* 11: 2140. doi:10.3389/fpsyg.2020.02140

Gallagher, S., Varga, S., and Sparaci, L. (2022). Disruptions of the meshed architecture in autism spectrum disorder. *Psychoanalytic Inquiry* 42(1): 76–95 doi.org/10.1080/07351690.2022.2007032.

Chapter 4 is a revised and updated version of Gallagher, S. and Daly, A. (2018). Dynamical relations in the self-pattern. *Frontiers in Psychology*, 9: 664. doi: 10.3389/fpsyg.2018.00664.

Section 6.5 draws from Gallagher, S. and Trigg, D. (2016). Agency and anxiety: Delusions of control and loss of control in schizophrenia and agoraphobia. *Frontiers in Neuroscience* 10: 459. doi: 10.3389/fnhum.2016.00459.

Chapter 7 includes a significantly revised version of Gallagher, S. (2021). Deep brain stimulation, self and relational autonomy. *Neuroethics* 14(1): 31–43. doi: 10.1007/s12152-018-9355-x. [with permission]; and a significantly revised version of Gallagher, S. (2018). The therapeutic reconstruction of affordances. *Res Philosophica* 95(4): 719–36.

Sections in Chapter 10 draw from: Ataria, Y. and Gallagher, S. (2015). Somatic apathy: Body disownership in the context of torture. *Journal of Phenomenological Psychology* 46(1): 105–22; and Gallagher, S. (2014). The cruel and unusual phenomenology of solitary confinement. *Frontiers in Psychology* 5: 585. doi: 10.3389/fpsyg.2014.00585.

List of Figures

List of Tables

Introduction

In 1937 John Dewey addressed the College of Physicians in St. Louis, advising them not to limit their treatment just to the body: "we must observe and understand internal processes and their interactions from the standpoint of their interactions with what is going on outside the skin." That is, we cannot understand bodily processes in isolation from the environment—an environment that is both physical and social. Rather, in the practice of medicine,

> we need to recover from the impression, now widespread, that the essential problem is solved when chemical, immunological, physiological, and anatomical knowledge is sufficiently obtained. We cannot understand and employ this knowledge until it is placed integrally in the context of what human beings do to one another in the vast variety of their contacts and associations.... A sound human being is a sound human environment.   (Dewey 1937, 54)

Forty years later, in his 1977 article introducing the biopsychosocial model, George Engel quoted Arnold Ludwig: "Psychiatry has become a hodgepodge of unscientific opinions, assorted philosophies and 'schools of thought,' mixed metaphors, role diffusion, propaganda, and politicking for 'mental health' and other esoteric goals" (Ludwig 1975, 60; cited in Engel 1977, 129). Engel was proposing a general systems approach to address such issues, and to reorder the work of psychiatry, and medicine more generally. Forty years after Dewey's lecture Engel was still seeking this more expansive or integrative idea of medicine as it pertained to psychiatry. Now, over forty years after Engel made his proposal, theorists are still wrestling with these issues (see, e.g., Syme & Hagen 2020).

For example, clearly counter to Engel's proposal for a biopsychosocial approach, there continues to be a strong movement toward transforming psychiatry into neuropsychiatry, despite the fact that there is no clear consensus about how precisely neurotransmitters or neuronal processes, or the pharmaceutical treatments that modify them, actually work. Furthermore, although multiple approaches to psychotherapy seemingly can claim success, there is a lack of understanding why such disparate methods (cognitive-behavioral versus psychoanalysis versus group versus movement and dance versus play versus narrative versus mindfulness approaches, to name a few) seem to work, or which of them should be preferred for any specific condition. As James Phillips puts it: "We really don't know why and how psychotherapy works" (2013, 193). Finally, as

The Self and its Disorders. Shaun Gallagher, Oxford University Press. © Shaun Gallagher 2024.
DOI: 10.1093/oso/9780198873068.003.0001

indicated in part by the increasing tendency to talk about spectrum disorders, problems about how to categorize psychiatric disorders and how to understand comorbidities have persisted for over a hundred years of theoretical debate.

To the extent that psychiatry is based on a particular understanding of the mind—of what the mind is and how it operates—psychiatric practice is never independent of epistemological and metaphysical assumptions. In a paper published in 2015, Josef Parnas and I pointed to a growing consensus that standard cognitivist or computational models of the mind, along with the most scientific explanations of mental disorders, underpinned by the latest theories of genes, neural processes, neurotransmitters, and cognitive modules, have simply failed to give us a good understanding of psychiatric conditions (Andreasen 2007; Legault, Bourdon & Poirier 2019). Pursuing these dominant models we end up at best with many unanswered questions, and, even worse, with mischaracterizations of the relevant phenomena.

In philosophical and psychiatric contexts, however, neither mind nor the conception of disorder is what it used to be. In the following chapters I propose, first, to rethink these notions in light of embodied and enactive models, or more generally, what has been called 4E cognition.[1] If we take seriously the idea that the mind is *embodied, embedded, extended*, and *enactive*, then we need to understand notions of mind and self in a way not captured by Cartesian-Lockean-Humean philosophies, or by contemporary cognitivist, internalist views. And if this is so, then, second, we also need to reframe the notion of psychiatric disorder or deficit.

In this book I develop an interdisciplinary perspective that follows in the spirit of what numerous authors have been calling an "integrative" perspective in psychiatry (Constant et al. 2022; Gerrans 2014; Maiese 2021; Sass et al. 2018; de Haan 2020). Engel's biopsychosocial model is an example of such an integrative approach (Engel 1977; 1980; Bolton & Gillett 2019). The scope of such integrative approaches, and specific frameworks for understanding integration vary, however (Maung 2021). Phillip Gerrans (2014), in his book on delusions, proposes a relatively narrow account of the "cognitive architecture" of delusions by integrating elements that are neuronal and phenomenological, with narrative generated in the brain's default mode network.[2] Even for delusions, but even more for the vast

---

[1] Enactive approaches to cognition emphasize the continuity between life and mind, and the action-oriented nature of perception and cognition (see Varela, Thompson & Rosch 1991; Gallagher 2017a). On such an approach, persons are agents understood as "precarious, self-constituted entities in ongoing historical development and capable of incorporating different sources of normativity, a world-involving process that is co-defined with their environment across multiple spatiotemporal scales and together with other agents" (Di Paolo, Thompson & Beer 2022, 3; also see Newen et al. 2018).

[2] The term "narrow" (versus "wide") is a term of art in philosophy of mind, signifying cognitive processes that are in the intra-cranial mind, the brain, or "in the head." "Wide" signifies the involvement of extra-neural, embodied, and ecological processes. Gerrans (2022), for example, provides a narrow account of addiction framed in terms of the way the self "is represented at multiple levels and in different representational formats" in the brain. Constant et al. (2022), in contrast, take a wide perspective that includes evolutionary, cultural, and computational processes, and frames the integration in terms of an integration of these different approaches.

variety of psychopathological phenomena, I'll argue that one needs to go wider and to scale out to include phenomena discussed in 4E approaches to cognition. Louis Sass et al. (2018) come closer to this view, combining phenomenological, social, and neurobiological factors; and Sanneke de Haan (2020) deepens this analysis by adding what she terms "existentialist" or self-relating dimensions. My approach aligns well with the integrative models proposed by Sass and de Haan, and especially with the latter's emphasis on the enactive perspective. Although our starting points and analyses differ, our conclusions end up closely aligned.

Mainstream psychiatry is characterized by a number of different approaches, including the integrative biopsychosocial model, but the most dominant approach is bio-reductionism or the medical model, which attempts to characterize disorders in terms of underlying (biological) mechanisms (Constant et al. 2022), most often characterizing psychiatric disorders as "brain circuit disorders" (Insel & Cuthbert 2015). This approach is exemplified by the continuing DSM reform and the recent development of the Research Domain Criteria (RDoC), which focuses on neuroscience. As Constant et al. (2022, 6) point out, the RDoC relies heavily on animal models, even though, "we have no animal models of many distinctive components of human experiences relevant to mental health and illness, such as narrativity, morality, racism, political violence" (also Baran 2019). In general, the mainstream approach tends to adopt two assumptions: the first, epistemological, namely, an explicit neo-positivist or behaviorist form of operationalism; the second, an implicit metaphysical position, namely physicalism (Parnas & Gallagher 2015). In this framework psychiatric symptoms and signs are defined from a third-person perspective, often in a context-independent way, and sometimes as reified (thing-like), mutually independent or atomic entities, without intrinsic meaning. This model, as Dewey was suggesting, isn't even adequate to the practice of somatic medicine.

In contrast, if we think of our human form of existence as embodied, enactively engaged, and environmentally embedded—and if we think that illness is a "complete form of existence," as Merleau-Ponty (1963, 107) suggests—then it's misleading to think of illness simply as something that happens in a brain or to an objective body—a purely physiological condition. More positively, the challenge is to develop a theoretical framework that will help to characterize the more complete picture (the positives as well as the negatives) of how the patient's *life* is different—a framework that supports both the concept of a *rich* diagnosis (Parnas & Gallagher 2015) and the kind of psychiatric practice needed to get such a rich diagnosis. The challenge, I'll argue, is to understand the human *system* of brain-body-environment as a dynamical *gestalt*.[3]

---

[3] The concept of a "psychopathological gestalt" has been proposed by Parnas (2012), who traces the concept back to Jaspers, who describes it as follows: "All research differentiates, separates, and studies individual particulars in which it tries to discover certain general laws. Yet all these individual particulars are taken out from what is in reality a complex unity. In grasping particulars, we make a mistake

On this view, a patient manifests not isolated *symptom-referents* but rather particular wholes of intertwined experiences, feelings, beliefs, expressions, actions, and social interactions, all of them permeated by the patient's embodied, habitual dispositions and by biographical (and not just biological) detail. A particular behavior or a particular feeling may be interpreted as a psychiatric symptom, but not in isolation from other factors or processes that belong to a synchronic context and a diachronic flow of self-related experiences and expressions.

If, in contrast to the dominant models, a 4E approach (or specifically an enactive approach) allows for a re-conceptualization of mind, brain, body, and environment, it should also allow us to think differently about how these notions play into psychiatric disorders. This in turn would suggest a different understanding of therapeutic interventions. In other words, if we think of mind and self-related phenomena and processes as distributed in a relational fashion across brain, body and (physical, social, and cultural) environment, then we may be able to understand why changes in any of these factors could push the system one way or another.

The broad hypothesis that I'll develop in this book is that psychiatric disorders are self-disorders. Although this is not a new hypothesis, I'll pursue it within a 4E, and especially, enactivist framework, and in a way that is non-reductionistic. The hypothesis extends the claim made by phenomenological psychiatrists about schizophrenia, namely, that schizophrenia is a disturbance affecting a very basic sense of self (Sass & Parnas 2003). Because the term "self-disturbance" can involve a variety of meanings, however, caution is required at this starting point. Sass and Parnas specify that by "self-disturbance" they mean disturbance in the basic sense of ipseity (sometimes referred to as the "minimal self"). Ipseity involves an intrinsic prereflective self-awareness, which, according to phenomenologists, generates a sense of "mineness," or "sense of ownership" (Gallagher & Zahavi 2021). As I am conscious of some object or event, at the same time, and as an intrinsic aspect of the same consciousness, I'm aware that *I* am experiencing it—that it is *my* experience. With this concept one is already broaching a set of controversies about the nature of the self, and about the nature of schizophrenia. One can ask, for example, does a focus on self or ipseity exclude other factors that may involve embodied, non-conscious processes or social–intersubjective relations. Doesn't schizophrenia (not to mention other disorders) also involve problems that have to do with cognitive function, behavior, social relations, and many other self-related aspects that seem to go beyond the concept of ipseity? Accordingly, to say that psychiatric disorders are self-disorders, *simpliciter*, seems an over-simplification.

Part of my task in this book is to resolve some of these issues. Indeed, from a philosophical perspective, any claim to explain something called "the self" immediately raises a host of problems. On the one hand, although many philosophers

---

if we forget the comprehensive whole in which and through which they exist. This [whole] never becomes the direct object of our study, but only does so *via* the particulars" (Jaspers 1997, 28).

and psychiatrists, as well as other theorists, are perfectly comfortable talking about "the self," when we push on what this concept actually means, almost any definition will be controversial. For example, that the self is socially constructed, and is nothing other than that construction (Gergen 2011); or that it is a product of narrative (Schechtman 2011), and nothing more; or that the self is strictly minimal, enduring at best for about three seconds before another self takes its place, and nothing more than that (Strawson 1997); or that the self is really a self-model generated by neuronal processes, but in itself isn't anything real (Metzinger 2004). These kinds of deflationary or reductionist accounts tend to be reactions against the traditional Cartesian notion of the self, understood as a substantial (soul-like) entity. That traditional conception has been challenged since the time of John Locke and David Hume, as well as in much more ancient traditions like Buddhism, and more recently through appeal to neuroscience.

On the other hand, and pursuing a different strategy, some philosophers prefer to avoid the phrase "the self" by pluralizing it with important modifiers. We thus find a multitude of variations, cataloged by Galen Strawson (1999, 100) as follows:

> [T]he cognitive self, the conceptual self, the contextualized self, the core self, the dialogic self, the ecological self, the embodied self, the emergent self, the empirical self, the existential self, the extended self, the fictional self, the full-grown self, the interpersonal self, the material self, the narrative self, the philosophical self, the physical self, the private self, the representational self, the rock bottom essential self, the semiotic self, the social self, the transparent self, and the verbal self.

Trying to improve on this list by addition or elimination would likely lead to terminological nitpicking, but from a neuroscientific perspective, we should add "the neural self" or "the synaptic self" (LeDoux 2002); or, with reference to self-referential processes in the cortical midline structures of the brain, what we might call "the midline self" (Northoff & Bermpohl 2004). Such a list could easily motivate the following question: "Which is it?"—which one is *the* self? Or perhaps, which one is the primary meaning of self? Or psychologists might ask: "Which is the authentic self?"

It's not clear, however, that one has to choose just one variation. Many of these concepts of self were developed in the plural. William James (1890), for example, distinguished between the physical self, the social self, and the private self, and all of them are part of what it means to be human. Continuing in this vein, Ulrich Neisser (1988) discussed five types of self-knowledge corresponding to the ecological self, the interpersonal self, the conceptual self, the extended self, and the private self. Despite the terminology suggesting a plurality of selves, however, Neisser (1991) carefully refers to them as *aspects* of self—e.g., the ecological aspect of self.

In this book I propose to defend a pluralist concept of self. I'll argue, in agreement with Neisser, that we should not think of these aspects as multiple selves; furthermore, we should not think of such aspects as aspects *of* "the self," as if they are simply modifying something that has its own independent existence. Rather, I propose that we think of these aspects as variable factors or processes that are organized in a certain pattern, and that what we call the self just is this pattern, and its possible variations. The self is not some entity, or some property of an entity; it's a pattern composed of processes, or more roughly, factors, elements, aspects, or variables—I'll use these terms interchangeably. In the following chapters I'll try to make this idea clear, and I'll try to indicate some advantages to thinking of self, or the *self-pattern*, in this way, especially in the context of psychopathology. In this regard, then, the broad claim that psychiatric disorders are self-disorders goes beyond any narrow conception of self, including just ipseity.

I've previously edited two interdisciplinary collections of essays on the topic of self. The first, *Models of the Self*, co-edited with Jonathan Shear, was published in 1999. The second, *The Oxford Handbook of the Self*, was published in 2011. In the introductions to each of these volumes I concluded with similar statements, and I think it is worthwhile repeating the same thing again here. The concept of self is a complex one. For that reason, one finds different and not necessarily commensurable characterizations of the self, depending on whether one is approaching it via introspection, phenomenological analysis, linguistic analysis, philosophical thought experiments, empirical experiments in psychology or cognitive science, developmental studies, psychopathology, or in ethical, social, or political analyses—methods and disciplines that operate on a variety of different assumptions. For this reason, taking an interdisciplinary approach can be problematic. One should not expect a neat triangulation. One is not always certain whether different characterizations of the self signify diverse aspects of some unitary phenomenon, or whether they pick out different and unrelated phenomena. At the same time, taking an interdisciplinary approach can be productive since we find a rich collection of insights that help us realize the complexity of the subject matter.

The first part of this book focuses on developing the concept of self-pattern, explaining what a pattern is, what is included in the self-pattern, how to deal with issues concerning coherence or identity, and how it relates to psychopathology. The second part includes further discussion of psychopathology and related therapeutic approaches, and some closely related issues that touch on a diversity of topics, such as AI and artificial enhancements, meditation practices, and the effects of torture and solitary confinement.

Before moving on to considerations about the self-pattern, however, I want to note that this wide integrative approach holds some implications for the issue of nosological classification in psychiatry. In 2017 I participated in a conference at the University of Freiberg on neurotechnological interventions in psycho- and neuropathologies. I presented a version of Chapter 7 in this book, asking how deep brain stimulation might affect the self-pattern. During some follow-up discussion it was suggested that the notion of the self-pattern could be the basis for rethinking the nosology of psychological disorders. I agreed with the general idea at that time; indeed, I was vaguely thinking along this line of specifying disorders in terms of typical correlating changes in self-patterns. Since that time, however, I've come to doubt the value or practicality of working out anything like a unique general nosology. My reasoning is connected with the complexity I've mentioned, and the requirement of using an interdisciplinary approach. These are issues that pertain more to hermeneutics and the philosophy of science, but let me say something briefly here to indicate why I am a nosological skeptic.

We can start by thinking of the project taken up by Emil Kraepelin near the turn of the twentieth century. In part, his project included a nosological classification of psychiatric disorders. As Stephan Heckers and Kenneth Kendler (2020) have indicated in an excellent historical survey of Kraepelin's project, his work underwent numerous transformations across the eight editions of his *Psychiatrie* textbook published between 1883 and 1913. One of his driving principles involved a rationalist-realist conception of convergence on what can be considered "a fact of the matter." He proposed an optimistic principle not unlike that found in the rational hermeneutics of someone like Chladenius (1752). Chladenius's famous example was a battlefield that, when described by different agents from different perspectives, seemingly yielded contradictory accounts. According to Chladenius, since there was only one battle, one fact of the matter, reason would be able to adjudicate the different reports of what actually happened in order to arrive a coherent story. The same idea is found in Kraepelin (1887) who proposes to combine the perspectives of anatomy, etiology, and symptomatology to define a particular illness. In the second edition of his textbook he writes:

> Were we to be in possession of a thorough and exhaustive knowledge of all details in one of the three fields, namely pathological anatomy, etiology or symptomatology of insanity, not only would each of them allow a uniform and thorough division of the psychoses, but each of these three groups would also—this requirement is the cornerstone of all scientific research—coincide substantially with the other two.
>
> (Kraepelin 1887, 211; translated A. Klee in Heckers & Kendler 2020, 382)[4]

---

[4] In the final edition we find a similar statement: "If we achieve the goal we have in mind, the recognition of the actual disease processes by means of our clinical descriptions, then the different delineation efforts, whether they occur from a pathological, anatomical, etiological or a purely clinical standpoint, have to finally coincide with each other. I view this requirement as the keystone for the scientific research of mental disturbances" (Kraepelin 1910, 14; translated by A. Klee in Heckers & Kendler 2020, 384).

According to Heckers and Kendler this remains a principle of current nosology, and today is typically considered to be governed by neuroscience: "[V]alidators will [ultimately] converge and psychiatric disorders will be defined at the level of the brain. . . . Researchers might start from very different vantage points, but their results will converge" (2020, 382–3). Kraepelin, however, also acknowledged the importance of attending to the natural course or development of the illness (the *natürliche Krankheitsvorgänge*), and being able to predict the general fate of the patient, as a way to get beyond what is sometimes the "baffling similarity" of symptoms in different disorders (Kraepelin 1893, 243).[5] Jaspers recognized Kraepelin's idea of convergence (toward a pure syndrome, or a unitary disease [*Krankheitsformen*]) as a Kantian ideal—that is, a piece of ideal theory that might guide diagnosis, but not an end that could be actually achieved (see Ghaemi 2009; Walker 2014).

Nassir Ghaemi (2009) makes clear the connections between Kraepelian nosology, the rise of psychopharmacology in the mid-twentieth century, and the DSM-3 (1980). On the one hand, a medicalization of psychiatry points to a determination of disease by etiology; on the other hand, for psychiatric disorders, etiology is often uncertain. The DSM-3 could not limit itself to etiology, and so it introduced other factors to guide diagnosis. The focus is meant to be the individual, not the disease, although subjective experience is still not adequately considered (on this point, Ghaemi cites Klerman et al. 1984). Moreover, for the clinician the point cannot be just diagnosis according to a classification (followed by automatic prescription of medication), but rather the use of clinical reasoning. A symptom is something to be interpreted—a sign that points to a set of disturbed processes.

On the one hand, Jaspers recognized the failure of Kraepelin's project:

> There has been no fulfillment of the hope that clinical observation of psychic phenomena, of the life-history and of the outcome might yield characteristic groupings which would subsequently be confirmed in the cerebral findings, and thus pave the way for the brain-anatomists. . . . The original question: are there only stages and variants of one unitary psychosis or is there a series of disease-entities which we can delineate, now finds its answer: there are neither.
>
> (Jaspers 1997, 568, 570)

He warns, "The chaos of phenomena should not be blotted out with some diagnostic label but bring illumination through the way it is systematically ordered and related" (1997, 20). On the other hand, as Ghaemi points out, Jaspers does

---

[5] In contrast to Gerrans, who interprets Kraepelin as a neuro-eliminativist, that is, someone who would reduce psychological symptoms to neuropathologies (2014, 13), Heckers and Kendler (2020, 386) argue that Kraepelin recognized that psychological states cannot be reduced to neural states.

provide a "classification scheme, heavily influenced by Kraepelin, remarkably similar to the nosology [of] DSM-III and ICD-9" (2009, 4). In effect, Jaspers provides an "ideal schema" (a Kantian ideal) that may in fact be a useful fiction, along with the caution that we need to face up to the idea that we will likely not resolve the different perspectives offered by just those disciplines Kraepelin listed: etiological studies, psychological structure, anatomical findings, and the course of illness.

Heckers and Kendler (2020, 386), provide the most recent update: "We are still searching for the best avenue to make progress in the nosology of psychiatric disorders" (see Jablensky 2016). Likewise, Clark et al. (2017), reviewing issues that pertain to etiology, discrete versus multi-dimensional classifications, boundary thresholds between disorder and non-disorder, and comorbidity in the DSM-5, the ICD-11, and the National Institute of Mental Health's Research Domain Criteria (RDoC), suggest that these classificatory systems remain "rudimentary" (also see Dalgleish et al. 2020; Syme and Hagen 2020).

What motivates my nosological skepticism is what Jaspers calls the "chaos of phenomena," which includes what Kraepelin calls the "baffling similarity" of symptoms in different disorders. That's what we find when we look straight-on at the clinical phenomena.[6] More theoretically, the issue is closely tied to questions about what we mean by mental disorder (Varga 2015). It's also an issue that involves who the practical consumer of the classificatory system is, since one classification that may serve clinical purposes doesn't necessarily serve research, legal, public welfare, or insurance administrative purposes (see Fulford & Sartorius 2009). De Haan also makes this very clear in her description of the contrast between clinical discussions about the everyday life of patients and scientific meetings where discussions are primarily about brains (2020, ix).

As Jaspers puts it, "It is difficult to bring diagnostic order…into shifting phenomena which continually keep merging into one another" (1997, 32). In the terms developed in the following chapters, the additional complication with finding order within disorder involves the dynamical integration, and the various overlapping modulations that can take place among some or all of the different variable processes or factors that come to constitute any self-pattern.[7] Symptoms

---

[6] As we'll discuss in Chapter 4, there is symptom overlap even when there is not a question of comorbidity. Thus, for example, studies using the Examination of Anomalous Self-Experience (EASE) found a significant number of symptoms similar to schizophrenia in cases diagnosed as depersonalization and panic disorder (Sass et al. 2013; Madeira et al. 2017; Værnes, Røssberg & Møller 2018; also see Sass & Pienkos 2013). As Sass et al. (2017, 10) suggest, "[M]utations of worldly experience (like mutations of ipseity or basic self-experience) typically have an overall or holistic character that defies ready operationalization into distinct features or factors." Such issues come to the fore in attempts to sort out something like the relationship between PTSD and dissociative disorders (see, e.g., Wabnitz, Gast & Catani 2013).

[7] As we'll see, the issue concerns the fact that the processes that make up the self-pattern are distributed across different temporal and spatial scales (e.g., brain, individual embodied agent, social environment). Even if we were to limit our analysis to brain dynamics we find difficulty in sorting

are not uniquely determined by a clear-cut disease process. Rather, they emerge and take shape in the dynamical organization or re-organization of the patient's self-pattern. Changes or disturbances in one process can be inextricably related to changes in other factors in the self-pattern, thereby transforming the self-pattern over the course of the illness. Symptoms are not static, nor do they form static and comorbid clusters. As signs, they reflect different orders and disorders in the self-pattern which, as Jaspers suggests, we should not try to blot out with some diag-nostic label.

To be more precise, what I hope to make clear is that a disruption of some process in the self-pattern is not simply a sign or symptom of a disorder; it is the disorder. In this regard, we should reject both strict naturalism, which claims a disorder to be a natural kind (some essential thing that exists independently of the subject's experience or social context), and any loose relativism that would hold it to be a mere socially constructed interpretation.

One can easily acknowledge that the concept of symptom has played a central role in psychiatry. But what precisely is a symptom? Denny Borsboom (2017) points out that the use of the term in psychiatry derives from the medical-biological concept:

> [T]he problems found in clinical practice have been categorized as symptoms, as exemplified in diagnostic manuals like the DSM-5 and ICD-10. Via the analogy with medical work, this use of the word 'symptom' suggests the presence of a 'disease', and this provides a suggestive answer to the question of why some people suffer from certain sets of symptoms, while others do not; namely, because they have particular kinds of diseases, to wit, mental disorders.   (2017, 5)

Borsboom goes on to explain an essential difference with respect to etiology between mental disorders and somatic diseases. He offers the example of a can-cerous lung tumor which causes the patient to cough, and to experience pain and shortness of breath. The tumor causes the symptoms that the observant physician uses to diagnose the disease. Although one might say that lung cancer causes the symptoms, that's an abstract way of putting it, since the physical tumor is the causal mechanism, the common cause that causes the symptoms. The cough, the pain, and the shortness of breath are real, existing physical things, but they are only symptoms when they are interpreted as such by an observer. There is a

---

things out. As Andreas Engel and colleagues indicate, "cognitive and physiological dysfunctions are present throughout the cortex in schizophrenia. This raises the problem of which mechanisms can account for such a distributed impairment. One possible implication of this finding could be that core deficits in schizophrenia arise out of the altered global dynamics....Accordingly, one strategy is to identify global coordination dynamics failures in schizophrenia" (Engel et al. 2010, 297). It turns out, however, that several disorders involve alterations in neural synchrony, so there remains the question of diagnostic specificity. Comorbid overlapping is still an issue even in the circumscribed framework of neuroscience.

specific etiology such that the physician doesn't cure the cancer by treating the symptoms—cough medication to treat the cough, pain medication to treat the pain, and so forth—rather, the physician cures the cancer by treating the tumor, which, in turn, relieves the symptoms. Lung cancer isn't just a collection of symptoms—it's the condition of having a tumor. In contrast, Borsboom suggests, a mental disorder refers to "a syndromic constellation of symptoms that hang together empirically, often for unknown reasons" (2017, 5). Etiology remains elusive, despite explanations that highlight brain processes.

Having said all of that, like everyone else I've just discussed, I won't be able to avoid referring to schizophrenia, or thinking that it is somewhat different from depression and other disorders. Nor will I try to avoid talking about what may be viewed as typical symptoms even if they manifest in different ways in different patients. My caution is simply to say that we should not expect that by characterizing different self-patterns we are offering a novel classification system for psychiatric disorders.

1

A Pattern Theory of Self

In this chapter I'll outline what I've called a pattern theory of self, which is a pluralist approach to questions about the self, following in the tradition of William
James (1890). I'll explain what I mean by a self-pattern, along with some background to the notion of a pattern theory. I'll then specify in some detail the various factors or processes involved in the self-pattern. I'll also consider some
philosophical issues and, finally, propose what I take to be some benefits of thinking of the problem in this way. In Chapter 2 I'll dig deeper into the question of
what a pattern is.

1.1 Pattern Theories

Although there are various theories or kinds of theories that have been referred to
as "pattern theories," in mathematics, for example (Grenanderm 1994), or in
studies of pain (Goldscheider 1894; Sinclair 1955), the notion of a pattern theory
of self, as I'll propose it, is inspired by two other, more recent, theories. The first
involves what we can call a pattern theory of emotion. This theory is a good one
to start with for two reasons: (1) it reflects a concept of pattern that is commensurable to the notion of a self-pattern, and (2) it contributes directly to the notion
of a self-pattern since, as I'll argue, *affect* or *affectivity* is one aspect that forms
part of the self-pattern. The second theory is Scott Kelso's dynamic patterns theory (Kelso 1995). Although Kelso's work is focused on more basic processes, it is
directly related to a pattern theory of self insofar as for Kelso a pattern is composed not only of various factors or processes, but also of their dynamical relations. That the same dynamical principles can be applied across numerous
phenomena, from brain processes to social processes, is made clear by Kelso and
his colleagues (e.g., Tognoli, Zhang & Kelso 2018; also Tognoli et al. 2020). I'll
discuss the dynamic pattern theory in Chapter 2, where it will help to head-off
some objections that consider patterns to be static arrangements, or simply a collection of elements. More generally, it will allow us to go into more depth in
regard to the concept of pattern and how it works.

The pattern theory of emotion claims that emotions are complex patterns of
bodily processes, experiences, expressions, behaviors, and actions—all of these
being factors that can make up an emotion-pattern. As such, emotions are indi-
viduated in patterns of characteristic features (Izard et al. 1972; Izard et al. 2000;

The Self and its Disorders. Shaun Gallagher, Oxford University Press. © Shaun Gallagher 2024.
DOI: 10.1093/oso/9780198873068.003.0002

Luhrmann 2006; Newen, Welpinghus & Juckel 2015). No one factor is sufficient, but taken together, a certain pattern of characteristic processes constitutes an emotion. Also, no individual feature by itself may be necessary to constitute an emotion. This means, as Newen, Welpinghus, and Juckel (2015) point out, there are borderline cases where it is not clear whether some complex pattern counts as an emotion.

J. L. Austin (1961, 77ff.) had suggested that a particular emotion, like anger, consists of a pattern of factors. Carroll Izard developed this idea under the title "differential emotions theory." What he meant was that a complex emotion consisted of a pattern of more basic emotions; and, likewise, depression, as an affective disorder, for example, consisted of a pattern of emotions. Newen et al. state the idea in an explicitly different way, namely, emotions (even basic emotions) are patterns of variables (that are not themselves emotions). We can think of such variables, such as neuro-hormonal, motoric, and experiential processes set up as evolutionary adaptations, as interactively related, so that emotions are constituted as dynamical interactions of such constituents, including organism–environment transactions. Think of discrete emotions as dynamically self-organizing in that "recursive interactions among component processes generate emergent properties" (Izard et al. 2000, 15). Thus, different emotions are constituted by different patterns of processes that yield behaviors that vary from one individual to another, and within individuals over time—where such behaviors/expressions are components of the emotion. Individual emotions may still combine or co-assemble with other emotions to form new emotion patterns that may stabilize over repeated occurrences.

Newen, Welpinghus, and Juckel (2015) provide a catalog of different features that may contribute to specific patterns that constitute emotions. They include:

(1) *Autonomic processes.* Here one might think of James's (1884) claim that an emotion is the perception of bodily changes that include autonomic nervous system (ANS) activity. For an emotion pattern, autonomic activity is only one possible constituent, and it may be experienced (i.e., the subject may be aware of autonomic effects) or not. Not every emotion has a distinct ANS pattern, and different emotions need not have different ANS patterns (Prinz 2004).

(2) *Actions or action tendencies.* Action tendencies (Frijda 1986) are bodily changes preparatory for actions that may be experienced as urges to perform a certain kind of action. Some emotions, for example, happiness, may or may not include this component; others may be typically associated with specific actions (e.g., freezing or fighting or fleeing in fear).

(3) *Overt expressions.* These may include expressive postures and movements, facial expressions, gestures, and vocal expressions (e.g., intonations,

screams, laughter). Such individual expressions may themselves combine into a typical emotion-related pattern, and again, such expressions are considered to be constitutive aspects of an emotion.

(4) *Phenomenal feeling.* This conscious or experiential component is often part of an emotion, although it is not necessary for every emotional occurrence. In some rare cases typical physiological, expressive, and cognitive aspects may be present without the phenomenal aspect (e.g., in subjects who are disposed to repress fear [Sparks et al. 1999]).

(5) *Cognitive aspects.* These include typical emotion-related attitudes, shifts of attention, and perceptual changes. Cognitive attitudes may include, for example, as Newen et al. suggest, belittling thoughts about one's rival in the case of jealousy, or a judgment that one has been treated unfairly in certain cases of anger. Such attitudes may or may not be manifested in behavior or in verbal reports. Shifts of attention, may include, for example, becoming alert to specific aspects of the environment in the case of fear.

(6) *Intentional objects.* These include the perceived, remembered, or imagined objects the emotion is about. As Peter Goldie put it, "This [intentional object] can be a particular thing or person (that pudding, this man), an event or an action (the earthquake, your hitting me), or a state of affairs (my being in an aeroplane)" (2000, 16–17).

I would add one other set of factors to this list:

(7) *Situational aspects.* John Dewey, in his critique of James, points out that emotions are not reducible to a set of bodily states, but also always include situational aspects. Because the body is always coupled to an environment, the unit of analysis should always be organism-environment, where, this relation defines the situation, such that the organism (or the experiencing subject) is itself part of the situation. These situational aspects are part of the emotion-pattern (Mendoça 2012). In this regard it is not just the intentional object, but also the situation reflected in the intentional structure of the emotion, that helps to disambiguate emotional expressions, and to make the response the emotion that it is. Importantly, situations are almost always social and/or cultural and such factors contribute constitutively to what an emotion is.

All of these aspects are variables that can take different values and weights in the dynamical constitution of an emotion. Some values are more or less likely to occur together. In this respect we can distinguish a typical pattern of affective aspects and values and define an emotion as involving some set of variations of that pattern. According to Newen et al., to say a particular feature is constitutive of an emotion does not mean that it is an essential component. Although there may be some minimal number of characteristic features and their values that are sufficient to constitute a particular pattern that counts as instantiating a particular emotion type (e.g., anger), one can have a token of the same type of emotion that lacks a particular characteristic feature. One typical pattern of anger, for example, may include a racing heart, faster breathing, aggressive action tendencies, an angry facial expression, a louder voice, a phenomenal feeling of heat and tension, a narrowed attention, a particular target, and a provocative situation (such as sitting in traffic having just been cut off by the driver in front of you). Not all instances of anger, however, involve aggressive action tendencies or a narrowed attention. One or more factors may be missing and there may still be a sufficient number and organization of factors that constitute the pattern as one of anger:

> A feature F is constitutive for a pattern X if it is part of at least one set of features which is minimally sufficient for a token to belong to a type X. 'Minimally sufficient' means that these features are jointly sufficient for the episode to be of type X, but if one of them were taken away the episode would no longer count as an instance of X.   (Newen et al. 2015, 195)

That is, a pattern can vary within limits defined as a minimally sufficient set, and still count as a particular emotion. Around a certain threshold, however, it can cease to be that emotion.

It is possible, of course, to include other aspects or characteristics in the list above. One may want to include more than just autonomic processes under a broad heading of embodied processes. For example, some specific brain processes may count as part of an emotion pattern. The idea that emotion can be understood as a pattern of this sort is also consistent with enactivist conceptions of emotion. Thus, Giovanna Colombetti writes: "emotional episodes correspond to specific self-organizing forms or second-order constraints—*emotion forms*, as I call them—that recruit or entrain various processes (neural, muscular, autonomic, etc.) into highly integrated configurations or patterns" (Colombetti 2014, 69).

I think this provides sufficient detail to indicate the kind of pattern theory that we want to consider. Let me also note that one of the advantages of this theory of emotion, as Newen et al. (2015) make clear, is that it becomes very easy to say that we can perceive emotions in others. If emotions are constituted by features that may include bodily expressions, behaviors, contextualized actions, and so forth, then emotions, or those specific features of an emotion, which are constitutive of the emotion, can be directly perceived, and such perceptions can be considered a form of pattern recognition (Gallagher 2008; Gallagher & Varga 2014).

1.2 Self-patterns

In a way that is similar to the construction of a pattern theory of emotion, I want to suggest that we can develop a pattern theory of self (PTS).[1] According to PTS, what we call self consists of a complex pattern of specific factors or processes (bodily processes, experiences, affective states, behaviors, actions, and so forth). Again, a pattern is a system of factors or processes that lacks any strictly necessary conditions, but rather consists of several jointly sufficient conditions. Some token instances can include most or all of the characteristic factors or processes, while others will consist of only a few.[2] A self-pattern operates as a complex system that emerges from dynamical interactions of constituent processes. Among the component processes that make up a self-pattern are processes that, like the components of emotion, are set up as evolutionary adaptations. Indeed, emotion-related processes themselves contribute to the constitution of a self-pattern.

To be clear, within the self-pattern there is no element that operates as a controlling agent. As Scott Kelso (1995, 1) indicates, "patterns in general emerge in a self-organized fashion, without any agent-like entity ordering the elements, telling them when and where to go." In this regard, there is no self within a self-pattern. There is no single element that by itself could count as a self. A self, of the sort that you are and that I am, just is a pattern.

A number of issues immediately arise on this view. One issue is this: What is it about a pattern of factors or processes that makes it a *self*-pattern, especially if there is no self-entity within the pattern? There are a lot of patterns in the world that are not self-patterns. Is there some particular element included in a pattern, or some particular arrangement of a pattern that makes it a self-pattern? In that case one may have to postulate one or more necessary or sufficient conditions involved in the self-pattern. I'll return to this question below.

Another issue: if we say that different selves are constituted by different patterns, but a pattern can change over time—that it can develop or perhaps be transformed by certain events—then questions arise about stability and self-identity over time. Although a self-pattern is not a thing, entity, or substance, one still requires some kind of identity conditions. On the one hand we need to

---

[1] Susan Schneider (2019) points to a somewhat underdeveloped version of the psychological continuity theory of personal identity found in Kurzweil (2005), which conceives of the self as a pattern of psychological or cognitive features, including memories. In contrast to what I am outlining here, this is what philosophers of mind would call a "narrow" pattern, completely reducible to psychological properties and ultimately to brain processes, or information patterns, modeled on a computational theory of mind (see Schneider 2019, 78ff.).

[2] This idea of pattern has some affinity to Morton Beckner's (1959, 22) definition of a polytypic concept. Thanks to Kenneth Schaffner for pointing this out. Also see Schaffner (1993, Ch. 3). One important difference, however, is that Beckner defines the polytypic concept as an aggregate; in contrast, a pattern, as understood here, is integrated by dynamical relations and is therefore something more than an aggregation of items.

consider questions about uniqueness, and argue for what we might call a finger-print principle (assuming that every self-pattern, on some scale, like every finger-print pattern, is unique). On the other hand, we need to account for the possibility of stability and continuity across changes in and of the pattern over time. We will address these concerns by thinking about the concept of a self-pattern as being anchored in a unique living body (being constituted in part by some embodied aspects) and as being characterized by a relatively stable (but changeable) set of dynamical relations among all of its factors. A self-pattern, in this sense, is a dynamical gestalt (see Chapter 2).

Another issue concerns the kind of theory that PTS is supposed to be. There are three possibilities. First, one can think of PTS as operating like a meta-theory that defines a general schema of possible theories of self, each of which would itself be a pattern theory. For example, one task of a meta-theory may be to iden-tify all possible factors that could be part of a self-pattern, without making claims about which of these factors are likely to be included (a question that may be answered differently by different particular pattern theories of self). Such a meta-theory would aim to provide a complete list of such elements, and to map out all possible relations that could exist among them without claiming that they neces-sarily exist in any particular case. Accordingly, for such a meta-theory, which is what I have started to describe, there would be no claims made about necessary or minimally sufficient conditions for constituting a self.

Second, any particular theory of self that attempts to identify some type or lim-ited set of factors that might compose selfhood can be a PTS, and one PTS can differ from another PTS by specifying different typical aspects and/or relations to be included as essential for a self-pattern. In this respect, one can think of a par-ticular PTS as defining the self at a general or abstract level, indicating, for exam-ple, that certain factors are necessary but not sufficient for selfhood. For example, some theorists may insist that to be a self requires reflective self-consciousness (ruling out non-human animals, infants, and coma patients), or a biological organism (ruling out angels and robots). Others may include items that are not standard components in the traditional conceptions of selfhood, such as techno-logical extensions. For example, Andy Clark's concept of a "soft self" could be viewed as a self-pattern; he characterizes it as a "rough-and-tumble control shar-ing coalition of processes—some neural, some bodily, some technological—and an ongoing drive to tell a story in which 'I' am the central player" (2007, 114).

Finally, one can think in terms of applying PTS in the specification of a token or individual instance of a self-pattern. This type of analysis is most relevant to understanding individual life stories and how various disorders, for example, depression or schizophrenia, play out in an individual's life. One might discover that the self-pattern of an individual with major depressive disorder, for example, exhibits some specific relations, values, or weights among factors that are typic-ally different from non-depressed individuals. Accordingly, if we are able to offer a better understanding of the differences, or recognize otherwise undetected deviations, then this pattern approach may work in the service of a psychiatric diagnostics. Generally speaking, in this and the following chapters, I employ all three types of pattern-theoretical analysis: a meta-theory to identify the possible factors that may be parts of a self-pattern; a particular enactive approach to understanding self-pattern processes that emphasizes their embodied nature; and, in the context of considering psychopathologies, a specific application of this theory.

What features can contribute to specific self-patterns? This is the meta-theoretical question. To philosophers it will come as no surprise that what gets included in this list is open to contentious debate. Moreover, how extensive this list is will depend on how far down one wants to drill into details. Keep in mind, however, that, when operating as a meta-theory, PTS does not attempt to identify necessary or sufficient conditions, so that a meta-theoretical analysis may be less contentious than trying to work out a more particular theory of self. We should also keep in mind the possibility that even in specifying a particular PTS, the self-pattern that constitutes an individual may lack a specific non-necessary characteristic feature and still be considered a self if a sufficient number of other elements that make up the pattern are still in place. For example, if autobiographical memory is thought of as a factor that typically contributes to a self-pattern, an Alzheimer's patient may be missing this element but still be considered a self, unless the particular PTS in question is a strict Lockean theory that would claim memory as a necessary condition for selfhood.

Here I'll provide a tentative, meta-theoretical list of factors, processes, or characteristic features that could count as contributing to the constitution of a self-pattern (summarized in Table 1.1). The list is not necessarily complete. The source of the list is a broad philosophical history that includes discussions of self and personal identity. For each element I offer some notes to indicate the scope of each process or factor (or set of factors). Such factors are variables that can take different values and weights in the dynamical constitution of a self-pattern. As I noted, a pattern exists not just as a collection of elements, but, importantly, as a set of relations among these elements. The specific value and weight each element has in the pattern will depend on its relations with other elements. We can think of the pattern as a dynamical gestalt where, if one factor (or value or weight relative to the whole) is changed above a certain threshold, some or all of the other factors (and perhaps the whole) adjust (see Chapter 3 for experimental methods that may allow us to test this idea). As the phenomenologist Maurice Merleau-Ponty puts it in discussing the nature of a gestalt, "what happens at each point is determined by what happens in all the others...this is the definition of order" (1963, 131). As in a living organism, such adjustments tend to maintain the whole as a continuing (albeit changing) pattern. The following processes may be considered part of a self-pattern:

Table 1.1 Elements of the self-pattern

Elements of the pattern	Brief description
Bodily processes	Includes core bio-systemic and autopoietic processes related to motoric, autonomic, endocrine, enteric, immune, interoceptive functions, allowing the overall system to maintain homeostasis necessary for survival, and to distinguish between itself and what is not itself.
Prereflective experiential processes	Includes prereflective self-awareness, a structural feature of first-person consciousness constrained by bodily factors; the sense of ownership (mineness) and the sense of agency, which can involve various sensory-motor modalities, such as proprioception, kinaesthesia, touch, and vision. These aspects form the experiential core of what is sometimes called the minimal self.
Affective processes	The fact that someone manifests a certain temperament or emotional disposition reflects a particular mix of affective factors that range from very basic and mostly covert or tacit bodily affects (e.g., hunger, fatigue, libido) to what may be a typical emotion pattern, a set of existential feelings, a background mood.
Behavioral/ action processes	Behaviors and actions make us who we are—behavioral habits and skills reflect, and perhaps actually constitute, our character. This is a classic view that goes back at least to Aristotle.
Social/ intersubjective processes	Humans (possibly some non-human animals) are born with a capacity for attuning to intersubjective existence; at a certain point in social relations a more developed self-conscious recognition of oneself as being distinct from others, a sense of self-for-others, and a sense of being part of a group or community.
Cognitive/ psychological processes	These are aspects emphasized in traditional theories of personal identity highlighting psychological continuity and memory, including one's conceptual understanding of oneself, beliefs, cognitive dispositions, as well as personality traits.
Reflective processes	The ability to reflect on one's experiences and actions—closely related to notions of autonomy and moral personhood, including the capacity to reflectively evaluate and form second-order volitions about one's desires.
Narrative processes	Self-interpretation has a narrative structure and recursively reflects (and often reinforces) the self-pattern. On some theories, selves are inherently or constitutively narrative entities.
Ecological processes	We tend to identify ourselves with our stuff—physical pieces of property, clothes, homes, and various things that we own, the technologies we use, the institutions we work in, and so forth. Our embodied-situated actions engage with (and sometimes incorporate) artifacts, instruments, bits, and structures of the environment in ways that define us and scaffold our identities. Situations shape who we are, and affordances define our possibilities.
Normative processes	Our extensive engagement with the environment includes social and cultural practices. These are not just what we do, but involve what we ought to do, and obligations that we keep or not. Constraints (and sometimes well-defined roles) imposed by social, cultural, institutional factors shape our habitual behaviors, and our self-conceptions of who we are, and who we think we should be.

Source: Author

1. *Bodily processes*: includes core bio-systemic and autopoietic processes related to motoric, autonomic, endocrine, enteric, immune, interoceptive functions, that is, processes which allow the overall system to maintain homeostasis necessary for survival, and to distinguish between itself and what is not itself—an extremely basic set of functions that both enable and constrain all kinds of biological organisms. Such processes involve brain and nervous systems, and include sensory-motor processes that underpin the body-centered spatial frame of reference, which in turn grounds a first-person perspective, and contributes to specifying possible actions in peripersonal space.

2. *Prereflective experiential processes*: Includes prereflective self-awareness, a structural feature of first-person consciousness constrained by bodily factors.[3] One's experiential life includes the sense of ownership (mineness) and the sense of agency, which can involve various sensory-motor modalities, such as proprioception, kinaesthesia, touch, and vision. These aspects form the experiential core of what is sometimes called the minimal self (Gallagher 2000a; Gallagher & Zahavi 2020; 2021).

3. *Affective processes*: The fact that someone manifests a certain temperament or emotional disposition reflects a particular mix of affective factors that range from very basic and mostly covert or tacit bodily affects (e.g., hunger, fatigue, libido) to what may be a typical emotion pattern (Newen et al. 2015), some mix of existential feelings (Ratcliffe 2008), or background mood.

4. *Behavioral/action processes*: Behaviors and actions make us who we are—behavioral habits and skills reflect, and perhaps actually constitute, our character. This is a classic view that goes back at least to Aristotle. John Dewey (1922, 24), for example, holds that habit forms our effective desires, furnishes us with working capacities, and rules our thoughts because "it is so intimately a part of ourselves. It has a hold upon us because we are the habit." This is a view reflected in Pierre Bourdieu's notion of *habitus* (1977) and that continues to be expressed in recent science: "Habits may define who we are" (Verplanken & Sui 2019).

---

[3] Jékely, Godfrey-Smith, and Keijzer (2021) have emphasized the importance of reafference for the phylogenetic emergence of a bodily sense of self. Reafference, including proprioception, for example, is an organic-organizational basis for a dynamical integration of body, action, and experience. "An organism has, or embodies, a body-self if it has a particular form of organization. That form of organization includes motility (of the whole or parts) and sensing, where action and sensing are tied together through reafference. The body-self then encompasses the devices and their activities that enable reafferent coupling between the animal's own actions and sensing. The body-self can thus include sensors and effectors, their activity or actions, and also the form of the body influencing reafferent coupling. In this view, brains, if they are present, are not the sole locus or even the centre of this self, but a part of the body that is characterized by this self" (3).

5. *Social/intersubjective processes*: Humans (possibly some non-human animals) are born with a capacity for attuning to intersubjective existence (Reddy 2008; Rochat 2011; Trevarthen 1979); at a certain point in social relations a more developed self-consciousness arises—a self-conscious recognition of oneself as being oneself as distinct from others, a sense of self-for-others (Mead 1913; Sartre 1956), and a sense of being part of a group or community. As Daniel Dennett expresses it: "In fact, we wouldn't exist, as Selves...if it weren't for the evolution of social interactions requiring each human animal to create within itself a subsystem designed for interacting with others" (2003, 47).[4] Or, again, as Charles Taylor puts it: "One is a self only among other selves. A self can never be described without reference to those who surround it" (1989, 35). Although there are various ways of thinking about the relations between self and others, ranging across nativist and empiricist views, the basic idea is that who I am, how I think, what I value (indeed, most aspects of my self-pattern), are very much shaped by my intersubjective interactions, and in some sense, and to some degree, my identity emerges from those relations. The term "intersubjectivity" is not unproblematic, and it does not capture everything of importance here. We also need to include extended and complex forms of social relations, such as the possibilities for and the constraints imposed on self-definition, introduced by collectives, groups, institutions, sociocentric cultures, and so forth (see *Normative factors*).

6. *Cognitive and psychological processes and states*: These are aspects emphasized in traditional theories of personal identity highlighting psychological continuity and memory (e.g., Shoemaker 2011), including one's conceptual understanding of oneself, beliefs, cognitive dispositions, as well as personality traits.

7. *Reflective processes*: The ability to reflect on one's experiences and actions—closely related to notions of autonomy and moral personhood, including the capacity to evaluate and form second-order volitions about one's desires (Frankfurt 1988; Taylor 1989). Reflection does not necessarily mean introspection, typically understood as a kind of isolated, internal observation of

---

[4] Many similar statements are to be found in a variety of theorists. For example, George Herbert Mead writes: "No hard-and-fast line can be drawn between our own selves and the selves of others, since our own selves exist and enter as such into our experience only in so far as the selves of others exist and enter as such into our experience also" (1962, 164). Or, as Julian Jaynes expresses it: "What your self is, and what others are, are part of the same thing and you really cannot separate it" (2019, d231). Likewise, Issiah Berlin (1969, 156) maintains that my "self is not something which I can detach from my relationship with others, or from those attributes of myself which consist in their attitude towards me." Before that, Edmund Husserl wrote: "Personhood is constituted only as the subject enters into social relations with others" (1973b, 175), such that my being as a person is a result of my "communicative intertwinement" with others (Husserl 1973c, 603). Annette Baier (1985, 84) gets to the heart of it: "A person, perhaps, is best seen as one who was long enough dependent upon other persons to acquire the essential arts of personhood. Persons essentially are second persons."

mental states. Rather, reflection can involve self-interpretation; it can be directed at situations that involve worldly events (Evans 1982, 225); and it may even be conducted by engaging in conversation with others.[5]

8. *Narrative processes*: Self-interpretation has a narrative structure and recursively reflects (and often reinforces) the self-pattern. On some theories, selves are inherently or constitutively narrative entities (Schechtman 2011). The conception of this narrative aspect ranges from an abstraction (Dennett's [1991a] concept of self as an abstract center of narrative gravity) to a complex accomplishment (Ricoeur's [1992] rich analysis of *ipse* and *idem* identity).

9. *Ecological processes*:[6] According to James (1890) we identify ourselves with our stuff—physical pieces of property, clothes, homes, and various things that we own, the technologies we use, the institutions we work in, and so forth. Our embodied-situated actions engage with (and sometimes incorporate) artifacts, instruments, bits and structures of the environment in ways that define us and scaffold our identities. Situations shape who we are, and affordances define our possibilities.

10. *Normative processes*: Since our extensive engagements with the environment also include social and cultural practices, they are permeated with value-determining norms. These specify not just what we do, but involve what we ought to do, and obligations that we keep or not. Constraints (and sometimes well-defined roles) imposed by social, cultural, institutional factors shape our habitual behaviors, and our self-conceptions of who we are, and who we think we should be. Christine Korsgaard (1996, 101) calls this a "practical identity"—"a description under which you find your life to be worth living, and your actions to be worth undertaking." Self-identity or the sense of who one is, is shaped by everything that comes along with one's profession, one's religion, social status, the various roles involved in marriage, in parenting, in friendship, and constraints imposed by gender, race, and economic circumstances, for better or worse. As Paul Ricoeur puts it, "To a large extent, in fact, the identity of a person...is

---

[5] It is also possible that reflective ability, to the extent that it involves an introspective stance, can introduce a philosophically troublesome distortion into the sense of self. Hans Jonas (1966, 186) writes: "In reflection upon self the subject–object split which began to appear in animal evolution reaches its extreme form. It has extended into the center of feeling life, which is now divided against itself. Only over the immeasurable distance of being his own object can man 'have' himself."

[6] The aspect I am calling "ecological" here is not the same as Neisser's concept of ecological, which he draws from Gibson's ecological psychology. Neisser means the ecological self-awareness involved in proprioception/kinaesthesia that gives us a direct embodied sense of self-movement distinct from other movement in the environment. On the concept of self-pattern outlined here, Neisser's notion of ecological would be part of prereflective self-awareness. The concept of "ecological relations" mentioned here does include the idea of affordance which is also drawn from Gibson (1977).

made up of these identifications with values, norms, ideals, models, and heroes in which the person...recognizes [him- or herself]" (1992, 121).

I'll have more to say about these various features (which we may think of as processes, factors, or variables that comprise the self-pattern)[7] and their relations as we go on, but here let me provide just a brief indication of some of the complexity involved in thinking about them as parts of an integrated pattern. We might think of some of these variables as overlapping or redundant. For example, some theorists may consider most of these features to be "embodied" and accordingly, it is not clear how to separate embodied aspects from, for example, affective or behavioral or cognitive aspects. If one accepts a pattern theory of emotion, for example, then affect already includes embodied, experiential, and cognitive aspects. Others may think that narrative processes overlap with cognitive-psychological and reflective factors. For example, Parnas and Zandersen (2018, 220) suggest:

The narrative self refers to features which characterize and individualize a person and which easily lend themselves to linguistic self-description (e.g., 'I have a tendency to act impulsively') and descriptions from the third-person perspective ('she is acting impulsively'). These features comprise biographical, characterological and cognitive characteristics and are heavily dependent on language and memory.

I think this individualizing capacity fits with the idea that narrative has a recursive-reflective function such that it reflects all of the other aspects of the self-pattern, and loops back into these other processes. The way that self-narrative and reflective ability interact, together with the role of affective and normative processes, provide the basis for what Sanneke de Haan (2020) calls the "existential stance," which includes some aspects of what Charles Taylor (1989) calls "strong evaluation," or a developed existential sense of understanding myself and of how I am faring. These functional configurations of narrative, reflection, affect, and normativity can lead to just the type of self-questioning and doubting of authenticity that one finds in some patients diagnosed with psychiatric disorders—"is this me or is it my depression?" De Haan suggests that self-understanding "aways takes place in a specific sociocultural context, and that how I understand myself is to some extent mediated by the narratives that are available to me in this context" (2020, 135)—which include the narratives that get promoted by others, including therapists, and those that express public opinion about psychiatric disorders—all

---

[7] I acknowledge the philosophically bothersome terminological promiscuity. What the best term is, I suggest, changes with the particular descriptive or explanatory context or purpose or perspective involved.

of which involve looping effects (Hacking 1995) that can impact the self-pattern (see Lindemann 2014).

This is neither functional overlap nor conceptual fuzziness, but rather the specific ways that the different processes of the self-pattern integrate or mesh (or sometimes fail to mesh), resulting in further configurations that make each of us who we are. It indicates the connectedness and the dynamical relationality involved in the pattern.[8] Accordingly, rather than focusing on the lines that divide one factor from another the focus should be on the lines that connect them.

Consider an ongoing debate about the nature of *prereflective experiential processes*, or what some phenomenologists call the "minimal self" (Gallagher 2000a; Ratcliffe 2017; Zahavi 2017). One question is just how much to include in this notion—how minimal should we make it? Dan Zahavi, for example, claims that the minimal self consists of the perspectival sense of mineness that I have for any of my experiences. When I perceive something, or when I feel something interoceptively, for example, this experience comes along with the intrinsic sense that this is *my* experience. The idea that this is an intrinsic feature of my experience means that it is part of the prereflective structure of that experience, and that it does not depend upon any higher-order reflective or cognitive process. This minimal experience of mineness is typically, and in part, proprioceptive in nature (including the kinaesthetic sense of movement), which means it can be found in pre-linguistic infants (and likely in some non-human animals). Generally speaking, through proprioceptive awareness I am able to sense that I am moving and where my limbs currently are relative to the rest of my body. The "proprio" in proprioception gives me a sense that this is *my* body, *my* movement—since, by its nature I cannot propriocept anyone else's body. The phenomenologist claims that prereflective self-awareness plays the same role for experience more generally. I cannot be prereflectively self-aware of anyone else's experience; and it is only because prereflective self-awareness is an intrinsic feature of my experience that when I introspectively reflect on some experience, I never find myself asking whether it is *my* experience.[9]

According to Zahavi (2017), as an intrinsic aspect of my experience, the sense of mineness does not depend on reflection, or on narrative, or on our intersubjective relations. I can be prereflectively self-aware, independently of my reflective

---

[8] This meshing may be reflected in the overlapping of neural processes. Albert Newen (2018), for example, notes that, (1) relevant to intersubjective factors, "interesting neural overlaps and shared neural activations" exist for self versus other (Decety & Sommerville 2003; Vogeley et al. 2004), (2) that the role of such overlapping neural activations is still an open question, but (3) in a "pattern account of the self we expect there to be an overlapping integration process which is then modulated by additional brain resources." For how this may fit with a predictive processing account, see Chapter 4.

[9] This is a principle referred to as "immunity to error through misidentification," which Sidney Shoemaker (1968) derives from Wittgenstein (1958).

capacity, or my narrative, or any social relation in which I may be involved. In contrast, and specifically in disagreement with Zahavi, some other theorists, such as Miriam Kyselo (2016), Matthew Ratcliffe (2017), and Anna Ciaunica and Aikaterini Fotopoulou (2017), contend that, for the human at least, intersubjective relations are so pervasive from birth onward that there is an intersubjective dimension involved even in minimal self-experience (for discussion on this point, see Higgins 2018; and, in relation to schizophrenia, Van Duppen 2017). Likewise, Marya Schechtman (2015) argues that once we acquire narrative competency our proclivities to understand ourselves in narrative terms is pervasive and, if in fact there is anything like a minimal self, narrative transforms it. Along this line, one might argue that in some sense all of the other factors in the self-pattern may in some fashion permeate and transform our minimal self-experience, affecting either its qualitative feel or its structural features. On this view, the minimal self and what one calls the sense of mineness could only be an abstraction from a much richer multi-dimensional experience.[10]

A pattern theory of self can adjudicate among these positions. That is, one can take the minimal sense of mineness to be an intrinsic structure of experience anchored in real bodily processes (like proprioception or interoception), without denying that as part of a larger pattern it is dynamically related to other processes, such as affectivity, narrative, and intersubjective processes, that may (to some degree, and in some cases more so than others) modulate one's sense of mineness and, as Ratcliffe (2017, 34–6) contends, even transform it into something more complex. If one can make a legitimate conceptual distinction between the minimal experiential aspect of the self-pattern and the other factors, that does not mean that existentially (or behaviorally) they operate in a separate or isolated fashion. The sense of mineness, rather than an abstraction, can be considered enriched by all of the various dimensions of experience that impinge upon it. Reciprocally, one could argue that the narrative at stake, and the intersubjective relations at stake, are experienced as *my* narrative and *my* intersubjective relations only because they are anchored in some way in the intrinsic structure of mineness. Thinking in this way at least provides a hint about how we should conceive of these factors and their dynamical relations (see Chapter 6). The pattern persists in the constantly re-adjusting reciprocal relations that exist between brain, body, and environment.

[10] Indeed, Zahavi (2011, 327) acknowledges this: with the possible exception of certain severe pathologies, for example, the final stages of Alzheimer's disease, he suggests, we "will never encounter the experiential core self in its purity. It will always already be embedded in an environmental and temporal horizon. It will be intertwined with, shaped, and contextualized by memories, expressive behaviour, and social interaction, by passively acquired habits, inclinations, associations, and so forth. In that sense, a narrow focus on the experiential self might indeed be said to involve an abstraction."

1.3 Philosophical Problems

This way of thinking of the self-pattern, of course, will not solve all philosophical problems. One may want to know which of these aspects are necessary or essential, and this will need to be specified by a particular theory. This brings us back to a question raised earlier. What is it about a pattern of factors or processes that makes it a *self*-pattern, especially if there is no self-entity or agent within the pattern? This turns out to be a difficult issue. There are many patterns in nature that we would not think of as self-patterns. My teacup consists of a pattern of elements, and we might say that there is a typical set of elements that make something a cup. Aristotle would have identified this as its form, which is closely aligned with its shape (*morphe*), but it is also the case that the material from which it is made is important. If the material is porous, it will not serve as a teacup. No matter what pattern instantiates a cup, however, it is not a self-pattern. So what differentiates a self-pattern from any other pattern? One approach would be to try to identify one of the component factors as decisive on this point.

For example, some might argue that an individualized bodily existence, understood as a living body, is a necessary and basic feature of a self-pattern. Surely, a self cannot exist unless it exists bodily. Setting aside some medieval questions about angels (who are species-patterns rather than self-patterns, see Aquinas 1485 for the latest research), and survival (although, according to some theologians personal survival may require resurrection and reuniting with one's body), if one says that bodily existence is a necessary (even if not sufficient) condition for the existence of a self-pattern, is that enough to say that what makes a pattern a *self*-pattern just is that it involves such a bodily existence?

Consider a version of Étienne Condillac's (1793) statue, a thought experiment that concerns sensory experience. We start with a statue made of stone in human form, without the possibility of movement or sensation. We give it life but leave it in a comatose state—no senses, no movement, no consciousness. As such this would not be sustainable life, but we can set that worry aside. If this living body were part of a spatial arrangement of juxtaposed objects that constituted (for us) a visual pattern, would this be sufficient to make that pattern a self-pattern? Clearly not. A pattern that involves a set of juxtaposed objects is just the wrong kind of pattern to be thinking about if we are trying to think about what makes a pattern a self-pattern. Also, of course, by self-pattern we don't mean just a visual pattern, or a spatial pattern, although there may be some visible and spatial aspects involved.

Alternatively, someone might argue, following our comments above, that a minimal experiential self-awareness is necessary to make a pattern a self-pattern, even if, on its own, a minimal experiential self-awareness is not a self-pattern. This would mean that there must be consciousness (a prereflective awareness) involved in a pattern of elements to make it a self-pattern. This doesn't seem right, however, since, most would agree, when I am knocked unconscious, or undergo anaesthesia, or fall into a coma, I don't cease to be a person or self. *In such cases*, it may be the *capacity* for consciousness that is relevant. We can add this capacity to Condillac's statue, and even actualize it and allow it to be conscious in some minimal way. In that case we should ask about how consciousness relates to the lived body, and what kind of pattern forms between the body and prereflective self-awareness. Let's give the statue interoception and proprioception, which are not only bodily processes, but may then allow it to be aware of its body, from the inside, so to speak, or as William James (1890) put it, to have a "warmth and intimacy" with itself.[11] For all of this to work properly one should also give the statue motor capacity and allow it to move. Now we have a pattern building up—a pattern that we might call a minimal self-pattern of sensory-motor processes that includes a form of self-awareness, and perhaps a sense of ownership and a sense of agency. But these elements don't come as a collection of separate processes or *partes extra partes*. They are mutually related such that one process does not run the same without the other. Likewise, this extends to the other processes of the self-pattern, as Dings and Newen (2021, 5) suggest in their characterization of the self-pattern as "dynamically modulated by the engagements of the embodied biological being with its social and physical environment" (2021, 5).

It might seem, then, that what makes a pattern a *self*-pattern is not any one particular element or set of elements, but the order or arrangement, or specifically, the dynamical connections among its parts or processes. I think this idea points in the right direction, but we need to be more specific by saying that the dynamical processes must be recursively self-organizing. This might seem circular in a logically vicious way if being self-organizing meant something like "organizing of a self." This is not what the phrase "self-organizing" means in this case. Rather, we should think of it in terms of a performative circle, which in enactivist philosophy is symbolized by the ouroboros. Here I want to follow some ideas laid down by Francisco Varela in connection with the concept of autopoiesis, where a pattern is viewed as a process of an identity constitution. By identity Varela means a particular kind of self-coherence. "It is not meant as a static structural description (it is a process), nor as carrying a mentalistic or psychological connotation." It is rather a process of "operational closure" (Varela 1997, §2), which involves a type of recursive dynamics. I won't say more about this here because we'll be in a better position to provide a clearer account in the next chapter. Here I am simply

---

[11] Perhaps just interoception would be sufficient to ground prereflective self-awareness, ipseity or the "minimal self." This can be made clear by considering what is something like the reverse of Condillac's statue thought experiment—Avicenna's Flying Man thought experiment in which we take away sensory input, proprioception, and kinaesthesia from a newly created human who is floating or flying in thin air. Avicenna argues that the flying man would still be self-aware without such sensory input from bodily senses. It's not clear, however, that Avicenna eliminates interoception.

indicating a particular direction that we can follow in seeking an answer to this question of what makes a pattern a self-pattern.

In whatever way we try to answer this question, it is important to note that the pattern theory of self, following a pluralist route, rules out reductionist and deflationary theories of self that would claim that the self is just X and nothing else. For example, a theory that would claim the self is just the collection of information that forms a narrative, and specifically the abstract center of narrative gravity (Dennett 1991a), and nothing else, would not be a pattern theory, since one abstract point does not constitute a pattern. Indeed, with respect to narrative, as PTS gets applied to individuals, it seems possible that one individual may experience life in a less continuous or coherent way than others do, thereby minimizing the narrative aspect, without denying that a self-pattern, or self-identity still exists (Strawson 2004). One may also lose a sense of agency, as part of one's first-person experience, as in some schizophrenic symptoms, without losing a sense of ownership or other aspects that define the prereflective experiential aspect of the self-pattern (see Chapter 6). One might lose the ability to recall one's past life, as in some cases of amnesia and Alzheimer's disease, and may also undergo character or personality changes. In such cases one's self-identity may continue to be supported by other factors, such as bodily processes, as well as by intersubjective relations, by a type of extended memory instantiated in narrative, including narratives told by others and/or ecologial aspects in one's surroundings (Baird 2019 provides some evidence for this; see Dennett 1996, 138; Heersmink 2022). The person is, as Hilde Lindemann (2014, 20) puts it, "held in personhood" by such factors.

This is not to say that such changes (with respect to narrative, agency, memory, or personality) do not result in a modulation of self-experience or self-identity, or more generally of the self-pattern as a whole, but rather, since self is not reducible to any one of these aspects, it is a modulation of the self-pattern rather than a complete loss of self. There may be various states of existence or pathologies associated with each of these aspects such that the aspect in question is eliminated or seriously modified, which in turn modifies the self-pattern.[12]

A reasonable view is that all of the factors listed in Table 1.1 can (but need not) be included in the self-pattern. It also seems reasonable to think that, at least for the human case, which is the one we'll be concerned with, some element (or elements) of the self-pattern should be regarded as necessary, such that if that element is removed, or its dynamical relations undermined, the pattern itself collapses and ceases to be a self-pattern. For the human being, as suggested above, a

---

[12] Changes in self-pattern, at least on the theory that I will defend, will (for principled reasons to be explained) always be a matter of degree, and always less than 100 percent. It may be possible to hold a particular theory in which changes in the self-pattern may be more radical, such that after such changes the individual is no longer to be considered the same person. This is one issue, among a number of issues that will need to be addressed by any particular PTS.

living body seems a necessary condition.[13] This doesn't mean that all aspects of the body need to be functioning or functioning properly, however.

In this regard, it may be helpful to look at a limit case. Consider a case in which an unknown male human body has washed up on a beach. He is still alive, but barely. He is taken to a hospital and put into intensive care. It turns out that he has suffered a severe spinal cord injury and is currently in a coma. How much of the self-pattern is still intact? Some of the relevant embodied elements still function. He is unconscious, however, so there are no occurrent experiential aspects in operation. Likewise no intersubjective interaction (something that would require response on his part), although others are caring for him; no behavior; no cognitive or psychological functions are manifest. Assume that we do not know who this man is, so, although we must assume that there is some narrative that comes with this body, not only is he unable to provide a narrative, no one else is either, except in the most minimal sense—"He's the man we found on the beach." In some minimal sense, he is still situated (now in a hospital) and there are normative structures in place, but he is not situationally coupled to his environment in a proper way. Nonetheless, we continue to treat him as a person and to keep him physically alive. The social-normative system may be important in providing him with the status of personhood.

In terms of necessary conditions, then, some may be inclined to argue that the living body counts, since if he were dead very little else would be intact. Yet, others may argue that even after a person's death there would still be a set of practices conducted by others, and a normative structure—there are proper and improper ways to treat dead human bodies, and in some sense we may still treat the now dead man as a (deceased) person and grant him a status that includes selfhood on some definition. If we set the detectives to work and find out more about him, and add more to his narrative, perhaps the case would be even stronger. Philosophers are easily led from this kind of case to consider others: Are historical figures, like Napoleon, still to be considered persons?[14] And some philosophers may raise questions about fictional characters like Hamlet, or about non-human animals, or about robots. These are all interesting questions but let me head off all such discussion and simply stipulate that in the following we limit our considerations to living humans who have at least some sustaining biological parts. In such cases I think it is safe to say that some embodied elements of a living human body will constitute a necessary component of a self-pattern, at least for the type of self we will consider.

---

[13] One might also think, however, that a non-living, robotic body may step in for a living body (see e.g., Georgie, Schillaci & Hafner 2019; Ryan, Agrawal & Franklin 2020).

[14] Ladyman et al. (2007, 229), conclude from their extensive account of a metaphysics of real patterns that "Napoleon is a real pattern"—see Chapter 2.

Some theorists may find it difficult to understand how ecological or normative factors can be included as part of a self-pattern. Someone might argue that a person or self is distinct from the environment she inhabits, or from the normative structures that may impinge on her. If we start with the idea that the individual must be conceived as an entity with strict boundaries that distinguish it from everything else then it's not clear how ecological factors can be part of a self-pattern. A different assumption, however, is that selves are relational (e.g., Guenther 2013), that is, that self-patterns are constituted by the relations that make them (as patterns) what they are, and (as persons) who they are.

This relationality is understood most easily in regard to intersubjectivity where, to some degree, our relations to others make us who we are. Charles Taylor points in this direction: "I define who I am by defining where I speak from, in the family tree, in social space, in the geography of social status and functions, in my intimate relations to the ones I love, and also crucially in the space of moral and spiritual orientation within which my most important defining relations are lived out" (1989, 35). More generally, unless one thinks that genes determine absolutely everything about an individual's identity, so that phenotype reduces to genotype, then who we are is not just constrained by environmental factors, but is constituted by a large set of relational variables that include specific types of coupling to environmental and normative factors.

Some version of this idea can easily be found in a number of philosophical traditions. Aristotle, for example, suggests that the goods that define our moral character include not only psychological and bodily goods, but external ones—wealth, friends, and children, as well as normative characteristics such as honor (NE 1099a31–b8; 1100a18–21; 1123b17–32). Of course, Aristotle is offering an explanation of happiness (*eudaimonia*) rather than a constitutive view of an individual self, but if we take happiness (or unhappiness) to involve a certain ordering of the soul (as Aristotle would say), then his analysis seems relevant to how we think of the self-pattern. Moreover, there are interesting arguments—arguments that run parallel to those regarding the notion of self—about whether one should consider external goods as merely causally relevant to happiness, or as constitutive of happiness (see, e.g., Roche 2014).

Another example that focuses more specifically on how factors that extend beyond the individual organism might enter into the constitution of a self-pattern can be explained in the very traditional terms of personal identity, which, as John Locke famously argued, depends upon one's autobiographical memory. If there is some truth in that claim, there is also some evidence from empirical studies that autobiographical memory, as well as self-narrative, depends not just on neural processes within the individual brain but on extra-neural, environmental, and intersubjective processes (see e.g., Heersmink 2017; 2021; 2022; Malafouris 2008; Milojevic 2020; Piredda 2020; Sutton 2009; Clowes 2013). These studies suggest that autobiographical memory, and thus some significant component of our psychological identity, can be viewed as extended or distributed, dependent on our interactions with others and our engagement with environmental artifacts. This idea is based not just on the stability that may be provided by such artifacts (think about how photographs or social media, or what Heersmink [2018] calls "evocative objects," may support memory preservation and activation; see Sutton 2009) but also on social interactions, cultural practices, and institutions. How I fit within a particular normative structure can determine how much or how little I can remember of my personal life. If the tasks I fulfill in my work environment are repetitive and unexciting, for example, I may remember less detail about my day-to-day practices, and that may shift what I do remember to moments of exceptional social interactions. This is not just about the content of my memories, but about the broad shaping of the kinds of things that I come to value, and remember, and form narratives about. Moreover, as Heersmink (2021) suggests, because autobiographical memories involve affective components, we can think of them, not only as cognitively extended, but also as affectively extended (see Krueger & Szanto 2016; Colombetti & Roberts 2015).

Similar considerations apply to behavioral and habitual aspects of the self-pattern. I already noted the relevance of Dewey's conception of intelligent habit. According to Dewey, habits are "functions of the surroundings as truly as of a person" (1988, 15). This is a concept further developed by Barandiaran and Di Paolo, for whom habits are "ecological, self-organizing structures that relate to a web of predispositions and plastic dependencies both in the agent and in the environment" (2014, 1), and by Roberta Dreon (2022) who defines habits in a relational way that shows how they are integrated with ecological, normative and intersubjective factors:

> [H]abits are more or less flexible channelings of both organic energies and environmental resources that are not only natural but also social and cultural, given human beings' marked degree of social interdependence. This idea is connected to a wider redefinition of the concept of behavior, which is not understood as the property of an individual or the way of being originated by a single agent, but rather as the result of mutual transactions—i.e., constitutive interactions—between an organism and the environment it is embedded in.
>
> [Dreon 2022, 94]

There are still plenty of other issues that could be discussed. At the level of meta-theory one can ask: How many different patterns are viable? If we rule out the situation in which just one aspect (i.e., narrative, or body, or memory) is claimed as sufficient for selfhood, since one element on its own would not constitute a (self-)pattern, is there some minimal number of aspects, or some specific combinations of aspects that constitute a viable pattern that counts as self? Is there a hierarchical relation among the aspects of a self-pattern? For example, if someone lacked certain experiential aspects, for example, a sense of agency or a sense of ownership, would she still be capable of self-narrative? Different answers to these questions define different variations of type-level pattern theories. There are further questions that I will address in the next chapter. For example, are not the elements that contribute to a self-pattern already patterns themselves, so that a self-pattern is more like a collection of patterns, and perhaps patterns within patterns? If so, how does one demarcate one pattern from another, and how precisely do they connect up to form a larger pattern? Before I explore some of these issues, however, let me say what I think are some benefits to appealing to the concept of a self-pattern.

1.4 Some Benefits of a Pattern Theory of Self

One benefit of PTS, understood as a meta-theory, is that we can more clearly understand how various interpretations of self may be compatible or in some cases incommensurable. For example, different definitions of personhood can be accommodated or can be viewed as different interpretations that place different weights on some aspects rather than others. John Locke, for example, defines person or self to mean "a thinking intelligent being, that has reason and reflection, and can consider itself as itself, the same thinking thing, in different times and places; which it does only by that consciousness with is inseparable from thinking, and, as it seems to me, essential to it" (1690, 318). We can see clearly that this notion of person focuses on cognitive-psychological aspects of self and ignores other aspects, although Locke also meant his concept of person to be a forensic one that involved taking responsibility for one's action.

Other definitions may emphasize bodily continuity, the importance of one's social role, or perhaps legal standing. Discussions of self always motivate cautions about making clear the different meanings that may operate in different disciplines. Some theorists define self as involving a complex form of self-consciousness that develops only when a child has language and conceptual thought; others contend that a more primary or minimal, prereflective sense of self is available from birth or very early in infancy. Some theorists hold that the self emerges gradually in development, on the basis of social interactions; others hold that there is a social dimension to self from the beginning of life. At the very least PTS, understood as a meta-theory, allows us to map out these different concepts of self, highlighting minimal experiential aspects in some cases, and narrative or higher-order cognitive capacities in other cases.

Indeed, a definition of self may differ according to the particular question under discussion—whether we want to understand the nature of personal identity, or moral personhood, or legal status, as opposed to the phenomenology of self-consciousness. I should note that generally, in this book, I use the terms "self" and "person" interchangeably. I acknowledge, however, that in some cases there may be interest in distinguishing personhood from self. But even this distinction differs from one theorist to another. Dan Zahavi, for example, distinguishes between self, understood as minimal self, and person, which he associates with narrative. Marya Schechtman (2007), in contrast, distinguishes between self, understood as the subject of experience who has a vested interest in its existence, from person, which is equivalent to an intersubjective forensic moral agent. For Schechtman, however, both self and person are conceived in terms of narrative processes. Evan Thompson (2020, 37) also distinguishes between self, understood as an independent entity—an owner of experience and action, denied by Buddhists—and person, as a phenomenological conception of a "multifaceted construction that includes modes of self-awareness." Jay Garfield (2021, 23) makes a similar distinction between a merely conventional conception of person, and the non-conventional concept of self rejected by Buddhists. It seems possible to disagree about where to lay the emphasis in defining self or personhood but continue to agree that more generally, self is composed of some pattern of factors that include all of these processes, some of which are relevant to the notion of personhood understood as a forensic concept, for example, and others which are not. When we focus on or emphasize a certain pattern or organization of aspects from a specific vantage point (an interpretation which may be tied to social roles, or to causal, legal, or moral responsibility, or to certain cultural practices, etc.), we can easily understand self-pattern to accommodate different concepts of person, or moral agent, or experiential subject, or physical individual, or mental entity, and so forth. PTS, as a meta-theory, remains neutral with respect to these inter-pretations, and in some respects defines the field of reference or common ground on which such debates about personhood or moral agency or other interpret-ations of self can take place.

Another advantage is that when one starts to investigate a particular process in the self-pattern, one begins to see, in its dynamical connections, that some aspects are both complex and distributed, or we might say, multi-dimensional. The sense of agency is a good example. In some basic way the sense of agency may be tied to motor control and the sensory-motor operations of the body, but it is also related to social and cultural norms and expectations (which may place limitations on agency), and to psychological/cognitive processes of reflective deliberation and decision-making. Something like the sense of agency is interwoven into several aspects of the self-pattern (see Chapter 6).

In this respect, a third advantage is that PTS may help to make sense out of some of the controversies surrounding the notion that self is related to specific neural processes. One such theory, developed by Georg Northoff and colleagues (Northoff & Bermpohl 2004; Northoff et al. 2006), claims that most self-referential processes involve activation in the brain's cortical midline structure (CMS), which includes the medial prefrontal cortex, the anterior cingulate cortex, and posteromedial cortices. One claim made in connection with this approach is that there is a common element that unites different aspects of self, an integrative glue that holds the pattern together, and that this common element is a neuronal processing of stimuli as self-referential (Northoff et al. 2006). On this view, the notion of self-referential is defined in terms of prereflective experience, which operates across a diversity of contexts, "auto-biographical, social, spatial," and so forth. It is also noted that in any particular case prereflective self-referential experience has an affective or emotional dimension. In this respect the notion of self-referential experience includes a number of aspects that can be accommodated by the concept of self-pattern (see Fingelkurts, Fingelkurts & Kallio-Tamminen 2021).

Experiments cited by Northoff et al. activate a large variety of brain areas— medial cortex, ventro- and dorsolateral prefrontal cortex, lateral parietal cortex, bilateral temporal poles, insula, and subcortical regions, including brain stem, colliculi, periaqueductal gray (PAG), and hypothalamus/hypophysis (Northoff et al. 2006, 441). These studies, however, compare only self- versus non-self-related tasks—that is, tasks where subjects had to discriminate between self and non-self.

Some critical studies, accordingly, challenge this view, arguing that processes in the CMS are not self-specific because activation in these areas also corresponds to non-self discriminations (Legrand & Ruby 2009), or to social cognition, and are related to the evaluation of others (Araujo, Kaplan & Damasio 2013). Moreover, prereflective experience is extremely difficult to operationalize in experimental settings. For example, Northoff et al. (2006), in discussing experimental data, shift the focus to processes that involve reflection or judgment, such as a trait adjective judgment task. For example, in a study by Kelley et al. (2002) subjects are asked to judge whether trait adjectives (e.g., "polite") more closely described "the participants themselves (self-referential), the current U.S. President (other-referential), or a given case (case-referential)" (Northoff et al. 2006, 441). Making this kind of judgment requires a reflective attitude, however, and it does not capture the prereflective aspect of self-awareness that defines self-referential experience. In effect, as Legrand and Ruby (2009) suggest, there are specific cognitive processes common to all of the tasks involved in the Northoff et al. review, namely a reflective process of differentiating self and non-self, involving more general or non-domain specific functions of inferential processing and memory recall. This means that the activated CMS areas are (1) not underpinning processes that are exclusively prereflective, and (2) not dedicated exclusively to self. That is, the *self-referential* processes at stake in these studies are not *self-specific* in the technical sense proposed by Legrand and Ruby as being (a) exclusively about self (and not about non-self) and (b) non-contingently (i.e., necessary for the process to be) about self. They suggest that only one thing actually meets the self-specificity requirements: the first-person perspectival nature of experience. First-person perspective is exclusively self-related (since it does not apply to the non-self) and non-contingent (since changing or losing the first-person perspective amounts to changing or losing the self/non-self distinction).

On the one hand, Legrand and Ruby want to specify one necessary condition of selfhood; on the other hand, this does not rule out that there are other relevant aspects of self that are important: "We do not claim that all there is to the self can be subsumed under a single process but propose that both basic and complex forms of self have to rely at least partly on self-specific processes" (2009, 279). Whether or not first-person perspective is a necessary condition of selfhood, the disclaimer about subsuming self under a single process is important.

The important move here is to admit that there are multiple processes that may count as self-related, even if not self-specific, and that they can be constitutive of self over and above first-person perspective. That sends us back to a pluralist approach, and it also opens up a theoretical space for the idea that processes associated with CMS may be relevant to the notion of self-pattern.[15] Indeed, Northoff et al. (2006; also Qin & Northoff 2011; Fingelkurts & Fingelkurts 2017; Fingelkurts, Fingelkurts & Kallio-Tamminen 2021) point to multiple processes that contribute to different aspects of self. These are processes in the verbal domain (as in trait adjective judgment tasks), spatial domain (egocentric versus allocentric perspective); memory domain (in relation to self-referential information); emotional domain (self-related versus non-self-related); facial recognition domain (self versus non-self); social domain (where, according to Northoff et al.'s simulationist approach, understanding of others depends on self-simulations); and domains that involve agency and ownership. Clearly, however, all of these domains can be mapped onto specific processes of the self-pattern. Processes that pertain to memory and face recognition clearly fall within the realm of psychological/cognitive aspects. Those pertaining to language (verbal domain) may also be cognitive or may include narrative aspects. Processes pertaining to the emotional domain belong to affective aspects, while social domain processes are clearly intersubjective. Those that pertain to spatial domain are closely related to first-person perspective which cuts across embodied and prereflective experiential processes and relates to the senses of agency and ownership. More generally, since all of these processes reflect a self/non-self matrix, they suggest that the embodied aspect of self/non-self differentiation may be interwoven into many of the other aspects of self-pattern. In this regard, it's notable that minimal self-referential awareness survives damage to critical areas in the CMS (Philippi et al. 2012).

Accordingly, to the extent that self-related phenomena do involve CMS activation, this reflects a self-pattern that includes a significant set of interconnected

---

[15] As I'll suggest in Chapter 4, this is important for understanding the dynamical relations within the self-pattern.

processes, but not all of the factors identified in Table 1.1. Does this analysis of the brain's CMS, then, lead to one particular specification of PTS? Whether the aspects reflected in self-referential processing in CMS constitute "the core of our self," as Northoff et al. claim, is of course open to debate. One could go more minimal and claim that the core is, as Legrand and Ruby suggest, a very minimal experiential aspect (first-person perspective), or the very basic aspects of self-awareness that survive damage to CMS areas; one could also go wider to include aspects that may go beyond CMS-related processes, such as ecological and normative aspects.

In regard to brain processes, other studies suggest that the self is both everywhere and nowhere in the brain (Gillihan & Farah 2005; Vogeley & Gallagher 2011). Although I think some of these studies raise important critical points about any attempt to reduce self to neural processes, the integrative approach pursued here does not rule out the idea that neuroscience can tell us something important about the notion of self and that neural processes may correlate in some complex, and perhaps ambiguous way with *some* specific aspects that are part of a self-pattern. I'll return to issues pertaining to such neural processes in Chapter 4.

What is clear, however, is that if ecological and normative factors, and perhaps other processes, enter into a definition of a self-pattern, then this suggests an important *proviso* on the type of approach taken by researchers who are looking specifically at neural processes that correlate with self-referential behaviors. The self-pattern is not reducible to neuronal processes, or to patterns of brain activation, although a self-pattern may certainly be reflected in such processes. This is the case not only for ecological and normative factors, but also for processes that relate to one's body, emotional, and intersubjective life, cognitive and narrative dimensions, and so forth. In each case more factors than just brain processes are involved. Although we can expect that brain processes will in some limited fashion reflect the way a self-pattern is ordered or disordered, who we are, or what self is, is more than the brain. In this respect, and at the very least, the pattern theory of self helps to map out more precisely what the possibilities are for a non-reductionist, non-deflationary theory of self that is also not inflated into a traditional Cartesian theory of the self as a substantial (soul-like) entity.

2

The Nature of Patterns

In this chapter I address some philosophical issues concerning the very concept of pattern, including the question: What is a pattern? What does it mean to say that some grouping of things constitutes a pattern, or that a pattern constitutes a self? One important question that we need to address concerns the difficulty involved in understanding a pattern in a non-reductive way. In this particular instance the question is how precisely we can take a scientific approach to what appears to be a very heterogeneous conglomeration—a motley collection that seemingly includes bodily, experiential, affective, cognitive, social, cultural, narratival, and normative aspects. How can such extremely disparate types of things somehow come together to form a pattern that supposedly constitutes a coherent phenomenon? I will propose that we should think of a pattern as an irreducible dynamical gestalt where parts or processes are organized in non-linear dynamical relations across a number of time scales. Three pattern theorists, Daniel Dennett, John Haugeland, and Scott Kelso, can offer some important guidance on these issues.

2.1 Dennett and Real Patterns

Dennett (1991b) starts his discussion of patterns with a question about whether beliefs, usually thought to be exemplar mental states, really exist. He suggests that this is not a yes or no type of question. He quotes Peter Smith, who is discussing Dennett's own notion of intentional stance (a way of explaining by attributing intentions to a system), and who suggests that Dennett: "insists that to adopt the intentional stance and interpret an agent as acting on certain beliefs and desires is to discern a pattern in his actions which is genuinely there (a pattern which is missed if we instead adopt a scientific stance)" (Smith 1988, 22). The intentional stance discerns a behavioral pattern, and we take this pattern to be what we mean when we say the other person has a belief. Is the pattern real? Dennett proposes that we should think in terms of scientific realism (rather than metaphysical realism)—X is real, even if it is an abstraction or abstract object, if it serves a productive purpose in science. Something serves a productive purpose in science if it gives us explanatory power that we do not get from a more basic account. The abstractum X is real if it cannot be reduced to or computed from all the facts about some lower-level account. A center of gravity is real on this view. If we can

The Self and its Disorders. Shaun Gallagher, Oxford University Press. © Shaun Gallagher 2024.
DOI: 10.1093/oso/9780198873068.003.0003

show that a pattern is real in this sense, and that a belief is a pattern in some secure sense, then a belief must have this kind of reality.

If a belief is a pattern—a pattern of what? Rather than neuronal pattern, Dennett opts for a pattern of behavior. Is that an objective pattern one can see in the light (as Gibson might say)? Or is the pattern something like an interpretive event—"the pattern is discernible in agents' (observable) behavior when we subject it to 'radical interpretation' (Davidson) 'from the intentional stance' (Dennett)" (1991b, 30). Indeed, Dennett seemingly wants to make the notion of pattern observer relative in the sense that he holds that "a pattern is 'by definition' a candidate for pattern recognition" (32).[1] Mechanisms of pattern recognition may differ in different animals (some animals may be able to see patterns that we cannot see), and may be affected by knowledge—expert knowledge will allow an expert to pick out patterns that others cannot see. Pattern-recognition can also be relative to the perceiver's interests:

> When two individuals confront the same data, they may perceive different patterns in them, but since we can have varied interests and perspectives, these differences do not all count as disagreements. Or in any event they should not.
> (1991b, 35)

Both patterns can be real in a pragmatic (instrumental) sense. That is, they can serve different purposes, or the same purpose differently. As Dennett makes clear, this pragmatism carries over into science. There is a pattern in a toy model, for example, that is oversimplified in comparison to the phenomenon that is being explained; but for purposes of explanation the toy model may do the job better than trying to work out the detailed pattern of the phenomenon. The same holds for the intentional stance in contrast to explanations in terms of design (explaining what a system is designed to do) or physics (explaining the architecture of the system).

But does this mean that something at the bottom of what appears to be a pattern has to be just that pattern for it to be perceived? Or can we say just that there has to be some arrangement (some pattern generation process) that allows for a pattern to emerge in such a way that it can be perceived by the right kind of perceiver? For humans with typical sense modalities set up by evolutionary forces, practically speaking, a large set of patterns can be recognized to the extent they serve survival, and so forth. A belief is a useful pattern that rests on "a reality diffused in the behavioral dispositions of the brain (and body)" (1991b, 45; Dennett

---

[1] At the same time he holds that "a pattern exists in some data—is real—if there is a description of the data that is more efficient than the bit map, *whether or not anyone can concoct it*" (1991b, 34, emphasis added)—the emphasized clause seems to indicate observer independence. This leads Haugeland and others (e.g., Ladyman et al. 2007, 205ff.) to note some ambiguity or equivocation in Dennett's essay.

is endorsing a view he finds in Paul Churchland, and rejecting Fodor's view that would put beliefs in the head, correlated to brain processes). This is Dennett's mild realistic view of pattern. He makes it clear that the opposite of the pattern is the random, that is, complete disorder.

2.2 Haugeland and the Elements

John Haugeland's (1998) insightful article is framed as a comment on Dennett's "landmark" essay on "real patterns." Haugeland offers insight because from the first he declares Dennett's essay to be not about beliefs or the intentional stance, but about "entities." On this construal Haugeland raises an important question. Does Dennett focus on patterns themselves, or on the elements (components) that make up the patterns? Haugeland's answer is that patterns and elements go hand in hand. This doesn't mean, simply, although true, that one does not have a pattern without elements, and an element does not count as an element unless it is part of a pattern. Rather, the point is that patterns and elements are relative with respect to the persistence that allows a pattern to stand out as such. From below, Haugeland explains, the pattern persists because its elements follow some kind of non-random regularity of behavior— processes occur in some kind of order. From above, a pattern persists because it has salience or relevance for purposes of predicting behavior of higher-order patterns of which it is an element. If patterns manifest this double or bivalent sense of being both a pattern relative to lower-level elements, and an element relative to higher-order patterns, the question becomes whether it's a case of patterns all the way down, or whether there are any really real (rather than pattern-real) elements at bottom.

Haugeland explains that these are two different ways of understanding the notion of pattern, which brings us back to what would count, in the context of understanding mental states, as Dennett's distinction between the physical (or possibly design) stance and the intentional (or what Haugeland might call more generally the pattern-recognition) stance. A physical or design stance (explaining something in terms of the non-random regularity of the behavior of its elements) motivates reductionist explanations and the anticipation that we will find real elements (e.g., molecules or neurons) or mechanisms at bottom obeying laws of nature. The intentional, or pattern-recognition stance depends on seeing a pattern as meaningful within a broader context. The problem for the physical or design stance is that often the elements are not well defined—the closer one looks, the more an element looks like a pattern that lacks a well-defined border. It flips into a recognition stance when you look too closely—and this seems to be the case even at the very bottom, that is, at the quantum level (see Gallagher 2018a). This, nonetheless, leads Haugeland to some optimism:

For if the independent identifiability of the elements of an orderly-arrangement pattern is problematic, and if, at the same time, the identity of a recognition pattern can be context dependent, then the one hand may wash the other. Rather than merging (so as to coincide), the two notions of pattern join forces, to mutual advantage. In this larger conception, the 'elements' of an orderly arrangement need no longer be thought of as *simple* ('elementary'), like bits or pixels, or even as independently identifiable. On the contrary, they might be quite elaborate, elusive, and/or subtle—so long as some relevant creatures are (or can learn to be) able to recognize them. This recognizability, in turn, can perfectly well depend, in part, on their participation in the arrangement of which they are the elements.   (1998, 275)

As it stands with the different stances that Dennett defines, they nicely fit his distinction between different levels—the subpersonal and the personal levels to be sure—the elements that subtend the pattern, and the pattern itself. Haugeland places quotation marks around "level" in one instance,[2] but otherwise continues to frame issues in "the larger, two-level picture" (1998, 276). Conceiving of elements and patterns in terms of levels typically leads, as Haugeland indicates, to a reductionist strategy consistent, for example, with mechanistic explanations. I think we may begin to move away from the ontological complications highlighted by Haugeland, by abandoning any strong, and certainly any ontological conception of level, and by adopting an ontological stance that looks for processes and dynamical connections, and that therefore treats levels as explanatory abstractions.

2.3 Kelso and Dynamic Patterns

The brilliant Irishman Scott Kelso, cites "the brilliant Englishman Alan Turing" on the concept of pattern: "Most of an organism most of the time is developing from one pattern to another not from homogeneity into a pattern" (Kelso 1995, 3). Likewise, I want to say that the type of pattern at stake in the concept of self-pattern is necessarily heterogeneous, and coming from heterogeneity, since it integrates very diverse phenomena. The integration, however, brings about some kind of coherence. One important question is how heterogeneous elements can be coherently integrated. Bodily, experiential, affective, behavioral, cognitive, narratival, social, worldly processes, plus normativity! Are these diverse factors integrated in a hierarchical scheme of levels? One could imagine the normative

---

[2] He writes: "Dennett's ambivalence between the two notions of 'pattern' is deeply connected with his initial vacillation between considering patterns and considering their elements; for both involve the same distinction of 'level'" (1998, 276).

floating on top of the behavioral, for example. Does the idea that all of these factors involve *processes* provide a common denominator? "Everybody knows that the world is made up of processes from which patterns emerge" (Kelso 1995, 3; also see Simondon 1958). In trying to work out how patterns emerge from heterogeneous processes, Kelso comes close to giving up the idea that we need to think in terms of levels:[3]

> Understanding will be sought in terms of essential variables that characterize patterns of behavior regardless of what elements are involved in producing the patterns or at what level these patterns are studied or observed....I will try to avoid dualities such as top-down versus bottom-up and macro versus micro because I think they can be misleading. What is macro at one level, after all, can be micro at another.   (1995, 2)

He nonetheless retains the notion of different levels of explanation, a notion also found in mechanist approaches. At the same time his account involves the complexity of self-organizing dynamical systems:[4] "Often mechanisms for a given phenomenon are sought on lower levels, in the interior workings of the system. That view may be flawed if lower levels also turn out to be governed by the same kinds of self-organized dynamical principles or generic mechanisms shown to be at work [at higher levels]" (1995, 134). Again, the closer you look at the elements the more you see patterns; dynamical relations rather than discrete elements or levels.

The problems to be solved in such a system concern integration (of the many and different kinds of processes or factors), adaptation ("how patterns are produced to accommodate different circumstances" or how they adjust to changing conditions [1995, 5]), and persistence or stability. This latter issue is critical for a self-organizing system in which, according to Kelso, there is no set of instructions to follow, no "self," "no agent inside the system doing the organizing" (1995, 8). Principles of self-organization have to solve these problems. Here, as I understand them, are the principles listed by Kelso that do some of the explanatory work:

(1) Interactions among the different factors are non-linear: "the whole is not only greater than, but *different* than the sum of the motions of its parts" (1995, 16).

---

[3] "Mind you, no value is meant to be assigned to the words 'higher' and 'lower' as if one level is better or more fundamental than the other. I simply mean the levels above and below where the cooperativity (pattern, structure) is observed" (Kelso 1995, 18).

[4] The idea of dynamic patterns with fields of prediction and control in the domain of psychology are prefigured in earlier research in theoretical biology (Rosen 1970; Maturana & Varela 1980) and cybernetics (McCulloch 1965). As we'll see, a "dynamic pattern" involves a non-linear, adaptive, dynamical causality involving processes of interdependent elements which are determined not only by their properties and fields, but also by their relationships and functions within the whole.

(2) Energy in the system is not uniformly distributed; it dissipates via those structures that tend to be efficient, reducing the degrees of freedom that contribute to behavior.

(3) This leads to an emerging pattern organized by order parameters (collective variables), "created by the coordination between the parts, but in turn [influencing] the behavior of the parts" (10); this is circular causality.

(4) Order parameters around nonequilibrium phase transitions may lead to loss of stability giving rise to new or different patterns; but this is balanced by some degree of stability due to order parameters that are not as near to transitions. This is sometimes called "metastability."

(5) Perturbations continually test the system, "allowing it to feel its stability" or to move toward new patterns.

(6) Control parameters (external constraints) or boundary conditions influence the development of new patterns.

(7) Order parameters may be simple or complicated, giving rise to behavioral complexity.

Kelso indicates that "the precise patterns that form may differ from one scale of observation to another, but the basic pattern-forming principles are the same" (1995, 25). I think the concept of different scales—specifiable different time scales as I'll suggest—is important. It leads to the claim that psychology "is not just applied physics, or for that matter, applied biology" (25); Dennett and Haugeland would agree that the intentional stance is something different from the physical or design stance. I note that none of this is far from Merleau-Ponty's rejection of reductionist views in regard to physical, biological, and the human orders in his first book, *The Structure of Behavior*. Under the influence of Gestalt psychology, he writes that even with respect to the physical order, the "genesis of the whole by composition of the parts is fictitious. It arbitrarily breaks the chain of reciprocal determinations" (Merleau-Ponty 1963, 50). As Kelso argues, such reciprocal determination, or what he terms "circular causality," is not reducible to simple feedback loops or comparator models, since "there is no reference state [in a dynamic pattern] with which feedback can be compared and no place where comparison operations are performed" (9).

All of this pushes toward the following question: What would an account of patterns that did not appeal to hierarchical levels look like?[5] The answer is

---

[5] A distinction is often made between ontological levels and explanatory levels with the idea that the latter does not entail the former. Still, explanatory levels come with implicit (if not explicit) ontological commitments. Levels of explanation seemingly imply something about the levels of the explananda. For example, when one says that a theory about molecules is lower level than a theory of neurons, that's because molecules are thought to be at a lower level. Oppenheim and Putnam (1958) clearly had both explanatory and ontological commitments. Thus, Eronen (2015, 48) writes: "The levels of Oppenheim and Putnam are not just an ordering of branches of science or theories; they involve 'things.' Oppenheim and Putnam assume that at each level there are certain types of things:

necessarily complicated. One reason is that explanations framed in terms of different levels have been very productive in science. Yet, it is also the case that there are different conceptions of levels. Philip Gerrans, for example, even as he attempts to integrate predictive processing with a mechanist approach in the psychiatric context, acknowledges something of a mishmash of levels:

> The notion of levels is ubiquitous, but not everyone uses it in the same way. It can refer to ordering relationships between theories . . . ; the objects of theories ordered by size or complexity, e.g., cells are smaller and less complex than the organs they make up; functional analyses, e.g., vision is a higher-level property than edge detection; or levels of mereological containment, e.g., parts are at a lower level than wholes. These uses can overlap. The notion of level relevant to [Gerrran's analysis] is that of mechanism. Higher levels correspond to the organization of components, lower levels to components.   (Gerrans 2014, 229–30).

In other words, he prefers a mereological conception. Yet, this would not be consistent with predictive processing, which is also an approach he favors. For predictive models, levels are not at all mereological, but include inter-level causal relations, and reference state comparators between higher and lower levels. That difference aside, the proliferation of different conceptions of levels is enough to motivate some theorists who employ the notion of levels to add some qualifications and to move away from the concept of hierarchy, especially in the context of understanding psychiatric disorders (e.g., Eronen 2021). Thus, for example, William Bechtel (2020) develops a mechanist view that favors a heterarchical set of neural control mechanisms, rejecting a hierarchical organization in favor of lateral constraints within a network:

> Control mechanisms do not have to conform to a hierarchy, and the hierarchical perspective is especially misleading in the case of organisms. Control mechanisms are added to organisms opportunistically in the course of evolution when they serve to facilitate the ability of the organism to maintain and replicate itself as an autonomous system. This does not impose any requirement of hierarchical organization.   (Bechtel 2020, 31; also see Bechtel & Huang 2022)

Likewise, James Woodward (2020) notes that "levels eliminativism"—"the thought that we would be better off avoiding level talk entirely"—is motivated by the fact that researchers operate with different conceptions of levels without

---

elementary particles at the lowest level, atoms at the next higher level, and so on. In this sense, the levels of organization are not just reflecting features of theories and sciences, but also features of the world." In this regard, even if one thinks of levels as metaphorical (Craver 2007, 177), or as a heuristic, it doesn't mean that they are ontologically neutral. Implicitly, if not explicitly, they reflect, as William Wimsatt (2007, 203) suggests, "the ontological architecture of our natural world."

always distinguishing them. Analyses that assume levels also tend to supports various reductive or mechanistic explanations (see Eronen 2015; 2021). Woodward, however, endorses the concept of levels because it continues to do some useful work in science. After discussing several different types of levels, he focuses on an interactionist conception of level, characterized by conditional independence. Conditional independence concerns explanation. If we can explain a phenomenon in terms of a higher-level variable, we don't need to explain it as depending on a lower variable:

> For example, if we are interested in the relation between thermodynamic variables, we don't need a detailed description of the behavior of individual molecules; their aggregate impact as expressed in terms of variables like temperature or volume is all that is needed.   (Woodward 2020, 428)

Accordingly, if I can explain a particular phenomenon in terms of temperature changes, there is no need to provide an account of subtending molecular changes. Woodward, however, goes on to suggest that the interaction conception of level is closely tied to the role of different spatial, temporal, or energetic scales in constructing causal models. Different scales matter specifically as they relate to the "strength and nature" of causal interactions.

The concept of scales, however, is different from the concept of levels.[6] Craver and Darden (2013, 162ff.), for example, assume this distinction in their discussion of integration. They distinguish between levels of products, levels of units, levels of causation, levels of composition, levels of mechanisms, and so forth. Differences in time scales, in contrast, involve differences in how we measure processes. Craver and Darden do discuss different temporal scales and intertemporal integration, indicating that "mechanisms often operate at and across different time scales" (182), although they would deny causal relations across different levels. They focus on relatively large time scales (evolutionary, developmental) and downplay the role of feedback by dividing processes into stages (172; see Section 2.4, below). Ladyman et al. (2007), call this "scale relativity," which they define as "the idea that which terms of description and principles of individuation we use to track the world vary with the scale at which the world is measured" (199). The fact that some process is observable only at a specific scale (e.g., X), however, doesn't mean that if it is not observable at a different scale (e.g., Y), it is not operating or having some effect at Y.

---

[6] Eronen (2021, 929) notes that "differences in time scales could be used to define levels, but scales are continuous, where the boundary between levels should be drawn may not have a clear answer.... The upshot is that defining levels in psychopathology is far from straightforward. The exact levels and their significance can vary strongly from context to context. In psychology, it is often unclear how part-whole or scale-based levels should be understood in the first place. This suggests that levels in psychopathology are best seen as heuristic idealizations that are helpful in making rough distinctions, but do not mark deep ontological features of the world."

In attempts to understand psychiatric disorders, Woodward notes, neat distinctions between levels or scales are complicated, because "the list of possible explanatory factors for some set of explananda may be very open ended and at different levels [by one or more different criteria]" (2020, 432):

> Arguably, this is the case for many explananda in psychiatry: many different causal factors—social or environmental factors, factors having to do with personality type, as well as genes and brain structure—are relevant to paradigmatic mental illnesses such as depression.   (2020, 432–3).

Nonetheless, appeals are made to the concept of levels in the biopsychosocial model, where Engel, considers the bio, the psycho, and the social as different levels organized in a "hierarchically arranged continuum," interconnected by "material and information flow" (1980, 536–7; see Figure 2.1). One finds appeals to different levels of explanation in network models of psychopathology (e.g., Borsboom 2017, 11), as well as in the Hierarchical Taxonomy of Psychopathology (HiTOP) model (Kotov et al. 2017), which attempts to identify psychiatric phenomena based on patterns of symptom covariation (Williams & Simms 2020). Likewise, again, in phenomenological (Fuchs 2012; Sass et al. 2018) and neurophenomenological (Nelson et al. 2020) approaches. Louis Sass, for example, worries about how to explain the relations among the various "component processes" that make up human existence—whether they should be thought of as hierarchical, causal, or constitutive. As he puts it, "these questions pertain to theoretical issues that are difficult or even impossible to settle, such as overall attitudes toward holistic explanation or the enigmatic mind/body problem (generally viewed as utterly insoluble)" (Sass et al. 2018, 725). Even if we acknowledge that the concept of hierarchical levels has been productive in discussions of diagnosis and treatment in psychiatry (see e.g., Holmes et al. 2021), there is still no consensus on the dimensions to be included, or how general or specific they should be.

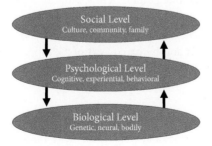

Figure 2.1 Biopsychosocial hierarchy of levels
Source: (Author; see Engel 1980).

To further motivate abandoning hierarchical level accounts, consider Coninx and Stilwell's (2023) discussion of Engel's biopsychosocial model, where they consider a number of general problems tied specifically to the concept of hierarchical levels, namely, that such models lead to reductionist, fragmented, and linear explanations. First, the tendency toward a *bio- or neuro-reductionist* strategy is reflected in "measurement choices, diagnostic focus, and treatment selection." Practically speaking, the biopsychosocial model is reinterpreted such that the biological level is treated as more basic—the "real or root cause" of psychological and social problems. Second, Engel himself suggests that each level needs to be investigated by different specialized disciplines—an investigator is generally "obliged to select one system level on which to concentrate" (Engel 1980, 537); this leads to a fragmented explanation. "Separate domains [thus] become the subject of independent research, diagnosis, and treatment while it remains largely unclear how they are connected. Engel's characterization of 'material and information flow' proves hardly informative" (Coninx & Stilwell 2023, 13). Elsewhere, I've referred to this as the "clunky robot problem" as it applies to theory formation—different teams of robotic designers work independently designing different parts of the system, and when it's time to put them all together to build the robot, they don't fit very well (Gallagher 2017a). Applied to theory building, this kind of fragmentation defeats the quest for an integrated theoretical approach. Finally, hierarchical level models tend to be implemented in a *linear* manner. "That is, uni-directional causal pathways are assumed between involved factors, which themselves are considered as insensitive to context or temporal unfolding and, thus, strictly decomposable....This picture seems empirically inadequate concerning the relation of processes within and across domains as they are dynamically intertwined along different time spans" which means that they are not easily differentiated or decomposable (Coninx & Stilwell 2023, 13).

In contrast to hierarchical levels, in my view, we should think of a pattern as an irreducible dynamical gestalt where parts or processes are organized in nonlinear dynamical relations across a number of time scales. Kelso considers this perspective to be opposed to what he calls the "machine stance" (1995, 35). It is also clear that this dynamical gestalt view is close to an enactive process view, most closely associated with Francisco Varela and a growing number of others (Di Paolo 2005; Gallagher 2017a; Hutto & Myin 2017; Thompson 2007; Varela, Thompson & Rosch 1991; and in the context of psychopathology, de Haan 2020, and Fuchs 2017; 2020). Evan Thompson expresses an important insight in this regard:

> In the process view, 'up' and 'down' are contextual-relative terms used to describe phenomena of various scales and complexity. There is no base level of elementary entities to serve as the ultimate 'emergence base' on which to ground everything. Phenomena at all scales are not entities or substances but relatively stable

processes, and since processes achieve stability at different levels of complexity, while still interacting with processes at other levels, all are equally real and none has absolute ontological primacy.   (2007, 441)

I think we can go further. Further even than what Woodward calls "level neutrality" (2020, 436). On his view, level neutrality allows us to define a level based on causal interaction, that is, a unique level defined by all processes that causally interact. Explanation can be confined to that level and can ignore other levels that are not part of the interaction. In that case, however, it's not clear that the notion of level is really doing any work. If the focus is on all processes that causally interact, without reference to other levels, this allows us to bracket talk about levels altogether, without explanatory loss. Rather than the vocabulary of "levels," we can use a vocabulary developed in dynamical/enactivist approaches. We can retain talk of metastability as a way to characterize dynamical coherence, and a set of closely related enactivist concepts: "organizational autonomy," "regional identity," "viability" (Kirchoff & Froese 2017; Ramírez-Vizcaya & Froese 2019) or "functional norm" (Nielsen and Ward's 2020; Maiese 2022, 98)—concepts that allow for adaptation, and can productively apply to a self-pattern that includes both bodily and social/cultural processes. To clarify the enactivist concept of a level-free pattern as dynamical gestalt, I'll contrast it with two other views: (1) a view associated with new mechanist explanations, and (2) a view of integration as an emerging fusion.

2.4 From Mechanism to Dynamical Gestalt

Here I follow up on Kelso's claim that in mechanist approaches explanations for a given phenomenon "are sought on lower levels, in the interior workings of the system," but that this may be problematic if what we find on lower levels are just more patterns that follow self-organizing dynamical principles (Kelso 1995, 134). According to what Varela and Goguen call a "fregean (sic) systems viewpoint" (1978, 316), a pattern is a phenomenon constituted by elements or parts that operate on a lower level and that are related to each other in a causal fashion. This fits precisely with the new mechanist view as proposed by Carl Craver (2007), and others. On this view, causal relations are *intra*-level relations only; constitutive relations are *inter*-level compositional or mereological, non-causal relations (Craver 2007; Craver & Bechtel 2007). Accordingly, one could think of a pattern as a whole, composed of parts or processes, each part or (partial) process defined as different from another part or process. The elements (individuals, properties, processes) that compose the pattern work together causally and come to be integrated so as to non-causally result in a specific pattern under certain background conditions. Lower-level properties can non-causally realize higher-order properties,

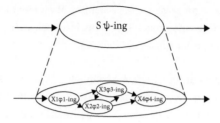

Figure 2.2 Schema of mechanism

Note: The micro-components at the lower level of the mechanism (X1–X4) engage in processes (φ 1-ing—φ 4-ing) that are causally related; these components constitute S, and the processes non-causally implement the higher-order process (ψ -ing).

Source: Redrawn from Craver (2007, 7).

and lower-level processes can non-causally implement higher-order processes. This kind of compositional inter-level constitution (where micro components at a lower level constitute macro components at a higher level) is non-causal, even if it involves productive intra-level mechanistic causal processes at the lower level (Figure 2.2).

Specifically, compositional (constitutional) relations, are "non-causal determination relations that are synchronous," and involve organized elements ("teams of individuals") all of which "are spatially contained within the constituted individual, and such that the properties of the individuals in the team realize the properties of the constituted individual and the processes grounded by the individuals in the team implement the processes grounded by the constituted individual" (Gillett 2013, 317–18). Something is a compositional constituent of an individual if it is a working part—i.e., if it contributes in a way "that non-causally results in the 'work' done by the relevant whole" (2013, 319).

Assuming that constitution relies on part–whole relations, there are two reasons why theorists such as Craver, Bechtel, Gillett, and other new mechanists distinguish between causality and constitution:

(1) The relation between part and whole cannot be causal, because causality involves mereological independence of cause and effect. For example, the handle of the teacup is part of the teacup, but it does not cause the teacup.

(2) Also, part–whole relations are contemporaneous relations; causality requires diachronicity.

To further clarify the analysis, Craver, in his book, *Explaining the Brain* (2007), notes the importance of mutual manipulability (MM) for defining constitutional relevance:

My working account of constitutive relevance is as follows: a component is relevant to the behavior of a mechanism as a whole when one can wiggle the behavior of the whole by wiggling the behavior of the component and one can wiggle the behavior of the component by wiggling the behavior as a whole. The two are related as part and whole and they are mutually manipulable.

(Craver 2007, 152–3)

At this point, however, some ambiguity emerges. The orthodox interpretation of constitutive relevance understands parts and whole to be spatiotemporally over-lapping entities such that their behaviors are not (and cannot be) causally related, even if they are subject to MM. Craver, however, explains the notion of whole-part mutual wiggling in terms of James Woodward's (2003) interventionist con-ception of causality.[7] This seems to introduce causality into the constitution relation, albeit causality of a circular or cyclic kind (see Woodward 2020, 440). MM, as defined on the notion of Woodwardian intervention, would pick out causal relations, but inter-level constitutional relations are not supposed to be causal. So, the question is: How do we save the constitution/causality distinction in Craver's model of mechanism?

I won't review the different attempts to address the causality/constitution prob-lem here (see Gallagher 2018b; Varga 2018, 115ff.). But one of these attempts is of interest because, although it stays within the framework of mechanistic levels, I think it leads to a more dynamical explanation, which answers the challenge of how to explain that different factors in a pattern are dynamically related. Beate Krickel (2017; 2018) shows how we can preserve part–whole relations as syn-chronically constitutive, but also allow for inter-level causal relations that are captured by an interventionist form of MM. On her account, the interventionist co-wiggling operates not between composite-working parts and whole, but between micro-level composite-working parts (or processes) and macro-level parts

---

[7] Woodward understands causality to be a probabilistic counterfactual dependence relation. In other words, X causally relates to Y iff an intervention on X makes a difference to the probability of Y, assuming appropriate background conditions. Causal relations are identified using interventions to show probabilistic dependencies between variables. Accordingly, this theory allows for causal rela-tions between a wide variety of factors—biological, psychological, social, and so forth—regardless of whether or not one thinks of such factors as existing on different levels. Let me note that an "interven-tion" in this context is meant to be an ideal or precision intervention, which means that one would want an intervention such that, when applied to the whole, it would directly wiggle just one part or element, holding fixed all other elements (thereby demonstrating that part's relevance to the function-ing of the whole), or such that, when applied to the one part it would directly wiggle the whole. Practically (experimentally) speaking, ideal interventions are very difficult to do. Eronen gives the following example: "one can change the behavior of the phototransduction mechanism by depolariz-ing the rod cell, and one can change the behavior of the rod cell by exposing the retina to a light stimulus" (2015, 48). It's not clear whether the intervention on the retina by changing the light stimu-lus (1) changes the retina as a whole (on the macro-level), that is, changing many processes in the eye, and not just the rods, in which case one loses precision, or (2) changes the retina by changing the behavior of just the rods, in which case it seems to be just an intervention on the rods rather than on the whole. For several other problems with the notion of levels in this kind of mechanist account, see Eronen (2015). For the application of interventionist causality in the psychiatric context, see Campbell (2016) and Woodward (2020). And for other issues involved in applying the interventionist causality model as applied to network theory of psychopathology, see de Boer et al. (2021).

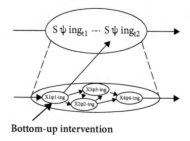

Figure 2.3 Krickel intervention
Source: From Gallagher (2018b), with permission.

(or processes) that are diachronically (rather than synchronically) inter-level related. One only needs to think of S ψ -ing as itself a temporal process, which makes it possible that an intervention on one lower-level process, X1φ 1-ing, for example, may wiggle, not the whole mechanism, but a temporal part of the S ψ -ing that is diachronically later than X1φ 1-ing (Figure 2.3).

This account requires that we allow for inter-level diachronic (and not strictly contemporaneous) relations that can therefore be causal, and that run along with compositional, non-causal constitutive relations (see Kirchhoff 2017 for a similar view). In terms of explaining a pattern, this means, at the very least, that we should not think of a pattern as something static or momentary. It is something that persists over time, and it may do so despite some changes in some of its compositional and temporal parts.

Pursuing this idea, we can step away from the mechanist view and move toward a genuinely dynamical conception of pattern of the sort that Kelso is after. This involves stripping away the notion of hierarchical levels—so a pattern is not at a higher level than the processes that constitute it; it just is, or is nothing more nor less than, and certainly nothing over and above the order or organization defined by the dynamical relations amongst the heterogeneous processes that make it up. This is what Varela and Goguen call a "system-whole," the constitutive relations of which are mutual and reciprocal and characterized by organizational or operational closure: "their organization is a circular network of interactions rather than a tree of hierarchical processes" (1978, 292).[8] Operational closure gives the system some degree of stability, which can be disrupted, but can also be re-established by compensatory adjustments. A pattern is the organizational closure of the processes that constitute it.

The organization, the dynamical arrangement, is key. On the enactive conception, an active biological system is constituted through processes of dynamical

---

[8] Note that Varela used the term "organizational closure" when writing with Maturana and in his early papers; he shifts to "operational closure" in his later work. Evan Thompson suggests that operational closure is more dynamic (2007, 45).

coupling, involving some set of causal interactions among processes that extend over brain, body, and environment, and may include elements, properties, relations, and processes that are not internal to the organism, or reducible to just the organism.[9] Although some aspects of a system can be characterized in synchronic terms, an account of an active system must include the kind of diachronic causal relations that explains the coupling between the different elements, and the constitution of the pattern. Constitution, on this view, is causal, specifically insofar as it involves a type of causality out of which emerges a relational, autonomous phenomenon.

It's important to understand the nature of this causality. It has been variously called reciprocal causality, circular causality (Kelso 1995; Fuchs 2012; 2020; Varela & Goguen 1978), or organizational causality (de Haan 2020). There are clearly reciprocal (two-way) or circular causal processes involved in the notion of pattern. But this is not a complete characterization of the causality involved. In a pattern, more than two elements may be involved in a more complex pattern of causality that can be circular, but can also involve multiple, non-linear or indirect interactions. One characterization of circular causality, however, retains the concept of levels. For example, Thomas Fuchs writes: "mental illnesses are marked by a disruption of vertical circular causality; that is, the interplay between lower-level processes and higher faculties of the organism" (2012, 331). On this view, circular causality just is a form of reciprocal, downward and upward relations between parts and whole (Fuchs 2020; also see Bolis et al. 2017 and Figure 2.4).

The term "organizational causality," suggested by Sanneke de Haan (2020, 119), might seem more appropriate. De Haan develops the notion of organizational causality as a way to address what she calls psychiatry's integration problem, which involves explaining how physiological processes are related to experiential processes (2020, 70), or more generally, how different perspectives (bio-psycho-social) can be integrated (2020, 2ff.). She suggests, following Paul Humphreys (1996), that this form of causality allows us to move away from the idea of levels or hierarchical arrangements.

---

[9] Evan Thompson characterizes a system in a similar way, emphasizing the autopoietic concept of autonomy. "What counts as the system in any given case, and hence whether it is autonomous or heteronomous, is context-dependent and interest-relative. For any system it is always possible to adopt a heteronomy or external-control perspective, and this can be useful for many purposes. Nevertheless, this stance does not illuminate—and indeed can obscure—certain observable patterns of behavior, namely, patterns arising from the system's internal dynamics rather than external parameters. An organism dynamically produces and maintains its own organization as an invariant through change, and thereby also brings forth its own domain of interaction.... A heteronomy perspective does not provide an adequate framework to investigate and understand this phenomenon; an autonomy perspective is needed" (Thompson 2007, 50). The concepts of internal and external are relative to where one sees the boundaries. This, in some sense, could be modeled as an enhanced General Systems Theory (von Bertalanffy 1950) which inspired the biopsychosocial model in psychiatry (Engel 1977).

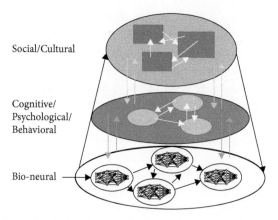

Figure 2.4 Reciprocal and circular causal relations between multiple levels
Source: Author (Modeled on Bolis et al. 2017).

On the one hand, this rejection of level- and hierarchical conceptions aligns well with what I have been arguing in this chapter (also see Gallagher 2020b; 2022; Gallagher & Daly 2018). The causal relations are neither bottom-up nor top-down. Moreover, I agree that the right conception of causality can lead to a better solution than the ambiguous mix of levels that we have seen in the theories discussed above. On the other hand, however, de Haan associates organizational causality with Humphreys' idea of emergence as fusion. The notion of fusion, however, is unhelpful; it's not commensurable with the idea of a pattern. Even if a pattern is constituted in some sense in the dynamical relations among its various factors and processes, those factors and processes remain distinct, although in some cases difficult to pull apart. In contrast, to explain emergence as fusion de Haan offers the analogy of a cake, where all of the ingredients, even if they start out as differentiated, once baked, become fused in such a way that one can no longer distinguish sugar from flour from flavorings, and so forth. In this regard she quotes Humphreys: "when emergence occurs the lower-level property instances go out of existence in producing the higher-level emergent instances" (Humphreys 1996, 10; de Haan 2020,118). Even if we bracket the talk of "levels," however, as de Haan wants to do, the various processes that constitute a pattern do not go out of existence, nor do they fuse to the point where we cannot discriminate among processes that are clearly affective or clearly cognitive, or clearly intersubjective, and so forth, even if such processes are dynamically integrated. In psychiatric practice we need a model of integration that does not subvert useful distinctions among the neurobiological, the phenomenological, the social, and the existential, to use de Haan's own list of perspectives.

Instead of fusion, we can think of organizational causality as involving dynamical transformations. When one factor is dynamically related to another factor, both factors are transformed or changed, but they do not disappear in the process. This is consistent with what de Haan maintains, namely that "we can no longer assume that parts or processes still have the same properties once they have become part of a whole" (personal correspondence; also see de Haan 2020, 116).

Within a self-pattern, for example, we still need to discriminate affect from narrative from cognitive processes, even if we do not want to think of them as operating on different levels, and even if they are in some way causally integrated or meshed and transformed in the process. Accordingly, emergence as a confectionary fusion seems too strong a characterization for the constitution of a pattern. A pattern is not a cake. Even if an individual's affective life changes by means of narrative therapy, for example, neither affect nor narrative go out of existence to form something else. We can acknowledge with de Haan that processes in the self-pattern change as they mesh with other changing processes, but this is not a fusion into indistinguishable processes. Indeed, when de Haan discusses psychiatric diagnosis and treatment, she reverts to the concept of complex patterns, framed in terms of network models (2020, 244ff.).

Although the term "organizational causality" works well here, to avoid the idea of emergence as fusion I'll refer to the idea of *dynamical causality*, where in some cases relations are non-linear, and transformational, but without levels and without fusion. In the case of dynamical causality an intervention above a certain threshold may result in changes to one or more factors, directly or indirectly, serially or in parallel, and include looping effects, all of which depend on parameters of flexibility in the pattern.

2.5 Enactive Constitution

The claim is that, on the enactive view, just these non-linear, dynamical causal relations constitute the active system as a holistic dynamical gestalt. We can find support for this in a number of authors. Anthony Chemero (2009) and Orestis Palermos (2014), for example, argue that the presence of just such non-linear relations, or the continuous mutual interaction loops which entail such relations, may count as an objective criterion of constitution. Also, consider that on the enactivist account the system is autopoietic and allows for the kind of recovery, repair, and reorganization (or restructuring) characteristic of biological systems. Leuridan (2012) cites Mitchell on the importance of such processes:

> Recovery and reorganization (also known as robustness) are both common and important phenomena: 'The capacity for robustness appears to be both ubiquitous and significant for biological systems. Indeed robustness gives evolved complex systems, including organisms and ecosystems, the ability to survive in an environment with changing internal and external conditions'.
>
> (Mitchell 2009, 71–2; Leuridan 2012, 405)

With respect to the concept of constitution, then, we can say that at the very least, there are several forms: synchronic compositional constitution (of the sort the new mechanists defend) and diachronic causal constitution (of the sort found in Krickel 2017 and Kirchhoff 2017).[10] Diachronic constitution, however, to the extent that it is still tied to a concept of levels, does not go far enough to satisfy the requirements of enactivism. Specifically, it does not capture everything we need in order to characterize the dynamical nature of the system. In this respect, the introduction of dynamical constitution across different time scales is important. As indicated above, time scales are distinguished from levels. For dynamical systems, non-linear relations across different time scales are essential. In contrast to mechanists who typically have in mind identical time scales (e.g., Craver & Bechtel 2007), the idea that there are diachronic inter-level relations that break with a strictly contemporaneous order and are subject to MM, motivates the need to consider different time scales.

In the system of brain-body-environment (which roughly is the system that generates a self-pattern) processes occur on several time scales. It's important to grasp how these time scales interrelate in order to understand how constitution can be, not only diachronic, but also non-linearly dynamic. To make this clear, I'll refer to a threefold distinction proposed by Francisco Varela (1999) among elementary, integrative, and narrative time scales—a distinction based on both neurobiology and phenomenology (see Gallagher 2017a for a more detailed account):

- The elementary scale (varying roughly across tens to hundreds of milliseconds)
- The integrative scale (varying roughly from 0.5 to 3 seconds)
- The narrative scale involving memory (above 3 seconds).

For our purposes here I'll focus on the elementary and integrative scales. The elementary scale corresponds to processes that involve neurophysiology, and many non-conscious bodily processes. On a dynamical systems interpretation, such processes synchronize (by phase-locking) and correlate to incompressible but complete subjective experiences on the integrative scale—an instance of prereflective consciousness, characterized by Husserl as the experienced living present (or what William James [1890] called the specious present). These processes integrate in fully constituted cognitive operations (an act of perception or memory, for instance). Motorically the integrative scale corresponds to a basic action (e.g., reaching, grasping). These time scales can be plotted on linear objective

---

[10] To be clear, I think Krickel's notion of diachronic constitution opens the door to considering a more enactive, non-mechanistic conception of dynamical constitution. Kirchhoff (2015) builds a concept of diachronic constitution that I think goes even more in this direction, and more rightly should be called dynamical constitution.

clock time, as indicated by the temporal specifications of milliseconds and seconds. Yet, objective time doesn't capture the significance of the relations among these scales, and it does not hold consistently as a rule across all three scales. The integrative time scale of conscious experience is not equivalent to the simple aggregate of intervals as measured on the elementary scale. For example, there is a form of elemental-to-integrative temporal relation such that from the perspective of the integrative scale, there is no experiential difference (one does not consciously experience the difference) between ten and twenty msecs as measured on the elemental scale. Successive elemental processes that fall within a thirty–fifty msecs time frame are typically experienced as simultaneous (Milton & Pleydell-Pearce 2016; Ronconi & Melcher 2017; Wutz et al. 2014). Accordingly, between the elementary and the integrative time scale, relations are not straightforwardly linear or additive such that one can simply sum up a number of elementary time periods or put them in a specific order to get to an integrated second or an experience of that same order. Because temporal integration is dynamically dependent on activation in a number of dispersed neural assemblies, it doesn't necessarily preserve an objective linear sequence that would reflect the neural events.

Consider another example. When a stimulus of fifty msec. is followed by a stimulus of 100 msec., the integrated event (i.e., the combined event experienced on the integrative scale) is not necessarily an additive sum of 150 msecs. "Instead, the earlier stimulus interacts with the processing of the 100 msec. interval, resulting in the encoding of a distinct temporal object. Thus, temporal information is encoded in the context of the entire pattern, not as conjunctions of the component intervals" (Karmarkar & Buonomano 2007, 432). The integration occurs according to dynamical, non-linear principles.[11]

The point is that relational phenomena as they are modulated across these different time scales are dynamically non-linear—processes that are not straightforwardly contemporaneous in their different time scales, but not simply diachronic if we think of diachronicity as involving mere succession. Accordingly, the enactivist notion of dynamical-causal constitution differs from both the mechanistic conception of contemporaneous, non-causal constitution and a merely diachronic (sequential/linear) causal conception of constitution.

On the enactive view we can think of the system as a set of elements engaged in processes that, across different time scales, constitute a dynamical gestalt.

---

[11] Other good examples involve intersensory integration (Foxx & Simpson 2002) and temporal masking (Bregman & Rudnicky 1975). Also see Dennett & Kinsbourne (1992); Gallagher (1998). Attempting to capture this idea, Varela, in his naturalized, neurophenomenological account, referenced Husserl's phenomenology of intrinsic temporality, the temporal structure of consciousness (Varela 1999; Gallagher & Varela 2003). The important point for Varela is that the biologically based system he describes captures the dynamical flow structure that Husserl was after, the constituting relations of which include diachronic relations that are nonlinear dynamical ones.

The dynamical processual relations among the elements that constitute the pattern make them elements of this gestalt. Any intervention (above a critical threshold) on a processual element will cause a change in the system precisely because it will be a manipulation of processes that are already in mutual dynamical reciprocal relations.[12] In such a system, a change in a part or process can change or constrain other parts or process elements. This defines dynamical constitution in terms of dynamical causality.

Because this kind of gestalt structure involves complex interconnections among its various processes, I mentioned that it is difficult to find examples of ideal or precision interventions. Here's an example of what I take to be close to a precision intervention which nonetheless tells us something important about overall structure. This is an experiment conducted by Kelso and colleagues (Kelso, Tuller & Fowler 1982; Kelso, Saltzman & Tuller 1986), who refer to it as a test of "pipe-block" speech. The system that enables speech in humans is complex. "For a baby to say 'ba' requires the precise coordination of approximately 36 muscles" (Kelso 1995, 40). An intervention on this coordinated system is made by a pipe (of the smoking sort) held between the teeth as one (adult in this case) speaks. The pipe freezes the jaw's movement but doesn't disrupt speech. In case this is viewed as a matter of practice, Kelso conducted an experiment that involved a more spontaneous adjustment that disrupted the action of the jaw during speech to see if the other parts of the system compensated for a novel disruption. Infrared sensors measured movements of the lips and jaw; wire electrodes recorded electromyographic (EMG) activity of various speech muscles. A prosthetic device allowed the experiments to manipulate jaw action.

> The results were stunning. When we suddenly halted the jaw for a few milliseconds as it was raising toward the final [b] in [b æ b] (rhymes with lab), the upper and lower lips compensated immediately so as to produce the [b] but no compensation was observed in the tongue [or speech muscles]. Conversely, when we applied the same jaw perturbation during the final [z] in the utterance [b æ z], rapid and increased tongue muscle activity was observed exactly appropriate for achieving the tongue-palate configuration for a fricative sound, but no active lip compensation.   (Kelso 1995, 40)

The intervention (stopping jaw movement) in one case selectively modulated lip movement to preserve the pronunciation pattern as a whole; and in the other case it selectively modulated tongue movement to preserve pronunciation of a different letter pattern. It's clear, of course, that there is more to the system than just these elements of tongue, lips, and jaw (consider what must be going on in Broca's

---

[12] For the relevance to psychopathology, and specifically to an understanding of ADHD, see Dengsø (2022).

area), and it's also clear that one could intervene in a way that would disrupt the pronunciation or verbal utterance by means of a different intervention on the jaw (or in the brain). But this shows the possibility of a precision intervention and the tight dynamical integration or synergy in this system capable of preserving important performance aspects of the pattern while making adjustments in other aspects that might be characterized as functional motor processes.

On this conception, we arrive at a way to characterize processes as involving holistic dynamical relations across brain, body, and environment consistent with an interventionist view of causality (Woodward 2003; see Section 4.2). Causal interventions above a critical threshold, in one time scale, or on one particular element of the system, will have an effect on the system, which may lead to recovery or repair, or, above a certain threshold, a reorganization of the pattern manifested by that system.

This approach does not require that systems are organized in terms of levels. Given the kind of recursivity involved in dynamical causal relations, even as they involve different time scales, the concept of level seems less important. In what sense is the activation of the genioglossus (tongue muscle) on a different level than a vocalization? Are motor processes in the brain on a different level than the contraction of the genioglossus or the jaw movement? All of these processes are bodily processes working together and organized in a set of dynamical causal relations. If we think of the system as a dynamical gestalt of brain, body, and environment, with an autopoietic (operationally closed) organization, we can still intervene (or propose interventions) to demonstrate the specifics of dynamical relations. In this respect, I think the enactivists would relax the assumption that ties us to viewing such systems as involving hierarchical levels.

2.6 What's in a Self-pattern?

What we take to be a pattern, as Dennett suggests, is tied to a process of pattern recognition which in turn is relative to our perceptual interests and intentions, which themselves may be cashed out in terms of behavior patterns. There is a certain causal order involved in a pattern. It's not a linear causality where one element or process bangs into another and produces a result that is something else. Rather a pattern involves an arrangement of processes in dynamical non-linear causal relations. Furthermore, it's not clear that there is a bottom or top to this set of processes.

In the example of Kelso's "pipe-block" speech experiment, is the pattern something reducible to just the arrangement of existing physical elements and their dynamical interactions? No, at least in the normal course of everyday events even if not in the precise experimental arrangement, since a further process is instantiated and becomes part of what that pattern is, namely, a speech act that, given certain complicated contexts, makes meaning and keeps all of the dynamical processes on a particular track. The experiment shows that the [b] or [z] sounds can be made in multiple arrangements of the apparatus of the speech system, and I suspect that they often are, even without artificial intervention, as when one is speaking in sentences where semantic emphasis, expressed by intonation, may be one variable, and the gesture of the tongue reflects a differential dynamics in order to create that emphasis and its correlative meaning. You don't need a pipe to change the dynamics; you can change the dynamics by changing the affective state of the speaker; or by adjusting the social circumstances to elicit a slightly different intonation.

Part of what Kelso shows in this and other experiments is that "the same behavioral patterns may be obtained from very different kinds of strengths of couplings among the components." Likewise, several patterns "may be produced by the same set of components and couplings" (1995, 64). This lack of one-to-one relationship between patterns and the elements that realize them, Kelso suggests, is "one of the basic differences between living things and mechanisms" (68).

There are a lot of technical terms that we can throw into an account that moves from the physical to the biological to the human or personal order. Entropy is equivalent to disorder, which is equivalent to (structureless) equilibrium, which entails too much free energy in the system. Order is equivalent to structure (sometimes referred to as negentropy), which entails more information in the system. Order-from-order may work for mechanistic accounts (for some theorists, biology is still a matter of mechanism); others look for order-from-disorder to account for life.

The kind of pattern that we want to conceptualize is more than just an arrangement of elements. A self-pattern is not a static pattern like the wallpaper in your room, or a piece of abstract painting hanging in a museum. It's more like a piece of music being played by a quartet or orchestra. It's a dynamic pattern of processes in which the ongoing relations among the processes matter. Perturbations or fluctuations are essential for the emergence of a specific order or pattern. Importantly, then, dynamical systems may be relatively stable, but respond to instability. We've known this about the brain, for example, for over a hundred years. An experiment by Layton and Sherrington (1917) demonstrated reversals and deviations of response in the body map of the motor cortex. Their point-by-point stimulation of this area showed fluctuating function—"the point that had previously yielded elbow flexion as its primary movement, that point now yielded abduction of thumb as its primary movement...and thumb and index movements as primary responses trespassed into the area that had previously yielded shoulder movement as the primary response" (1917, 141). For them, this demonstrated "expression of the functional instability of a cortical motor point" (145). This doesn't mean that the brain is disorganized; it means it is *dynamically* organized and context sensitive (in the sense that it is sensitive to repeated stimulation over time). "It's not a static keyboard playing out a motor program" (Kelso 1995, 262)—it's more like a flexible stringed instrument where vibrations and bendings yield precise, or precisely imprecise patterns of sounds, or like vocalizations capable of nuanced intonations that produce improvised patterns of determinate meanings.

It will seem counterintuitive to philosophers who are used to working on questions that concern personal identity that instability, and not just relative stability, may be important in a self-pattern. Consider, for example, the philosophical angst that David Hume voiced when he was unable to discover anything stable in his experience because what we call self is supposed to be just that—something stable that remains identical over time:

> If any impression gives rise to the idea of *self*, that impression must continue invariably the same, thro' the whole course of our lives; since *self* is suppos'd to exist after that manner.... [What we find, however, is] a bundle or collection of different perceptions, which succeed each other with an inconceivable rapidity, and are in a perpetual flux and movement.... [N]or is there any single power of the soul, which remains unalterably the same, perhaps for one moment. The mind is a kind of *theatre*, where several perceptions successively make their appearance; pass, re-pass, glide away, and mingle in an infinite variety of postures and situations. There is properly no *simplicity* in it at one time, nor *identity* in different; whatever natural propension we may have to imagine that simplicity and identity. The comparison of the *theatre* must not mislead us. They are the successive perceptions only, that constitute the mind....   (1739, 251–3)

A self-pattern is neither a unitary or stable impression, nor a mere bundle of such impressions, since it includes more than mental impressions, and is more than a bundle or aggregate; rather, it's characterized by an integration of heterogeneous factors. Some degree of stability, and some degree of instability in a pattern allows for change and flexibility such that the pattern rarely undergoes a radical break.

Here I return to the question raised in the previous chapter: what makes a pattern a *self*-pattern. I suggested there that the answer involves a kind of recursive dynamics among all the elements or processes, rather than any one element or set of elements. Varela characterizes these dynamics as involving self-generating operational closure, which not only does not rule out interaction with the environment, but rather is a necessary condition for such interaction. Such recursive dynamics describe an autonomous system:

> [An] autonomous system is defined as a system composed of several processes that actively generate and sustain an identity under precarious circumstances. In this context, to generate an identity is to possess the property of operational closure. This is the property that among the conditions affecting the operation of

any constituent process in the system there will always be one or more processes that also belong to the system. And, in addition, every process in the system is a condition for at least one other constituent process, thus forming a network

(Di Paolo 2009, 15).

Di Paolo, Thompson, and Beer (2022, 14) explain this further: "the processes that constitute an operationally closed network relate to each other such that they form a mutually enabling set of relations. They do so under precarious conditions, meaning that in the absence of these mutually enabling relations, the same processes would tend to run down. No component is, in other words, strictly self-standing in the absence of the whole network." In this regard, operational closure involves "a circular reflexive interlinking process, whose primary effect is its own production," such that it gives rise to "an emergent or global coherence, without the need of a 'central controller'" (Varela 1997, 73). As he puts it, it is a selfless self.[13]

Varela has in mind here a characterization of a living organism of any kind, but he notes that "Different organisms differ in the kinds of multifarious identity mechanisms they have, due to their unique evolutionary pathways" (Varela 1997, 73); furthermore: "Every class of entities has an identity which is peculiar to them; the uniqueness of the living resides in the kind of organization it has" (84). My specific interest here is the human self-pattern, and I'll leave aside the interesting question of whether all organisms, including non-human animals, have their own kind of self-pattern. If they do, it will be because they involve not only operational closure, but a sufficient number of factors to constitute a pattern. The human self-pattern will be dynamically complex given its different "running redefinition" of its constituent processes (1991, 96). Varela rightly insists that since the identity (or self-identity) that we are considering is neither substantial nor abstract, "the role of historical coupling and contingency is not secondary but inseparable" (1997, 74). He cites the work of Richard Lewontin, (1982), who describes a set of processes which stand in relation to each other, such that one "cannot exist without the other, that one acquires its properties from its relation to the other[s, and] that the properties of [such processes] evolve as a consequence of their interpenetration" (Lewontin 1982, 2, 3; see Varela 1991).[14]

---

[13] In close alignment with Kelso (see above), for Varela, there is no center or localized self: "the whole behaves as a unit and for the observer it is as if there was a coordinating agent 'virtually' present at the center. This is what I meant when referring to a selfless self—we could also speak of a virtual self: a coherent global pattern that emerges through simple local components, appearing to have a central location where none is to be found, and yet essential as a level of interaction for the behavior of the whole unity" (Varela 1997, 95). In this context, however, we should not take talk of a "virtual" self to mean that the self-pattern is not real (see below).

[14] In this regard I don't take autopoietic operational closure to reflect a hylomorphic theory in any standard sense. Even if one is able to descriptively abstract the form or organization from the specific materials or material constraints of the system, there is no ontological claim about this abstraction. It's not that it is just the form that is important, and the material indifferent (such that the system could be multirealizable in any kind of material), despite some machine-related

This conception involves looking at the self-pattern from the systems-perspective (from the outside, so to speak). In contrast, if it is possible to look at it from a first-person or phenomenological perspective, the question about self-identity is already answered by the fact that there is a first-person perspective which emerges from the systemic relations that exist amongst the elements or processes that make up the pattern. This is not to suggest what turns out to be a controversial claim (see Chapter 6), that the first-person perspective of prereflective experiential self-awareness, which includes most basically a sense of ownership or mineness, is the sufficient anchor for any pattern that can be considered a self-pattern. Rather, the point here is more about the recursive relations that exist among the different factors of the self-pattern.

I'll summarize the principles (derived from Varela 1991 and 1997) that I take to support the notion of recursivity at stake:

1. A self-pattern involves a recursive "meshwork" (Varela 1991, 80), or more precisely, a meshwork of recursive processes. We can think of this recursivity as characterizing the relations amongst the elements or processes that constitute the pattern. This includes bodily existence, to which Varela attributes an autopoietic-like self-organization (he highlights the immune system) (1991, 80), which also involves organism–environment relations. Likewise, prereflective experience involves a kind of reflexivity that integrates proprioceptive and kinaesthetic bodily processes from which emerges a "cognitive perceptuo-motor" organization. As I'll suggest in the following chapters, narrative processes reflect (or represent) all of the other processes that make up the self-pattern, such that self-narrative is shaped by those processes, but also further contributes to the coherency of those processes. In effect, there is a redundancy of recursivity (a multiplicity of recursive processes) built into the pattern.[15]

2. There is a further recursivity involved in action and behavioral habits. This can be explained by appealing to Ezequiel Di Paolo's (2005) addition of adaptability to the general characterization of the autopoietic. Adaptability

wording to that effect in Maturana and Varela (1980). The material makes a difference to the form and one cannot treat them separately. Accordingly, one should not think that the starting point is top-down with relational form, or bottom-up with just the material. Rather the specific features of the material processes do enter into the determination of the relations that define the system. I think this interpretation of autopoiesis escapes the critique levied by DiFrisco (2014), or more generally, the critique of Simondon (2005). Di Paolo, Cuffari, and De Jaegher (2018) understand the notion of autopoiesis to be consistent with Simondon's own view of self-individuation. Also see Meincke (2019) and Di Paolo (2021).

[15] Varela and Goguen (1978, 293) note that this notion of recursivity is called by different names in different disciplines: *feedback* in systems engineering/cybernetics; *self-reference* in logic and philosophy, *autonomy* in philosophy and biology, *recursion* in logic and computer science, *self-reflection* or *reflection* in psychology, and a form of *looping* or *re-entry* more generally.

is balanced by habit. Frank Lorimer, a student of John Dewey, views habit as intrinsic to organic life such that it maintains itself within the natural environment; habits involve patterns of "organismic tension" (Lorimer 1929, 13), which characterize the dynamics of organic-environmental systems. The "fundamental principle of habit formation [is] individual organismic adaptation in relation to actual conditions which tend to disturb organic equilibrium" (1929, 12; see Dreon 2022, Ch. 4).

3. Varela emphasizes coherence and the stability of autopoietic organization, tied to operative closure (Varela & Goguen 1978). "For as long as it exists, the autopoietic organization remains invariant. In other words, one way to spotlight the specificity of autopoiesis is to think of it self-referentially as that organization which maintains the very organization itself as an invariant" (Varela 1991, 84). In this respect, the organization maintains a signature pattern. Despite constant flux, "the pattern remains." We'll discuss this later in terms of what, in discussions of personal identity, is termed *idem* identity. It is also clear, however, that within this coherence there can be structural change and adaptation. Patterns vary over time, and this may be due precisely to dynamical adjustments and the phenomenon of adaptivity. Change relates to *ipse* identity (see below and Chapter 5), and it relates to what we suggested above about the importance of perturbations or fluctuations in the self-pattern.[16] This dialectic of stability-instability facilitates a kind of fragility, flexibility, and possibility of change in the self-pattern. In this regard Varela uses the metaphor of jazz improvisation (1991, 97; 1997, 84).

4. On a view that goes beyond mechanistic accounts (as well as traditional vitalistic accounts), Varela suggests that "the local and the global are braided together explicitly through . . . reciprocal causality" (1991, 84; 1997, 78), or, what I am calling dynamical causality. It is dynamical causality, precisely because it involves "multi-directional multiplicity" typical of complex systems (1991, 93), and not just a simple dyadic reciprocity.

5. As we noted above, operational closure does not preclude organism–environment interaction. Varela indicates that the notion of operational closure "emphasizes that closure is used in its mathematical sense of recursivity, and not in the sense of closedness or isolation from interaction"

---

[16] In autopoietic theory the distinction is made between "organization," which is invariant, and "structure," which may vary over time. "Autopoiesis is the description of a class of systems, i.e., a description of the organization that defines this class. Concrete autopoietic systems may be instantiated in a wide variety of structures, and a given structure may belong to more than one class of organization (Fido is a dog, a mammal, a living organism). Structures may also change over time, even if the organization is invariant (Fido was a puppy, is an adult hound, will be a lazy senior)" (Di Paolo, Thompson & Beer 2022, 13; Beer 2020; Maturana & Varela 1980). With respect to a self-pattern, I take this distinction to correlate with Ricoeur's *idem–ipse* distinction (see below).

(1991, 93; 1997, 82). In fact, in earlier work Varela (1975) proposed a mathematical formalism, derived from the work of George Spencer-Brown (1969), that captures the recursivity involved in autopoietic systems.[17]

Varela's notion of a selfless self is consistent with Kelso's notion that within the pattern there is no self, understood as a substantial agent that controls the pattern. Varela wrestles with this idea, however, especially in the context of thinking of self as person, and our ordinary experience of self as if it were something substantial. In this respect, as noted above, he suggests the idea of a virtual self that emerges from the dynamical pattern—"a non-substantial self can nevertheless act as if present, like a virtual interface" (1991, 100). This would be an illusory self, which he explains in the following way: "What we call 'I', ourselves, can be analyzed as arising out of man's recursive linguistic abilities and their unique capacity for self-description and narration.... Our sense of a personal 'I' can be construed as an ongoing interpretative narrative" (100). This view, however, leads to the idea that the self is an emergent property of the self-pattern, existing on a different level. Indeed, Varela is inclined to use terminology of upward and downward relations, between local and global processes, that comes close to the mechanistic talk of levels which I have suggested we avoid. I think we can circumvent all of this simply by saying that what we call the "self" just is the self-pattern. We'll see that narrative does play a recursive role in constituting this self-pattern, without having to say that something over and above the pattern emerges as an illusory self. If the self just is the self-pattern, it's not illusory.

Further with respect to the idea expressed in the third point above, that there is both coherency and change, invariance and flexibility, stability and instability in the self-pattern, we can think more generally that despite changes in some features, the general parameters of a greater part of the self-pattern tend to remain intact, even if modified. For example, by entering and exiting particular social or normative contexts (being among friends, or meeting strangers, in the pub, at a religious service, at a football game, and so forth) a person may engage in different behaviors of intersubjective interaction where different aspects of their personality and different affective profiles emerge. These changes may lead to small changes in some other aspects of the self-pattern, but the overall arrangement and the overall set of relations hold steady. In the case of a more dramatic overall change involving adaptation or compensation there is nonetheless an observable continuity in the pattern. We'll consider such changes due to psychopathology, and different therapies and practices in later chapters. A not so

---

[17] Varela (1975; Varela & Goguen 1978). Also see, Louis Kaufmann (1987) and Soto-Andrade et al. (2011). There is much more to find and to endorse in Varela's essays, including his notion of a double dialectic that brings forth not only self-organization in the organism, but simultaneously brings forth a world in sense-making (Varela 1991).

dramatic example of this is development across a life span. There can be varying degrees of change in cognitive ability, personality, behavior, and even in bodily details, but what persists is some recognizable continuing set of features or processes. Varela talks about minor "breakdowns in autopoiesis" that get repaired in sense-making: "every breakdown can be seen as the initiation of an action on what is missing on the part of the system so that identity might be maintained" (1997, 80).

Judgments about such continuity through change are, of course, made by different stakeholders in different contexts and on different time scales. An encounter between old friends is one thing; raising a child, or living with a family member is something else, and our own self-perceptions are even more changeable, as Hume acknowledged (even to himself). This is part of the recursivity built into such changes in the sense that such diachronic changes are part of what forms the self-pattern, and we would be surprised (or dead) if no such changes occurred.

Just here philosophers want to raise questions about continuity, unity of self, and identity over time. If the self is a pattern, and the pattern changes, then doesn't the self change? Yes, as selves do. Paul Ricoeur (1992) addresses this issue by making a distinction between *idem* identity (that which remains relatively the same, persists across time) and *ipse* identity (that which makes me who I am in relation to another, even as I change over time). These are two different problematics addressing two different questions. As Marya Schechtman (1996) puts it, this is the distinction between the question of reidentification—what makes a person the same from one time to another?—and the question of characterization—what makes a person the person she is? As will be clear in the following chapters, to the extent that there are multiple questions about identity, the notion of a self-pattern offers resources to answer all such questions. Moreover, even in cases of radical change in *ipse* identity, which may be found in psychopathology, or in recovery from psychopathology, understanding the changes in terms of the self-pattern will give us a way to understand and characterize such disorders.

Admittedly, trying to explicate the holistic character of the self-pattern is, as de Haan et al. (2013, 6) suggest, "tricky business." Nonetheless, focusing on dynamics is the way to start mapping out how various factors in a self-pattern relate to or mesh with one another. Accordingly, it is only through empirical, clinical, and phenomenological studies, rather than a priori definition, that we will be able to sort out how the dynamics of the self-pattern work, and how they may be different in pathological cases, or become readjusted in cases of clinical treatments. In the next chapter I'll outline a threefold method, involving theoretical analysis, empirical investigation, and dynamical modeling, as a way to address the tricky business of explaining the holistic character of the self-pattern.

2.7 A Note on Network Theory

Let me conclude with a note about some important differences between the pattern theory as developed in these chapters, and the network theory of psycho-pathology (Borsboom 2017; Borsboom & Cramer 2013). One can easily think that the pattern theory is consistent with some aspects of the network theory, according to which a disorder is constituted by a network of symptoms. Both views are anti-reductionist; they emphasize that psychopathology is "massively multifactorial not only in its causes but also in its constitution" (Borsboom, Cramer & Kalis 2019, 10); and they both appeal to Dennett's concept of "real patterns." Indeed, if we understand symptoms to be anchored in an enactive system that includes brain-body-environment extended over time, the theories seem very consistent, even if the concept of *self*-pattern is missing in the characteriza-tion of the network.

Although this is not the place to work out a detailed account of differences between enactive approaches and more standard cognitivist approaches in phil-osophy of mind and the cognitive sciences (see Gallagher 2023, for such details), these are the kinds of differences to be found between a pattern theory, informed by enactive views, and network theory, which, as it has developed, retains some basic assumptions that are tied to more standard cognitivist approaches. If net-work theorists sometimes seem to lean in an enactive direction (e.g., "we should expect to find interactions between symptoms to be grounded in an even more complex set of biological, social, and cultural factors involved in psychopath-ology" [Borsboom et al. 2019, 10]), their analysis begins and continues with the standard functionalist and representationalist assumptions of cognitivist theories, and they focus on folk-psychological attributions of rational mental states (see Slors, Francken & Strijbos [2019] concerning the limitations of treating this as a rational system). Cultural and historical variations are said to impinge upon the symptom network structure through mental state content, and in some cases, the cause of one symptom may be "the mental representation of [another] symptom" (Borsboom et al. 2019, 9). In the attempt to allow for interactions between psychological and biological processes, they appeal to reciprocal causal relations between a "mereological ordering in levels" of a mechanistic sort (2019, 10), even if there is no claim that one level is the most basic. Much of this, however, is inconsistent with the enactive perspective that underpins the notion of self-pattern.

Furthermore, network theory's focus on symptoms tends to ignore processes. Elbau, Binder, and Spoormaker (2019), for example, make this point, although they take processes narrowly to mean brain processes. Pattern theory, in contrast, focuses on processes, and significantly, on a wider set of processes—extended to include, for example, ecological, socio-cultural, and normative processes—in order to understand symptoms. Network theory does acknowledge that "symptoms do not arise out of the blue, but arguably result from dynamical interactions among experiences, feelings, and behaviors in daily life" (Bringmann et al. 2022, 3); still the variables of choice remain symptoms, and other factors that may be causally constraining are treated as falling outside of the system (Roefs et al. 2022). The difference between a symptom-focus and a process-focus of the sort found in the pattern theory, will be clear from the analysis of communicative processes in ASD where it is not enough to identify a symptom (e.g., a deficit of social interaction), and ask how it relates to other symptoms, but requires an investigation of how wide variations of processes of social interaction, across individuals and contexts, operate across the spectrum (see Section 3.6).

As network theory has developed, theorists have identified several problems and have attempted to resolve them. Many of the problems concern methodology, which for network theory ranges across the use of sophisticated statistical tools, to the use of interventionist causality and mechanistic models, and includes issues concerning the selection of nodes in the network, how to integrate data across different time scales, different levels, and different kinds of variables, and how to study changes in networks (Bringmann et al. 2022; Borsboom & Cramer 2013; de Boer et al. 2021). These are all complex problems, and it is likely some of them are relevant to studies and applications of the self-pattern (see Chapter 3).

De Boer et al. (2021), for example, suggest that network theory wants to establish causal explanations, and not just statistical correlations. Accordingly, they suggest that a Woodwardian interventionist strategy would serve this end. They then list a number of issues that make the straightforward application of interventionist causal analysis difficult in the context of psychopathology. The main one is that it is difficult to know if interventions on symptoms are precise enough to not influence other variables in the network. As de Boer et al. allow, imprecise (or "fat-handed") interventions can still be useful, and this would be the case in both network theory and pattern theory. This raises a related issue, however:

> [C]an we actually take for granted that psychiatric symptoms are distinct and non-overlapping entities? It is necessary to properly define target variables in order to perform suitable interventions. Although proponents of the network theory assume that symptoms [some of which are defined as mental states] are defined at the right level of detail and specificity . . . it has also been argued [by Woodward 2014] that it is difficult to actually pinpoint individual mental states as suitable targets for intervention.   (de Boer et al. 2021)

This is especially a problem if psychiatric symptoms are characterized by feedback loops, which, as de Boer et al. point out, they typically are. For pattern theory, however, it is not the symptoms themselves that do the work; rather, symptoms point, like signs, to disruptions or disturbances in the processes and dynamical relations that constitute the self-pattern. The approach outlined in the next chapter is an attempt to explain how we can gain more precision and specificity about those processes and dynamical relations.

3

A Threefold Method for Studying Self-pattern Dynamics

In this and the following chapters I'll focus on several factors of the self-pattern for purposes of exploring in more detail how those factors are dynamically related, and how they may be affected in various disorders. In this chapter I'm primarily concerned to outline a methodological approach that will allow for a detailed analysis of how these relations are typically ordered and sometimes differently ordered. I'll consider, as an example, the case of autism spectrum disorder (ASD). Relevant to ASD, I'll focus on bodily, experiential, cognitive, affective, intersubjective, and social factors in the self-pattern. In line with the idea that we should not attempt to define a priori either the relevant factors that belong to the self-pattern or their dynamical relations, I want to outline an empirical approach to such details. In the following sections I'll gather some tools that have been developed in several other areas of research in order to craft a threefold method that will allow for this detailed analysis. The first part of this threefold method is adapted from performance studies where questions about skilled action are addressed using the model of a "meshed architecture" (Christensen, Sutton & McIlwain 2016). A second part depends on some insights from our previous discussion of new mechanist analysis and manipulations aligning with interventionist conceptions of causality (see Sections 2.4 and 2.5). And the third part rejoins Kelso's dynamical analysis of patterns, and specifically his coordination dynamics approach.

3.1 Mapping the Self-pattern in a Meshed Architecture

It should already be clear that the self-pattern, by definition, is not an isolated phenomenon that is in any way cut off from the world. If there is no controlling agent or self within the pattern, that is, if no one of its elements by itself constitutes a self, this does not mean that the dynamical gestalt of the self-pattern as a whole is not agentive in a way that allows us to speak of an individual embodied agent capable of engaging in action and interaction with the world and with others (I'll discuss this in more detail in Section 5.1). The relational coupling with the world that exists in the self-pattern means that the individual agent is situated

The Self and its Disorders. Shaun Gallagher, Oxford University Press. © Shaun Gallagher 2024.
DOI: 10.1093/oso/9780198873068.003.0004

in a rich physical, social, and cultural environment. The notion of a meshed architecture is meant to capture the structure of this self-world relation.

The idea that the self-pattern is a dynamical gestalt means that the various processes and factors involved in the pattern are dynamically related to form a whole. This holistic view of the self-pattern involves a number of philosophical issues, as we discussed in the previous chapter, but practically, for psychiatry, it presents additional challenges both in regard to diagnosis and therapeutic interventions. One needs to say precisely what process or factor, or what set of processes or factors, in any particular case, is problematic, and how it might be addressed. The model of a meshed architecture borrowed from performance studies, allows for a mapping out of relevant factors, and how they are situated in the self-pattern. I take this to be a first step in a three-step approach to gaining an explanatory grasp of specific disorders.

Let me start with a few important provisos concerning this first step. The first proviso is to emphasize that it is just a first step rather than a finished product. It is meant to be a heuristic to help map out the relevant processes and to set up the next two methodological steps. Second, as originally introduced in performance studies by Christensen, Sutton, and McElwain (2016), the meshed architecture involves a concept of operational levels that we are trying to avoid, "a broadly hierarchical division of control responsibilities" (2016, 43). In working out what I'm calling an "enhanced meshed architecture" (EMA), I propose to move beyond this concept of hierarchical levels. Finally, my aim is not to provide a detailed account of the various debates about the nature of expert performance (see Gallagher 2020c; 2021a), but rather to put the model to use in the context of an analysis of the self-pattern relevant to the study of psychopathology. Accordingly, I'll short-circuit the debates in the performance literature and simply present the EMA and a brief background, which I understand to be consistent with an enactive approach that can generalize to explanations of embodied-situated-social cognition (Gallagher & Varga 2020), and in this case, relevant to psychiatric disorders.

In performance studies, one problem is to explain how complex cognitive processes, such as memory and attention, can guide or control what are construed as automatic motor processes in skilled performance (e.g., in athletics, dance, theater, or musical performance). Performance in many cases is fast and seemingly automatic, yet it is also context-sensitive and strategic in a way that suggests there is an "interpenetration of thought and action" (Sutton et al. 2011, 80):

> Skill is not a matter of bypassing explicit thought, to let habitual actions run entirely on their own, but of building and accessing flexible links between knowing and doing. The forms of thinking and remembering which can, in some circumstances, reach in to animate the subtle kinaesthetic mechanisms of skilled performance must themselves be redescribed as active and dynamic.
>
> (Sutton et al. 2011, 95)

One proposal is that cognitive control must counteract automaticity and introduce flexibility into motor control. When we think of it in this way, the central question is this: How precisely does thought "reach in" to the body-schematic processes of skilled performance?

Christensen, Sutton, and McIlwain (2016) answer this question by developing the model of a meshed architecture which describes the integration of perceptual and cognitive elements (which they take to be higher-order processes) with body-schematic motoric processes (they consider as lower-order). On this hybrid view performance is neither fully automatic nor fully cognitive. They propose a division of labor in the *meshed* functioning that, as indicated, involves "a broadly hierarchical division of control responsibilities, with cognitive control usually focused on strategic aspects of performance and automatic processes more concerned with implementation" (2016, 43). This description, however, reflects an overly intellectualist arrangement portrayed as a type of vertical alignment between higher-order cognitive processes controlling lower-order motoric processes, with different degrees of integration between the higher and lower processes. Top-down cognitive control can be "smooth," "adaptive," or "effortful" (2016, 52). Accordingly, this divides the vertical into two poles: cognitive at the top, descending to do its job; automatic bodily processes at the bottom receiving instructions when necessary.[1]

An alternative, more enhanced version of the meshed architecture is possible. EMA allows that cognitive processes can be a matter of degree, ranging from thoughtful, reflective consciousness to a thin performative prereflective awareness, with different gradations in between, involving, for example, selective target control, conscious monitoring, or a sense of one's rightly configured body. The phenomenology of performance may thus be complex and varied, such that performers may shift across a full register, from explicit conscious control to implicit prereflective consciousness, to a spontaneous attunement of body-schematic processes, improvising in some cases to adjust to changing conditions. To get a fuller explanation, however, we need to add three aspects that are not accounted for in the original model: (1) *intrinsic control*—an enactive view that takes motor processes to be integrated with cognitive processes from the start; (2) an important role for *affectivity*; and (3) a complexity introduced by what we can call the *horizontal axis* (Gallagher 2021a; Gallagher & Varga 2020). This structure of vertical-horizontal axes operates as a heuristic that we can then drop in favor of a more dynamical model.

---

[1] Several competitor theories similarly confine the analysis of skill, expert performance, or know-how to this vertical axis, ranging from the highly intellectualized view of Stanley (2011) to what are advertised as more hybrid views (e.g., Fridland 2017a; Montero 2015; Pacherie & Mylopoulos 2021; Papineau 2013). All of these views pose high-order cognitive control against low-order automatic processes.

3.1.1 Intrinsic Control in Bodily Processes

Body-schematic, motor control processes are attuned by practice and provide the agent the freedom to pay mindful attention to relevant surrounding factors—to heedfully focus on selective target control if that is required. Practiced and habitual movements, together with variations in heedful and targeted (attentive, perceptual) awareness, are constrained and enabled by a consolidation of fine, detailed body-schematic processes. But such processes should not be viewed as fully automatic. Jonides et al. (1985), for example, explicitly argue that motor control processes overall do not automate. Evidence from kinematics suggests that body-schematic processes are perfectly specific, adaptive, and highly dynamical such that they adaptively attune to differences in situations (environmental conditions, object positions, initial and unfolding body postures) and agentive intentions. To align with a particular action intention or goal, there are, in fact, lots of moving parts that require controlled integration, across varying time scales, many of which are too fast for conscious control. In contrast to an intellectualist view that insists on the automaticity and "perfectly general" nature of such processes (e.g., Stanley 2011), however, body-schematic processes are neither fully automatic (blindly pre-set, like a reflex, to do the same thing in each circumstance, regardless of differences), such that in varying circumstances they require top-down cognitive guidance (e.g., Papineau 2013, 184), nor perfectly general; they rather include a specificity that involves an "enormous number (which often reaches three figures) of degrees of freedom" (Bernstein 1984), as well as a complex temporal organization involving anticipatory processes across skeletal geometry, kinematic phase constraints, muscular geometry, and the dynamics that characterize the relationship between kinematics and geometry (Berthoz 2000; Gallagher & Aguda 2020). These complex processes come to intelligently align with a particular intentional trajectory, *not automatically* (clicking into place in a machine-like fashion), but rather, in a way that is flexibly attuned to the particularities of the situation.[2]

We can think of this attunement as a form of habit, developed when the body "acquires the power of responding with a certain type of solution to a certain form of situation" (Merleau-Ponty 2012, 143). Habit involves an intelligent response, where intelligence is built into the movement. Instead of blind automatic repetition, habit is an open and adaptive way in which the body learns to

---

[2] Ellen Fridland (2017b) argues that some automatic processes are intelligent. My point is slightly different. I claim that not all processes that have been considered automatic are automatic in any straightforward way. According to John Bargh (1994, 3), for example, there are no processes that are purely automatic by the four-criteria standard, that is, (1) unintentional, (2) unconscious, (3) uncontrolled/uncontrollable, and (4) attention-independent or effortless.

cope with familiar or unfamiliar situations.[3] Intrinsic control involves motoric processes that are already context-sensitive, smart, open, and adaptive, such that they can even elicit or shape or enable the required cognitive elements that may be contingently incorporated into the mesh. Rather than thinking that cognition in some way penetrates or controls automatic processes (Fridland 2015), we should think that sensorimotor processes regulate the activation of specific cognitive processes when they are needed. In such cases mindfulness is not simply imported from the "top"; it's already built into the "bottom," and, again in some cases, such habitual processes may be what guide any need for more reflective cognitive processes.

Skills and habits can persist even in pathologies where forms of memory that are more cognitive are lost, as in cases of dementia. Christian Tewes (2021) cites a patient of Thomas Fuchs who in advanced stages of dementia is still able to skillfully play football with his grandchildren (Fuchs 2017, 301). As Tewes explains, this is not automatic behavior but "situation-specific embedded action patterns that depend on attention to and implicit understanding or know-how of the respective social context" (2021, 383). Such skill is also strongly linked to previous life experiences even if, as in the case of dementia, these life experiences cannot be explicitly recalled by the subject.

3.1.2 Affectivity

In addition to the reciprocal integration of cognition and body-schematic attunement, other factors play an important role in performance. This includes affect, which in the broadest sense includes emotion processes, but also more general and basic bodily states such as hunger/satiation, fatigue/well-restedness, pain/no pain/pleasure.[4] Affect, including "existential feelings" (Ratcliffe 2012a), and what Michelle Maiese (2018) calls "affective framing," shapes our ability to cope with the surrounding world (Colombetti 2014). Along with skills and habits, affect introduces possible modulations of functional integration with that world. Affect

---

[3] This contrasts to views of habit that understand it to be a matter of mere repetition, as found in, for example, Ryle (1949, 30), or Pacherie and Mylopoulos (2021, 649): "It is of the essence of merely habitual practices that one performance is a replica of its predecessors"; or standard views in psychology that "characterize habitual actions as automatic, inflexible, and stimulus-driven" Pacherie and Mylopoulos (2021, 649). Like Merleau-Ponty, John Dewey (1922, 42) distinguishes between intelligent and routine habit. "Repetition [i.e., automaticity] is in no sense the essence of habit.... The essence of habit is an acquired predisposition to *ways* or modes of response.... Habit means special sensitiveness or accessibility to certain classes of stimuli, standing predilections and aversions, rather than bare recurrence of specific acts."

[4] Automaticity is often characterized as being effortless (e.g., Fitts & Posner 1967; Shiffrin & Schneider 1977). Clearly, however, degrees of effort correlate with degrees of fatigue or pain the performer may be experiencing, which may in fact modulate details of how body-schematic processes structure a movement—in which case, such processes are not so automatic but rather adaptive.

may work differently in different types of skilled actions, where important differences may have to do with the way that affective factors are integrated with motoric/agentive factors, the kinetic and kinaesthetic feelings associated with body-schematic processes,[5] and how all of these processes integrate with environmental constraints and affordances.

Affect/emotion may involve expressive movements and gestures, an important component of intersubjective communication. It may also be involved in different mixes or integrations of expressive and instrumental movements in different contexts of performance. The body schema, in this respect, does not carry on independently, delivering technically proficient movement, to which we then add an expressive style motivated by specific emotions that may be occasion relative. Rather, affective processes directly shape body-schematic processes—slowing down or speeding up such processes, for example, or leading to the adoption of certain initial postures that may influence performance or how agents are functionally integrated with the world. Affect and body-schematic processes are integrated—still pictured as part of the vertical mesh in expert performance—but they also allow for an integration attuned to targets and environmental features located on a horizontal axis (see Figure 3.1).

3.1.3 The Horizontal Axis

EMA incorporates a form of horizontal integration. Ecological, normative, cultural, and intersubjective aspects of the physical and social environment, including

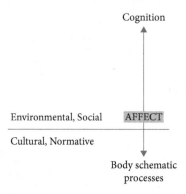

Figure 3.1 Vertical and horizontal axes of the meshed architecture
Source: From Gallagher and Varga (2020).

[5] Christensen et al. (2016) suggest that negative emotional arousal (e.g., fear) can interfere with performance. Hatfield and Kerick (2007) also point out that emotional reactivity, which involves autonomic and endocrine functioning, can result in changes in kinematic, motor activity.

physical and social affordances play a role in this regard. On this view, what makes performance what it *is* is not entirely internal to the performer.[6]

As one engages in a particular action (or performance) one's agency (or sense of agency) may be modulated (causally influenced) by affect, but also by the quality and quantity of affordances available. When, for example, the performer "can 'feel' that her motor system has the right configuration" (Christensen et al. 2016), this configuration is just the right one to mesh with the specifics of the performer's physical and social environment. This is a form of "interkinaesthetic affectivity" (Høffding 2019, 244; see Høffding & Satne 2019; Salice, Høffding & Gallagher 2017). Neither body-schematic processes nor affective processes are isolated from the agent's environment; rather they are attuned to both stabilities and variations in environmental factors, including other agents. The performance, and the cognition involved in it, are situated, that is, functionally integrated with the environment, which is not only physical, but also socially, culturally, and normatively defined.[7]

3.1.4 The Self-pattern as a Meshed Architecture

The notion of a meshed architecture has application beyond performance; for example, in defining situated cognition (Gallagher & Varga 2020) and in clarifying intersubjective interactions in regard to social cognition (Gallagher, Varga & Sparaci 2022). With respect to the self-pattern, it offers a pragmatic heuristic in the service of mapping or diagraming relations. In this regard, the distinction between vertical and horizontal axes offers a way to start thinking about how different processes and factors integrate or mesh, even if conceiving of the self-pattern as a dynamical gestalt implies a holistic rather than a hierarchical arrangement of factors.

If it is standard to think of cognitive, reflective, and narrative processes as top-down, and to think of bodily, affective, and experiential processes as bottom-up,

---

[6] Simon Høffding's (2019) analysis of musical performance provides some good examples: the musical instruments, the performance space, and the music itself shape the musical performance. The style of music, whether one is playing from a score, whether improvisation occurs—such factors define different dynamics. For example, the individual performer affectively resonates with and through the music. Playing the musical notes initiates a resonance between the sounds one creates and the musical sounds in the environment made by other musicians. Also see Ryan & Gallagher (2020).

[7] To continue with the example of musical performance, playing in a concert hall or in a church may be quite different from performance in a stadium or a pub or in the open air. When playing music with others, who those others are, how skilled they are, and how long we have interacted with them will have an impact (Clarke, DeNora & Vuoskoski, 2015). If one is playing music with others, there will be an intersubjective and affective resonance between an individual's performance and the performance of other musicians. This may be mediated by the music itself, by conscious, non-conscious, and/or non-verbal perceptual cues in the others' embodied performance (see Høffding 2019; Høffding & Satne 2019). In some cases there may also be resonance between the performer and the audience. The concert hall and the people I'm making music with elicit a specific feeling and style.

the EMA allows us to think of them as integrated processes on a more level playing field, so to speak. In any particular instance, bodily processes will have an intrinsic influence on many of the other factors; affect may also play a pervasive role in shaping experience and our cognitive/reflective/narrative practices.

As I noted in the introduction, some integrative approaches remain narrow in the sense that all of the important processes are conceived of as happening "in the head." I gave the example of Phillip Gerrans (2014) analysis of delusions. He attempts to explain the "cognitive architecture" of delusions by integrating elements that are neuronal and phenomenological, with narrative generated in the default mode network. These are all conceived to be arranged in top-down inferential processes on a vertical axis, and specifically in the hierarchical order of predictive processing. It's not clear, however, that we should carry over the predictive processing assumption about hierarchical arrangements into characterizations of the different factors of the self-pattern. On a dynamical gestalt view, for example, it's not clear why we should think of sensorimotor processes as on a more basic or lower level than cognitive or social processes (unless we have already made some reductionist assumptions, or have decided a priori that relations in the self-pattern have to be hierarchically arranged). Sensorimotor, cognitive, and social processes can be aligned or integrated in non-linear arrangements across different time scales, involving dynamical causal relations. Moreover, for the vast variety of psychopathological phenomena, including delusions, we need to go wider and to scale out to include the horizontal axis, which, in terms of the self-pattern means ecological, intersubjective, social, cultural, and normative factors. In this particular case we can be geometrically Cartesian, thanking Descartes for giving us a starting point in a coordination system where all of these factors can be plotted with different weights and on points that can shift both vertically and horizontally, from one case to the next, or from one situation to the next, specifying, for example, weighted value and degree of coupling (see Figure 3.2).[8]

If we think of the mesh as a dynamical gestalt constantly adjusting to changing situations, we may still be able to get a bearing on what factors might be heavily weighted and duly or unduly influential in any particular case. But further explanation requires an account of the dynamical relations that exist among all of these elements so that we start to think of the mesh as a set of processes in which vertical and horizontal are clearly just explanatory abstractions. To be able to specify these precise relations, however, we require two other parts of the method.

---

[8] In this case, the vertical Y-axis would not signify high-order versus low-order processes, but could measure, for example, the degree to which a subject is conscious of the various factor-effects. The horizontal X-axis might then signify the degree of strength or dominance for any particular factor in any particular instance.

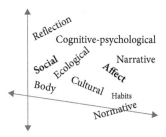

Figure 3.2 A Cartesian gestalt
Source: Author.

3.2 Imprecise Interventions

Much of what we need for the second part of this methodological approach follows on from our discussion of Woodward's conception of an interventionist notion of causality in contexts of both experimentation and therapy (in Sections 2.4 and 2.5). I'm using the concept of intervention in a broad sense to characterize any possible event or change that could influence a particular factor or process. In a gestalt arrangement, a change to one variable, above a certain threshold, will likely cause changes in other variables in the system. That includes any change in brain, organism, environment, or in any particular habit or practice. These may be changes in a life circumstance (e.g., a traumatic experience, the loss of a life-long partner), or in a controlled experiment (e.g., the presentation of stimuli that would alter a person's mood), or in a therapeutic context (e.g., medicating or changing cognitive or motoric habits). Life, or the experimenter, or the therapist intervenes on a particular process. Above a certain threshold, we would expect that such an intervention could have significant effects on the processes or factors in the self-pattern.

If we want to understand how changes in one factor can lead to changes in other factors, or more holistic changes in the pattern, we could aim to devise experiments that precisely target one particular process to see what else might "wiggle" as the result of that change. This can be more than just a wiggling of an internal mechanism (e.g., a drug effect on neuronal processes)—it can be a "smiggling" where for example, an intervention on a social factor, or a therapeutic intersubjective practice, can lead to a rearrangement of the entire gestalt (see, e.g., Bundesen 2021). Intervention methods of wiggling, smiggling, changing, adding, or subtracting, could allow us to identify the relations that are enabling, constraining, or that involve dynamical causality and are, in that sense, constituting. Precision interventions (where all factors other than the process being tested are held fixed) are generally difficult, and more so in psychiatric contexts (de Boer et al. 2021). Imprecise interventions, however, are still useful, especially when multiple interventions are possible. Experimental science tends to work that way—in most cases no one experiment provides the precision of an airtight conclusion, but with more experiments, higher degrees of precision can be attained.

As an example, consider therapeutic interventions on body-schematic processes to address psychomotor retardation, deviant gait and posture in major depressive disorder (MDD). In a meta-analysis Reed and Ones (2006) reviewed 158 studies showing that positive affect is increased by engaging in physical exercise (e.g., walking). Studies have also shown that depression affects how self-related information is processed, biased toward the recall of affectively negative self-referent material and reduced processing of positive information. Johannes Michalak and colleagues (Michalak, Rohde & Troje 2015; Michalak, Michnat & Teismann 2014) conducted intervention experiments in which they caused alterations in posture or gait patterns. Such alterations led to changes in the subjects' recollections on self-referent positive versus negative words, demonstrating that "biased memory towards self-referent negative material can be changed by manipulating [posture or] the style of walking" (2015, 124). They thus conclude that "changes in the grossmotor system affect processes that are relevant in the aetiology of depression.... Bodily aspects such as posture or movement patterns (e.g., gait characteristics) might be more than epiphenomena of psychopathology but also might contribute to an escalation of distorted processes in psychological disorders" (Michalak, Michnat & Teismann 2014, 523; also see Wilkes et al. 2017, and Varga 2019, 146ff. for discussion).

Consider also that changes to ecological arrangements can result in changes to other factors in the self-pattern. One can think of this broadly in terms of "cognitive niche construction" (Sterelny 2010), where we design environments in ways that enhance our cognitive or affective processes, or in terms of the scaffolding function of designed environments where one can "manipulate the scaffolded by manipulating the scaffold" in order to make a difference (Varga 2019, 52). In therapeutic contexts manipulation of the environment may be facilitated by the use of virtual reality (VR). Specifically, the use of VR and mixed reality in clinical environments allows for the creation of (virtual) affordances to facilitate or support embodied, interactive, and affective therapies (Freeman et al. 2017; Röhricht et al. 2014). Psychotherapeutic applications of VR can address a variety of anxiety disorders, phobias (Emmelkamp et al. 2002; Rothbaum and Hodges 1999), eating disorders such as anorexia (Riva et al. 1999), as well as PTSD (Difede et al. 2007). Avatar-based therapy has been used for treating patients with schizophrenia to control a hallucinated voice (Rus-Calafell et al. 2018). VR has also been used to diagnose and treat schizophrenia (Freeman 2008; see Chapter 8 for further discussion).

In addition to changing postures or movements, or changing affect, or changing ecology, this interventionist logic can help to make sense of a therapeutic experiment designed to understand capacities for social cognition in the case of ASD. Tager-Flusberg and Anderson (1991), informed by the standard views of social-cognitive problems in autism as involving deficits in theory of mind (ToM) (e.g., Baron-Cohen, Leslie & Frith 1985), studied conversational ability in children with ASD. They hypothesized that impairment in conversational ability may be due to deficits in ToM development. Hadwin et al. (1997) then tested this hypothesis, training children with ASD on tasks that employ ToM abilities for understanding mental states in others, focusing on beliefs, emotional states, and pretense. We can consider this an experimental test of a therapeutic intervention. Hadwin et al. compared conversation abilities prior- and post-training using four categories:

1. Simple answer—a child simply provides a one-word reply to a question and does not further engage in conversation
2. Developed answer—child is able to produce utterances that involve two or more sentences
3. Echolalic or repetitive answers
4. Unclear responses—non-sequiturs.

After training on ToM tasks, the children did learn to pass tasks concerning emotional and belief understanding (but not pretense). They improved their ToM skills on these tasks. However, there was no corresponding advance in social communication skills. Specifically, no improvement in the development of conversation and no increase in the use of mental state terms in speech were found (Hadwin et al. 1997, 533). The majority of children with ASD remained in the simple answer category and did not improve.

What this suggests is that intervening on cognitive factors to improve ToM abilities doesn't wiggle conversational ability or improve social interaction. Informed by a different set of data about deficits in sensory-motoric processes in ASD (see Gallagher & Varga 2015 for review), one could design a different experiment to ask whether early intervention to improve motor coordination would have any effect on conversational ability or social interaction. I'll return to this possibility below (Section 3.4.3).

Simply put, after identifying factors relevant to a particular condition, and mapping them out using the EMA, we can test such factors by interventionist methods to discover whether and how such factors are causally related. An intervention on one factor (neuronal, cognitive, social, etc.) may shift things around, perhaps bestowing more weight on other factors, revealing causal relations that range from simple one-way causal relations to reciprocal, circular, or non-linear dynamical relations. Contra the narrow integrationist view, an intervention can be more than just a manipulation of an internal mechanism (e.g., a drug effect on neuronal processes)—it can be a change in an environmental or social factor, or in bodily, or narrative practices, or, as may be the case in therapeutic contexts, some combination that can rearrange the entire gestalt.

3.3 Coordination Dynamics

The third component of the methodological approach I am outlining is based on the work of Scott Kelso and colleagues on dynamical patterns, some of which was discussed in Chapter 2. According to Kelso, "Dynamics is a language for connecting events from the genetic to the mental" (Kelso & Tognoli 2009, 106). If we think of the motley collection of processes and factors that make up the self-pattern, then the dynamic processes that define their relations may be the common element that allows us to explain how they are ordered or disordered. Kelso and his colleagues have proposed a method of dynamical analysis called "coordination dynamics." Although much of their work focuses on brain dynamics, and they frame their analysis in hierarchical and reductionist terms of top-down and bottom-up arrangements, their approach generalizes to any complex dynamical system and can apply to patterns understood as gestalts or complex systems. A complex system such as a biological, ecological, or social system, is typically bound together by coordination between dynamical processes operating at different spatio-temporal scales (Kelso 2009; Zhang et al. 2020). The measuring of coordination dynamics allows researchers to get into the fine details of dynamical processes and to develop explanatory models of how they are ordered. The method involves recording continuous time-varying processes as they unfold, and then analyzing the dynamical structure of such processes using time-series analysis. This allows for a precise measuring of behavioral coordination by evaluating the synchronized patterning of system components as they change over time (Fitzpatrick et al. 2016).

Coordination dynamics as a form of topology can mathematically capture the integration of local information with global information (Thom 1975). It's a quantitative approach maintaining the same system of measurement across different scales in order to analyze patterns of coordinative structures. Rather than tracking individual state variables, coordination dynamics studies "the topological features of the spatiotemporal patterns generated by virtue of their interaction" (Zhang et al. 2020, 2). This type of analysis has focused mainly on rhythmic coordination, involving phase-locked synchronization and metastable coordination dynamics. In the latter case, phase relations are formed intermittently, rather than permanently, and this helps to preserve a diversity of processes (segregation) which are nonetheless linked (integration) (Kelso 2014). One can see this, for example, in social interaction, which requires both the autonomy of individual agents, and an interactional coupling that generates meaning (De Jaegher et al. 2010).

Different causal factors will have different weights in their relative contribution, some elements presumably playing more important causal roles than others (see Section 4.4). In the self-pattern, as we indicated, if one factor (or value or weight relative to the whole) is changed above a certain threshold, some or all of the other factors (and perhaps the whole) adjust. It is also in the dynamics that one will be able to measure different weighting patterns—including different connection weights between different factors (see, e.g., Kelso, Saltzman & Tuller 1986; Saltzman & Munhall 1989). Such measurements will have significance for both explanation and for the tailoring of treatment.

One relevant example is the study by Ramseyer & Tschacher (2011) which shows that non-verbal synchronous coordination of body movements between therapist and patient reflects therapeutic outcome. More generally, affect can modulate such dynamics. For example, participants coordinate to a higher degree when they like their communication partner (Zhao et al. 2017). Likewise mean-ingful joint or collaborative actions can elicit higher degrees of synchronized movements. For example, participants' bodily movements show higher coordin-ation when engaged in a positive conversation than when having an argument (Paxton & Dale 2013). This kind of "complexity matching"[9] is also evident in instances of joint deliberation (Brennan & Hanna 2009), and several experiments have shown significant synchronization in body-schematic processes (Soliman & Glenberg 2014—see Section 7.5 for further discussion), and more generally (Marmelat and Delignières 2012), during joint actions. Indeed, similar dynamics can be seen in individual body-schematic processes (e.g., coordination between left and right hands during a task) and in dyadic (intersubjective) processes in which participants used their dominant hands while standing next to each other (Schloesser, Kello & Marmelat 2019).

Kelso and his colleagues are able to diagram meaningful changes in dynamical patterns as transitions in topological recurrence plots:

> Overall, topological recurrence plots reveal local and global transitions of coordination patterns in the data that elude traditional methods....Such irre-ducibility of certain topological properties may tap into the very nature of col-lective transitions in multiscale coordinative structures....The relational quantities in such patterns constrain each other and form [more complex] structures which may not be discernible by examining each quantity individu-ally....[T]he ability of topological portraits to capture global properties is a key to detecting transitions in collective patterns that are not just an accumulation of pointwise changes....In other words, topological portraits capture emergent features in the collective dynamics that are not reducible to the sum of its parts, tapping into a key feature of complex systems.   (Zhang et al. 2020, 10–11)

The patterns to be studied can be behavioral patterns (such as those involved in social interaction, e.g., Tognoli & Kelso 2015; Tognoli et al. 2020), or neuronal activation patterns in the brain (Tognoli & Kelso 2014). This approach, which has

---

[9] Schloesser, Kello, and Marmelat (2019, 260) define complexity matching as the measure of the "degree to which two measurement series have similarly structured long-range correlations." See Abney et al. (2014).

focused on tracing the same dynamical principles across brain, body, and social interaction, is meant to be integrative, not only revealing dynamical details in the meshing or integration among different variables, but also providing an integrated theory of such patterns. This kind of analysis identifies "emergent phenomena where the whole is not only greater than the sum of its parts, but different too" (Tognoli et al. 2020).

The relevance of this method for the study of social interactions in the context of psychopathology can be seen in the suggestion of Leong and Schilbach (2019, 636): "disordered social interactions play a pervasive role in many, if not all, psychiatric disorders.... [T]hese disorders may result as much from an 'interaction mismatch' across persons as from the breakdown of individual brains." With respect to social cognition in specific, Dumas, Kelso, and Nadel (2014) suggest that "the case of autism provides a test bed for an integrative approach." Following this suggestion we can see how this threefold set of tools—the enhanced meshed architecture, experiments based on interventionist notions of causality, and the analysis of coordination dynamics—can help us drill down into the dynamical processes characteristic of the self-pattern in ASD.

3.4 Autism as a Test Case

If the model of a meshed architecture can identify which processes or factors to ask about, an interventionist strategy to test for causal or constitutive relevance can show us how factors are actually meshing, and the application of coordination dynamics can fill in some of the details of the dynamics to give us a more complete model. Let's consider ASD as a test case for this sort of analysis.

3.4.1 ToM and Social Cognition

Theoretical and empirical considerations suggest the testable factors of the self-pattern relevant to understanding ASD. Compared to typically developing children, one of the primary differences found in children with ASD involves social cognition and intersubjective interaction. As mentioned in Section 3.2, a standard approach is to consider such problems in social cognition to involve deficits in theory of mind (ToM), specifically in abilities to "mindread," that is, to make theoretical inferences about another person's mental states (Baron-Cohen, Leslie & Frith 1985; Frith & Happé 1999), or deficits in the ability to simulate the other's mental states, possibly due to a disruption in the activation of the neuronal mirror system (Iacoboni & Dapretto 2006; Oberman & Ramachandran 2007; but see Hamilton 2013 and Heyes & Catmur 2021 for important qualifications).

Such views are informed by empirical studies that show children with autism fail to pass false-belief tasks (Baron-Cohen, Leslie & Frith 1985; Yuk, Anagnostou & Taylor 2020). In the classic experiments, typically developing (TD) children at four years of age, on average, but not children of less than four years, are able to distinguish between how things really are in the world and what other people may falsely believe about such things. Around this age (if not earlier—see Baillargeon, Scott & He 2010), we begin to recognize that other individuals have their own sets of beliefs and intentions that inform their behavior, and we are able to explain or predict their behavior based on these mental states. Significantly, however, individuals with ASD fail false-belief tests even at mental ages significantly higher than four years. Individuals with autism are thus said to lack a theory of mind, and this cognitive deficit explains their lack of social responsiveness and understanding. Such views informed the experiments by Hadwin et al. (1997), discussed above (in Section 3.2). In those experiments the intervention targeted specific cognitive abilities associated with ToM, but, as noted, failed to improve social communicative interaction.

3.4.2 ASD and Affectivity

According to ToM approaches, the important factors in the self-pattern are cognitive and intersubjective processes. It is likely, however, that other processes are involved. Peter Hobson (1993), for example, has argued that affective processes are directly relevant in ASD. He cites empirical developmental studies that show the importance of affective relatedness in the infants' developing capacities for social interaction as early as the first year of life: "very young infants have perceptual-affective responsiveness to some aspects of another person's affect-related expressiveness and behavior, even though they may not be able to discriminate specific 'meanings' in abstracted expressions until the middle of their first year" (1993, 232). Affective relationality is, according to Hobson, the basis for primary intersubjectivity (Trevarthen 1979) and manifests itself both behaviorally and experientially. He argues that deficits in affective relationality, and its concomitant effect on intersubjective interactions, lead to the cognitive difficulties seen in ASD, rather than the other way around:

[S]uch limitations in the capacity for affectively patterned subjective experiences that are co-ordinated with the experiences of others, and corresponding disability in relating to the affective attitudes of others vis-à-vis a co-referenced world, might seriously constrain autistic children's understanding of 'minds' and communication, and through this restrict their ability to symbolise.

(1993, 227; see Hobson 1990)

In addition, actions are communicative in relation to *how* they are being performed. Daniel Stern introduced the term "vitality form" ("the felt experience of force in movement with a temporal contour and a sense of aliveness, of going somewhere" [Stern 2010, 8]), to capture how the dynamics of perceived action style in everyday interactions convey relevant information. Vitality forms are hardly ever perceived by children with ASD when attempting to imitate others, possibly affecting social skill learning (Hobson & Lee 1999). Further investigations specifically targeting vitality forms strengthen this conclusion by showing difficulties even in basic vitality form recognition during the observation of others' actions (Krueger 2021; Di Cesare et al. 2017). The notion of vitality form can be integrated into the notion of affect or affective attunement as described in the enhanced meshed architecture (see Trevarthen & Delafield-Butt 2013).

This speaks to both the integrated relations of different aspects (affective, cognitive, intersubjective) of the self-pattern, and a certain order in the meshed architecture. In working out the meshed relations within the self-pattern, however, one does not need to take a deficit in affective relationality to be the core or generative deficit in autism (Greenspan 2001). More generally, taking ASD to involve a particular disorder of the self-pattern means that there may not be any one deficit (whether affective, cognitive, or social) that can be identified as the core deficit (see Happé & Frith 2014; 2020). Rather, if ASD involves an intertwined pattern of deficits, then problems with affective relationality, as well as problems with social cognition, may be part of that pattern, and may be modulated by other processes. Bird and Cook (2013), for example, acknowledging that ASD may be associated with disordered emotion processing and deficits of emotional reciprocity, argue that there are wide variations in this regard across the spectrum. They suggest that when deficits in affective relationality are observed, they may be due to a frequently co-occurring alexithymia (a condition involving reduced ability to identify or describe one's own emotion, resulting in reduced empathy and impaired ability to recognize emotions in others). Also, it may be alexithymia that interferes with the passing of false-belief tasks if the task involves identifying an emotion. Whether it is best to distinguish complications arising from alexithymia from social impairments in ASD (Bird & Cook 2013), or to think that difficulties in emotion processing, and lower accuracy with facial emotion recognition in people with autism, are due to alexithymia rather than core features of ASD (Kinnaird, Stewart & Tchanturia 2019; Ola & Gullon-Scott 2020; Sivathasan et al. 2020), may require further research (see Mazefsky et al. 2013; Oakley et al. 2022), and can be complicated by other issues that involve sensorimotor problems, and processes that involve cultural and normative factors.

3.4.3 Motor Control

Impairments in the production and recognition of bodily affective expressions, and in the communication of feelings, broaden to communicative behavior generally, including problems with gesture. Thus, individuals with autism "rarely make gestures such as showing, giving or pointing in order to share awareness of an object's existence or properties, or comprehend such gestures when they are made by others" (Hobson 1993, 242). Klin et al. (2003), following an enactive model, show that individuals with autism fail to follow another's pointing gesture in some cases, and this may be tied to a lack of expertise in social perception, related to differences in visual focus when viewing complex social situations. Their experiments show that individuals with autism direct their gaze to aspects of the environment, or to other people in ways that miss socially salient information, for example, focusing on a person's chin instead of on their eyes.

This may also be linked to evidence that in ASD, besides cognitive and affective factors, there are some deficits in bodily processes that involve sensory-motor performance. Studies of individuals with ASD show that sensorimotor problems (specifically disrupted patterns in afferent and proprioceptive sensory feedback) can interfere with motor control (Brincker & Torres 2013; Torres 2013; Torres et al. 2013). These may involve postural instabilities, atypical gait, mis-timing of motor sequences, motor coordination problems, problems with anticipatory postural adjustments, and expressionless faces (Cattaneo et al. 2008; Cook, Blakemore & Press 2013; Fabbri-Destro et al. 2009; Gallese, Rochat & Berchio 2013; Hilton et al. 2012; Whyatt & Craig 2013), all of which scaffold effective social interactions and thus have implications for primary intersubjectivity (Gallagher 2004b; Gallagher & Varga 2015). For example, some studies have shown that children with ASD have difficulties in predicting *why* an action is being done by another person based on kinematic cues and this may reflect difficulties in the children's own motor planning (Cattaneo et al. 2008; Boria et al. 2009; Sparaci et al. 2014).

Other studies have shown that infants at heightened risk and later diagnosed with ASD at thirty-six months show a slower progression in the development of gross motor skills such as unsupported sitting and walking (Leezenbaum & Iverson 2019; West et al. 2019) and fine motor skills such as grasping and functional object use (Sparaci et al. 2018). Being able to grasp and manipulate objects while sharing them with others has been shown to support communication and in particular word learning in typical development (Yu & Smith 2012; Pereira, Smith & Yu 2014). Several studies now suggest that differential development of motor skills may have cascading effects on vocabulary acquisition, gestures, and social skills, suggesting a rather different account of the origins of problems in social interactions compared to traditional ToM approaches (Bhat, Landa &

Galloway 2011; Cook, Blakemore & Press 2013; Iverson et al. 2018; Sparaci et al. 2018; West et al. 2019).

3.4.4 Vertical and Horizontal Meshing

Iverson and Wozniak (2016) suggest that communicative delays and atypicalities in intentional and symbolic communication in children with ASD should be considered as extending beyond the individual since they have an impact on social partners and the communicative environment understood in a broader sense. In terms of the enhanced meshed architecture described above, this would involve the horizontal axis, and a context-related dynamic interplay between the communicator and his/her social and material environment, including artefacts, instruments, and established practices in communicating with other people. Likewise, the intrinsic dynamics that involve motor control and affectivity, on the vertical axis, includes the development of habits and basic skills, which, may be relevant to social communication, and are often important for participating in joint action and for processes involved in intersubjective interaction.

García-Pérez et al. (2007) suggest that children with ASD show a deficient propensity to engage with the bodily expressed attitudes of others (also see Hobson & Lee 1998). Children with ASD are less likely than matched controls to spontaneously respond with speech or gesture, to make eye contact, to engage in joint attention, joint action, or social referencing (Dawson et al. 1990; Kasari et al. 1990; Sigman et al. 1992). And as mentioned above, they may also be impaired in perceiving the vitality forms in the other person's communicative style (Di Cesare et al. 2017). It's important, however, not to lose track of the other side of the conversation. It's not only the children with ASD that show a deficient propensity to engage with the bodily expressed attitudes of others, those in conversation with the children do so as well. The reciprocal dynamics that constitute the conversation collapse on both sides. As Victoria McGeer (2001) notes, the burden of understanding is typically distributed between the participants who are trying to understand each other. Failure on one side may be reinforced by failure on the other side.

Furthermore, social impairments in autism are not limited to disruptions of dyadic (face-to-face) coordination dynamics. They can also involve a failure of people with autism to comfortably inhabit built environments and social institutions that are organized to accommodate neurotypical styles of engagement. It's not just about eye contact or the timing of conversational responses (which may involve processes in a very short time scale—measured in seconds or parts of a second), but it may also include the amount of lighting or background music used in public spaces, social arrangements or cultural practices that may be upsetting to some individuals with ASD, or even disruptive to development (on a longer time scale that may be measured in years). Negotiating such material and social/normative, neurotypical environments may have a long-term impact on their embodied interactions with others within these spaces, and their "habits of mind" (Krueger & Maiese 2018) or ways of being in the world. It may lead to or reinforce what are sometimes observed in ASD, namely, "highly structured and regimented life routines that avoid novelty and the inherent unpredictability of typical social life" (Klin et al. 2003, 345). Similar things can be said about what Constant et al. (2022, 7) call "practical causality" (or looping effects) in the medical or psychiatric context—that is, changes in behavior caused by virtue of being classified or labeled autistic. Classifying someone as autistic may in fact change expectations and behavior.

In the case of ASD, disruptions seemingly occur along both axes of the EMA. On the vertical axis the verbal accomplishment of thought seems impaired in conversation when most responses are simple answer-type replies. This impoverishment of expressed thought may not be divorced from the various anomalies involved in sensory-motor processes that can disrupt the intrinsic control processes involved in nonverbal and gestural performance (Klin et al. 2003). Likewise, problems in the affective dimension may disrupt the possibility of smooth dynamics amongst these factors as well as with factors on the horizontal axis. The deficient interactive response of others to people with ASD may not only reinforce disruptions to interkinaesthetic affectivity, but may also signal a change in normative expectations that accompany most social and cultural practices. Indeed, the integrative meshing of what we called the whole dynamical gestalt of intersubjective interaction seems to be differently aligned in the case of ASD.

3.5 Experimental and Therapeutic Interventions

Intervention into this complex, integrated self-pattern can happen in numerous ways. In Section 3.2 we saw a clear, albeit unsuccessful, but nonetheless telling example in training on ToM tasks (Hadwin et al. 1997). Psychological therapies that target emotional awareness or provide emotion recognition training, however, may improve social communication in ASD (Cameron, Ogrodniczuk & Hadjipavlou 2014; Cooper, Loades & Russell 2018). It is also possible to intervene by training motor control processes via procedural learning (Gidley Larson & Mostofsky 2008; Sparaci et al. 2015; Wek & Husak 1989). Moreover, one could think that intervention would be possible by changing the behavior of the conversational interlocutors. Of course, it may be that improved therapy requires interventions on multiple factors.

Problems with affective relationality identified by Hobson and others, together with the problems involving proprioceptive feedback and motoric behavior mentioned above, as well as developmental delays involving purposeful actions (object exploration and functional actions) beginning in infancy, and their possible cascading effects on later language development (Sparaci et al. 2018), may all play a part in disrupting nonverbal aspects of conversation pragmatics. Wimpory et al. (2000), for example, have shown that very young children with ASD show impairments in nonverbal communication that can disrupt timing in intersubjective engagement, frequency of eye contact and turn-taking, as well as referential looking and pointing. Nonverbal cues are important for the smooth flow of conversation.

The study by Hadwin et al. (1997) showed that an intervention training on ToM tasks did not improve the conversational abilities of children with ASD. An experiment by García-Pérez, Lee, and Hobson (2007) gets us closer to what may be some more basic problems in the conversational ability of autistic children, and points to a tight meshing of affect, motor control processes, intersubjectivity, and factors that define the horizontal axis (see Harrison & Tronick 2022; Larkin et al. 2017). García-Pérez et al. showed that subjects with ASD "made fewer head-shakes/nods (but not smiles) when the interviewer was talking" (1310).[10] A principle of social interaction, reflected in detailed analyses of the distributed semiotics of conversational processes (e.g., Goodwin 2000), is that it involves two-way, context-rich interaction. In this respect García-Pérez et al. also studied the responses of the conversational partners, the interviewers who interacted with the children with ASD. It turns out that they also made fewer head-shakes/nods when the children were talking compared to their typical conversation style. In this regard the dynamics of the conversation itself, as a whole, changes when the interkinaesthetic affectivity of the interaction goes off. This kind of affective disruption was reflected in significant differences measured as "subjective" ratings of (a) affective engagement and (b) the smoothness of reciprocal interaction (as rated by two evaluators blind to diagnosis, rating emotional connection during the videotaped conversation and the flow of the conversation on scales of 1–5).

Consider also, a study by Kostrubiec et al. (2018), who reference Kelso's coordination dynamics approach. The researchers compared twenty ASD versus twenty-one typically developing children (eight to fourteen years of age) on motor coordination in intentional motor tasks, and correlated this to Socio-Adaptatif Quotient (SAQ) scores that measure communication ability and socialization (e.g., saying "please," "thanks," or "excuse me"). They found no notable differences in a simple, perceptual-motor coordination task; but children with ASD showed increasing deficits in more demanding interpersonal coordination tasks when coordination patterns were intentionally requested by the experimenter

---

[10] Although a study of adolescents with ASD conducted by Capps, Kehres, and Sigman (1998) found more headshaking and nodding in response to yes or no questions, the subjects were less likely to nod while listening to their conversational partners talk. They concluded that "children with ASD demonstrated limited involvement in the co-construction of a shared conversational trajectory through nonverbal as well as verbal channels" (1998, 337).

(consistent with other studies—e.g., Fitzpatrick et al. 2016; Marsh et al. 2013). This result also correlated to poor SAQ scores. Improved performance in older ASD children, however, suggested that therapeutic intervention would be beneficial. This led the researchers to the following hypothesis: "This leaves the hypothetical and to-be-tested possibility that by manipulating [motor coordination] parameters in ASD children, their coordination abnormalities could be reduced, and their social deficits, perhaps, alleviated" (Kostrubiec et al. 2018). It is surely more complicated, however, since there were increased deficits in coordination *when socially interacting with the experimenters,* and since in other disorders—for example, ADHD—anomalies in motor coordination do not lead to similar social deficits. This suggests not a one-way or one-to-one causal relation, but some more nuanced (dynamical, non-linear) relation between social interaction and motor coordination.

The therapeutic intervention might also be based on considering the communicative practices of the experimenters as they interact with children with ASD. Context is also important, and communicative interactions may be very different outside the lab, in the home, when, for example, children with ASD are interacting with parents (see Henderson 2020 for an insightful ethnographic study). Indeed, considering that there may be deficiencies in several factors, the reference to Kelso's coordination dynamics approach is apropos.

3.6 The Dynamics of ASD

Embodied and enactive perspectives on social cognition emphasize the importance of movement coordination of one's body with the other person while performing actions (social-motor coordination) (Gallagher 2020a; Zapata-Fonseca et al. 2016; 2019). As noted in previous sections, children with ASD have difficulties in social communication skills, some of which may be due to motor deficits (found in 50 percent to 80 percent of children diagnosed with ASD) (Baillin et al 2020; Isenhower et al. 2012; Kaur et al. 2018). Fitzpatrick et al. (2013) suggest

> social motor coordination both in the form of imitation and in the lesser known phenomenon of interactional synchrony, is important for maintaining critical aspects of successful human social interaction, including interpersonal responsiveness, social rapport and other-directedness...positive self-other relations...and verbal communication and comprehension.
> (Fitzpatrick et al. 2013; citing research by Bernieri et al. 1994; Lakin & Chartrand 2003; Miles et al. 2009; Shockley et al. 2009)

Social synchronization is an important component of interpersonal interaction, across a wide diversity of situations, including emotional arousal, imitation, joint attention, parent–child exchanges, mutual gaze, shared attention, and empathy (Kinsbourne & Helt 2011; Trevarthen & Daniel 2005). A breakdown or significant modulation of such synchronization or entrainment across many of these contexts are reported in children and adolescents with ASD (e.g., de Marchena & Eigsti 2010; Fulceri et al. 2018; Macpherson et al. 2020). In the case of stable coordination patterns, the variability of relative phasing (the phase relation between movement patterns) between two or more individuals reflects the strength of coupling or alignment. Higher variability, as found in ASD, reflects weaker coupling.

Using coupled oscillator modeling,[11] Fitzpatrick et al. (2016) showed that adolescents with ASD demonstrate less interactive synchronization in both spontaneous and intentional social coordination, corresponding to lower sensitivity and decreased attention to the other person.

> Adolescents with ASD demonstrated a disruption of both spontaneous synchronization and intentional synchronization.…[T]he ASD group [compared to typically developing adolescents] had weaker spontaneous synchronization…when participants were viewing each other's pendulum.…ASD participants synchronized less well under conditions in which synchronization occurs spontaneously in the presence of perceptual information of the social partner and in situations when there is an explicit social goal to coordinate with another person (e.g., intentional synchronization).

The researchers suggest two possible interpretations of these results, namely that the synchronization problems of adolescents with ASD involved problems with either attention or motor control. Di Cesare et al. (2017) suggest that it may also involve lack of perceptual sensitivity to variation in vitality forms, but that this too may be due to motor atypicalities in ASD (also see Fitzpatrick et al. 2017; Kaur, Srinivasan & Bhat 2018).

An alternative method using coordination dynamics to study nonlinear dynamics of human social coordination, including behavioral measures of social interaction (and interpersonal synchrony) in people with ASD, employs a research tool called the Human Dynamic Clamp (HDC). This set-up allows a dynamic bidirectional interaction in real time between a human and a virtual avatar (modeled on human–human interaction) (Dumas et al. 2014; Kelso et al. 2009).

---

[11] This task allows for the study of both intentional (following instruction) and spontaneous interpersonal coordination. Two people coordinate handheld pendulums swinging them "from the wrist joint in the sagittal plane (using radial-ulnar abduction–adduction). This methodology has demonstrated that the strength of interpersonal synchronization…can be understood in terms of a dynamical model of synchronization.…Using such a dynamical model to understand how synchrony breaks down in social deficits has the distinct advantage of allowing one to infer which dynamical components of the model are underlying the impairment" (Fitzpatrick 2016, 3; also see Marsh et al. 2013).

Using this method, Baillin et al. (2020) studied behavioral aspects of interpersonal synchrony in ASD, considering several variables, including motor control and emotion recognition.

Noting that children with ASD have difficulties in coordinating their body during social exchange (see the research cited above), Baillin et al. showed lower motor skills among ASD participants suggesting a significant link between motor skills and social-cognitive skills among a population of children and adolescents. The low score on motor ability was a significant factor distinguishing the ASD from the typically developing individuals.

Social interaction is not unidirectional, of course. We know that there is a difference between a one-way coupling, for example when a participant is responding to the movement of a computer-generated avatar who is not responding to them, and a two-way interaction (see Oullier et al. 2008). As indicated above, one's own response may depend on how one's interlocutor or social partner responds. The use of coordination dynamics should also be able to throw light on this. The degree to which social partners contribute to entrainment in joint coordination may differ. The results of the above experiments suggest that persons with autism may adapt their movements less to those of their partner. But it is also possible that (1) the social partner compensates for this by adjusting their own movement, or (2) that the partner shows less entrained attunement when coordinating with an individual with ASD.[12] There is some evidence of differences in people's motoric response to others they perceive as psychologically different. For example, Brezis et al (2017) report that an experimenter, who was not blind to the diagnosis, interacting with subjects with ASD, moved more slowly than when interacting with typically developing participants (also see Rainteau et al. 2020). This is a question that calls for further experimentation and clarification that does not simply focus on the subject with ASD, but on the relational dynamics of interacting that is two-sided (see De Jaegher 2013; Morrison et al. 2020). Generally speaking, interaction is reciprocal in the sense that in typical social encounters understanding is distributed between the person trying to understand and the person who is trying to make herself understandable (McGeer 2001).

To conclude, these studies of interactional dynamics in ASD can yield significant detail about the precise nature of disordered communication and interactive practices. They clearly motivate further experiments and more comprehensive therapeutic interventions that can help to define the dynamical relations existing among motoric, affective, intersubjective, cognitive, and ecological factors and their disruption in ASD (see Alonim et al. 2020; 2021, for just such a comprehensive

---

[12] This is sometimes called a "double empathy" problem (Milton 2012); communication and interaction problems are not driven solely by the autistic person; the non-autistic partner often exhibits difficulty communicating in specific interactions (Edey et al. 2016). Peper, van der Wal, and Begeer (2016) point to a possible strategy to measure these differences developed by Słowiński et al. (2016).

approach). This, in turn, would allow us to map more precisely the meshed architecture of the self-pattern in the context of social interaction.

To summarize, we've seen that the integration problem in psychiatry is tied to conceptions of causality and explanatory levels in our understanding of mind and human social existence more generally. In this chapter I proposed a threefold method for exploring the dynamics of integration within the self-pattern, based on a concept of dynamical causation and a non-hierarchical (level-free) notion of gestalt. In these terms I've explored ASD as a test case. This approach supports an analysis that both distinguishes and integrates the various factors and processes that contribute to differences in social engagement found in ASD. The model is different from, on the one hand, most standard explanations of autism in terms of ToM or any one factor. It rather focuses on a pattern of dynamically intertwined factors. On the other hand, this model is also different from the model of a fused integration (de Haan 2020), which would necessarily fail to capture or discriminate the specific factors that contribute to this pattern. In this regard:

1. We can give up explanatory concepts of levels or hierarchy;
2. but still use interventionist analysis to identify causal relevance—non-linear/dynamical causality that allows useful distinctions to be made between various factors/processes, and at the same time, can account for their integration; and
3. provide a dynamical systems explanation that can sort out in some detail the dynamical relations that define the self-pattern.

4

Dynamical Relations in the Self-pattern and Psychopathology

In the previous chapters the dynamical nature of the self-pattern was emphasized. And as we've seen in Chapter 1, the notion of a self-pattern, as developed in the pattern theory of self (PTS), acknowledges the importance of neural dynamics, but also includes extra-neural elements and extra-neural dynamics. PTS however, has been criticized for failing to explicate the dynamical relations among elements of the self-pattern. Although we have been emphasizing the role of dynamical causality in the self-pattern, I'll continue to address this issue by showing that the dynamics of a self-pattern are reflected in three significant and interrelated ways that allow for investigation. First, a self-pattern is reflectively reiterated in its narrative component. Second, studies of psychiatric or neurological disorders can help us understand the precise nature of the dynamical relations in a self-pattern, and how they can fail. Third, referencing predictive processing accounts, neuroscience can also help to explicate, in a non-reductionist way, the dynamical relations that constitute the self-pattern.[1]

The pattern theory affirms that selves are only ever apprehended as situated in a meaningful world; it accommodates change and adaptation to context; and at the same time, it acknowledges a coherent organization as the locus of experience and self-ascription. On this account, dynamical self-patterns involve and are revealed in self-narratives, which track situated actions, but also reflect regenerative self-organizing processes and the various disruptions of those processes in anomalous or pathological experience. Such patterns and disruptions are also reflected in dynamical neural processes. Self, as reflected in terms of such neural and narrative processes, is not a fixed entity but is rather an ongoing production which brings a real but contingent coherence to an evolving stream of sensations, thoughts, emotions, desires, memories, and anticipations.

I'll begin with some comments on an alternative to the notion of a self-pattern, namely Thomas Metzinger's notion of a self-model. Metzinger's concept of self-model is primarily oriented to processes in the brain. Although he indicates the relevance of brain processes and their dynamical connections for an understanding of the concept of self, he also contentiously proposes that "[n]obody ever *was*

---

[1] The account I give in this chapter was first sketched out with Anya Daly (Gallagher & Daly 2018; also see Daly & Gallagher 2019).

The Self and its Disorders. Shaun Gallagher, Oxford University Press. © Shaun Gallagher 2024.
DOI: 10.1093/oso/9780198873068.003.0005

or *had* a self" (2004, 1). To be clear, with this assertion Metzinger is rightly rejecting accounts that explicitly endorse or implicitly underwrite substantively "real" Cartesian selves. There are, however, some challenges that Metzinger's account needs to address. First, if a self is not real the way a substance is real, it is also the case that the self is *not non*-real in the way an illusion is non-real (Metzinger 2009, 209). Accordingly, one needs to specify in what way we may talk about the reality of the self.

Second, according to Metzinger, the phenomenal self is generated in a process involving neuro-dynamics, from which subjective self-awareness emerges. The key challenge for this approach is to explain precisely how a self-model is related to or generated in the brain. As I suggested in Chapter 1, and as I'll show in more detail in the following section, there seems to be no agreement about what specific brain processes are relevant to a self-representational system, or whether there are specialized or exclusively self-specific areas in the brain. This could very well motivate an appeal to more general predictive processing models. Indeed, Metzinger's original proposal already sketched such a model (2004, 51–2), and more recently he has moved further in that direction, endorsing the idea of an automatic and continuing minimization of prediction errors, a process in which the brain monitors the body and immediate environment for potential unexpected events (Metzinger 2013; 2014; Wiese & Metzinger 2017; also see Limanowski & Blankenburg 2013; Seth 2013).

Third, I note that the notion of a self-model is an attempt to explain the phenomenal self—that is, the phenomenal sense of or experiential aspect of self. Although it is important to give an account of the phenomenology of self, it is not clear that this is all there is to a self, or that self is something that can be reduced to its phenomenal appearance. In this respect, from the perspective of pattern theory, this identification of self with just one aspect of the self-pattern amounts to a mereological fallacy, taking just one aspect or part to be the whole.

An alternative way to think of a self is to consider it as irreducible to brain processes or to phenomenal experience, although neither of these aspects are irrelevant to self. The alternative to the self-model is the notion of a self-pattern, as proposed in the previous chapters. In addition to neural processes, the self-pattern depends on a variety of extra-neural bodily processes, and ecological processes that are social and cultural, such that, in part, it is generated in the organism's relations with its environment. On this view (as indicated in Section 2.1), the self has the scientifically useful reality of a pattern.[2] Still, although the

---

[2] Some theorists suggest that the idea that a self just is a pattern means that it succumbs to the "self-illusion" hypothesis. Bruce Hood (2012), for example, makes this claim, although he explains: "[y]ou only exist as a pattern made up of all the other things in your life that shape you. If you take each away, 'you' would eventually cease to exist. This does not mean that you do not exist at all, but rather than you exist as the combination of all the others who complete your sense of self" (Hood 2012, 215). It's not clear, however, why that means you exist as an illusion. Also see Madsen (2017) for a similar claim.

brain is not the sole generator of the self-pattern, mapping of self-related brain function may help to demonstrate the dynamical nature of self-patterns. In this respect, some version of the predictive processing model might provide a means to clarify these dynamical relations. I return to this issue in Section 4.5.

In this chapter, then, after reviewing some issues concerning self and brain, I'll answer some objections that have been raised concerning the dynamical relations among different elements of a self-pattern. I'll argue that there are three ways to track the dynamical relations in a self-pattern: first, through narrative; second, through the study of psychopathology; and third, through predictive processing as a version of brain dynamics.

4.1 Neural Patterns and the Self

A number of approaches have attempted to relate neural processing to the concept of self. Karl Popper and John Eccles (1977; Eccles 1989; 1994), for example, defended a dualist view that treated the self as an autonomous entity that interacted with neural processes, and purportedly controlled them: "The self-conscious mind acts upon…neural centres, modifying the dynamic spatio-temporal patterns of the neural events" (Popper & Eccles 1977, 495). This non-reductionist, Cartesian view, however, did not represent either the philosophical or neuroscientific consensus of the time, and still does not. It did motivate a debate between the philosopher Mario Bunge, who defended an emergentist view, and the neuroscientist Donald McKay, who, although starting "from our immediate experience of what it is like to be a person" (1978, 601), staked out a position between materialism and dualism (Bunge 1977, 1979; MacKay 1978, 1979, 1980). MacKay argued that since each change in experience corresponds to a change in brain activity, there is both first-person data and third-person data about the conscious self. Importantly, for MacKay, despite the high degree of correlation between these data sets, one set is not reducible to the other set.

In these various discussions the concept of self was never clearly defined. Since the 1970s, however, there have been both clarifications and complications introduced around the notion of self as it is discussed in both philosophy and neuroscience. And there have been important qualifications made regarding correlations between brain and self. For example, Joseph LeDoux (2002, 31) has pointed out that theories of the self "are not usually framed in ways that are compatible with our understanding of brain function." This idea is echoed by Northoff et al. (2006, 453): "Neither the historical nor modern psychological approaches are obviously isomorphic with any known brain analysis." The lack of a perfect correlation between self and brain thus results in worries such as those expressed by Apps and Tsakiris (2014, 85–6): "recent reviews of this literature have concluded that the absence of a unifying theoretical framework has resulted in a largely incoherent picture of the circuits and mechanisms which are engaged during self-recognition."

Such thoughts have not stopped the continuing analysis of how various aspects of self relate to brain, however. Much of this research asks how specific brain areas correlate with self-related phenomena. Thus, for example, autobiographical knowledge, personal beliefs, self-conceptions, and the recognition of our own face have been grouped together as related to left hemisphere activity (Turk et al. 2003; see also Kircher et al. 2000). At the same time there is evidence that "processing of self-related information (e.g., autobiographical memory, face self identification, theory of mind) is related to activity in the right frontal cortex" (Platek et al. 2003, 147). Representations of both the physical and phenomenological aspects of self, and "self-representation in general" is said to involve the right lateral parietal cortex (Lou et al. 2004, 6831), while the "self model…a theoretical construct comprising essential features such as feelings of continuity and unity, experience of agency, and body-centered perspective" (Fossati et al. 2003, 1943) involves activation of the medial prefrontal cortex in both hemispheres. Tisserand et al. (2023) show how the insula plays an important role correlated with multiple aspects of the self.

As we've seen (Section 1.4), cortical midline structures (CMS) have been shown to process information related to self. In particular, activation of the ventromedial prefrontal cortex (VMPFC) has been repeatedly observed when subjects think about themselves (Northoff & Bermpohl 2004; Northoff et al. 2006) and when they make judgments about their own personalities (D'Argembeau et al. 2007; Gutchess et al. 2007; Heatherton et al. 2006; Johnson et al. 2002; Kelley et al. 2002; Ruby et al. 2009). Lesion studies also show that damage to the VMPFC leads to deficits in self-awareness (Stuss, Gallup & Alexander 2001; Stuss et al. 2001). Northoff and colleagues thus argue for a unitary neural network or system responsible for all self-related phenomena. The putative CMS self-system, however, covers quite a large set of brain regions (including ventro- and dorsomedial prefrontal, anterior and posterior cingulate, retrosplenial, and medial parietal cortices). It involves a multitude of connections between CMS and subcortical areas, reflecting the possible role of subcortical areas related to an embodied self (Northoff & Panksepp 2008). Disruptions in such network connections are likely involved in psychiatric disorders such as schizophrenia (Nekovarova et al. 2014). The distinction between prereflective, embodied processes and self-referential cognitive processes, but also their connection in terms of neural dynamics, have also been explored experimentally using the psychoactive effects of psilocybin as an intervention that disrupts self–other differentiation or self-coherency, most clearly in self-referential processing (Duerler et al. 2022; Smigielski et al. 2020).

As discussed in Chapter 1, the large number of cortical areas that correlate with self-reference or self-experience suggests that there is no specialized brain area, *simpliciter*, responsible for generating "the self" (Gillihan & Farah 2005).

LeDoux notes the complexity: "different components of the self reflect the operation of different brain systems, which can be but are not always in sync" (2002, 31). It is also likely that no area of the brain is exclusively self-specific (Legrand & Ruby 2009). According to Craik et al. (1999, 30), "every significant activation in the [self condition] was also found in either the [other person condition] or the [general semantic] condition, or both" (also Gillihan & Farah 2005, 94). Moreover, most of the cited studies focus on self-referential tasks, that is, tasks that take the self or self-aspect to be part of the object of consciousness—for example, thinking about myself, judging my personality traits, self-face identification. As Legrand and Ruby (2009) make clear, this focus misses prereflective self-awareness, in which I am not aware of myself as an object, but am self-aware in a non-observational way, as the experiencing subject. Neisser's (1988) notion of ecological self-awareness is an example of this kind of prereflective self-awareness. The fact that I always perceive from a first-person (egocentric) perspective suggests that there is always a proprioceptive sense of this self-related perspective implicit in my experience. Metzinger's self-model accounts for this distinction between self-referential (self-as-object), and prereflective self-awareness (self-as-subject) in terms of a distinction between phenomenal self-model, equivalent to the *content properties* of a self-representation available for introspection, and functional self-model or "minimal phenomenal selfhood" (MPS), where the latter includes elements like the body schema and first-person perspective—basic aspects of prereflective bodily processes (Blanke & Metzinger 2009; Limanowski & Blankenburg 2013).

Rather than finding a common, well-circumscribed brain area of self-referential activation, then, these various studies indicate a complex diversification of activations for a variety of self-related experiences, but with no area ever activated exclusively for self—a self that is seemingly everywhere and nowhere in the brain. This led Vogeley and Gallagher (2011) to offer a caution:

> To achieve clarity in neuroscientific studies of self it is incumbent on researchers to define the precise aspect of self under study. Selves are experiential, ecological, and agentive; they are often engaged in reflective evaluations and judgments; they are capable of various forms of self-recognition, self-related cognition, self-narrative, and self-specific perception and movement. In many of these activities, selves are more 'in-the-world' than 'in-the-brain', and they are in-the-world as-subject more so than as-object. (2011, 129).

4.2 The Problem of Dynamical Relations

The notion of self-pattern attempts to capture both the plurality of factors involved in self and the idea that the self (as an agent) is more "in-the-world" than "in the brain."[3] As indicated in the previous chapters, the self-pattern is not an additive collection of components, but a set of dynamically interrelated factors and processes arranged in a dynamical gestalt. Thus, an intervention that affects one factor can involve modulations in the other factors. Adjustments in one aspect, above a certain threshold, will lead, via dynamical interactions, to changes in others. For example, very basic aspects of self-experience, such as the sense of agency, can be modulated by more complex, relational aspects, such as social, normative factors that involve culture, gender, race, health, and so forth, and by specific intersubjective factors that can either diminish or enhance one's autonomy and sense of agency (Carel 2016; Gallagher 2012a; Gatens 1996; Leach-Scully 2012; A. Murphy 2008; Weiss 1999; Young 1980).

Although I've emphasized the dynamical nature of the self-pattern, such that particular elements or factors are to be considered dynamically interwoven with other elements, one important criticism of PTS has been that there is so far no explanation of these dynamical relations. Thus, for example, Miriam Kyselo (2014, 1) writes: "Once the diversity of self related phenomena is acknowledged [as in PTS], we also need to understand how the elements of a collection of relevant self features interrelate. A pattern approach to the self acknowledges diversity but lacks integration, offering no account of the individual as explanatory whole" (also see Beni 2016). Likewise, Sanneke de Haan and her colleagues suggest that the main weakness of PTS is that:

> [I]t is just a list; a heaping of aspects, without an account of how they relate. There are no considerations on their potential ordering, hierarchy or structure. But in the case of psychiatric disorders and their treatment the relevant questions precisely pertain to this structure, to the relation between aspects of the self.   (2017, 5–6)

Both Kyselo and de Haan are concerned about how PTS might explain various pathologies. As Kyselo rightly suggests, researchers in cognitive science as they set up experiments, and psychiatrists as they evaluate patients and attempt to understand pathologies of the self, need to have a conception of the self as an explanatory whole. On the one hand, it's not enough, of course, to simply say that the self-pattern is a dynamical gestalt, and that the different elements of the self-pattern are dynamically related. On the other hand, this is not something that one can determine a priori, or simply by adopting a particular theory. Rather, we need precisely the empirical and clinical studies of psychiatric or neurological

---

[3] The phrase "in-the-world" is found in the phenomenological philosophy of Heidegger and Merleau-Ponty. It signifies a structural characteristic of human existence rather than a geographical location. It's meaning relates, in part, to concepts such as "situation" in John Dewey (1938), where the agent is not only always situated, but the situation is always defined relative to the agent; Gibson's notion of "affordance" (1977); or Koffka's (2013) gestalt notion of "behavioral environment."

disorders mentioned by Kyselo to help specify how something like the dynamical integration of a self-pattern can occur, how it is ordered and how it can become disordered. Accordingly, PTS remains consistent with Kyselo's suggestion that an embodied-enactivist approach may be able to offer an integrative perspective on the self as a whole. Given that we should not be satisfied with a set of a priori generalities about the dynamical relations, providing a method to do the kinds of empirical and clinical studies, as indicated in this and the previous chapter, is certainly part of what is needed.

From the perspective of PTS, it is not the case that one needs to add something extra to the specific pattern dynamically formed by the interrelations of the various elements in order to identify the coherency or structure behind the diversity; rather coherency or structure will be reflected in the pattern constituted by these interrelations. Dynamical connections in the pattern get reflected in three significant and interrelated ways that allow for investigation. First, a self-pattern is reflectively reiterated in its narrative component. That is, self-narratives reiterate the other processes and their dynamical relations in a way that will allow us to make sense of these relations. Second, as already indicated, the dynamics of a self-pattern are revealed in the way that they break down in pathology. Empirical, clinical, and phenomenological studies of psychiatric or neurological disorders can contribute to sorting out the precise nature of the dynamical relations in a self-pattern. Third, neuroscience can also help to explicate the dynamical relations that constitute the self-pattern. In taking the notion of a self-pattern to be the basis of a non-reductive approach to understanding self, the intent is not to exclude neuroscience, or to downplay the importance of brain function, as it relates to many of the bodily, experiential, and cognitive factors that make up a self-pattern. Indeed, as Fingelkurts and Fingelkurts (2017) suggest, changes in neurophysiology can "index" changes in the self-pattern, complementary to the way that narrative reflects such changes. In this respect, however, given the issues raised in the first section of this chapter, it will be more productive to look, not at specific brain areas or supposed neural representations to find correlations, but to look more generally at dynamical processing and brain function.

4.3 What's the Story with Narrative?

One way to understand the narrative aspect of self is to take it as an opening onto the landscape of the self-pattern and a way to map, retrieve, disclose, or express the dynamical relations among the various other factors of the self. Self-narratives in some sense reflect, explicitly in content, or implicitly in form, all of the other processes of the self-pattern (Gallagher & Daly 2018).

To show how this works, consider an example from Frith and Metzinger (2016). They discuss the case of regret, which, as they propose, involves a form of self-knowledge. This kind of self-knowledge takes a narrative form in which I, as the narrator, can give an account, and evaluate my past action. Assuming that I have made the wrong choice sometime in the past, I come to regret that choice, and this is something that manifests itself in my self-narrative. What gets reflected in my narrative in this respect are changes or adjustments in a variety of aspects of my self-pattern.

For example, the minimal experiential aspects of the self-pattern include the sense of agency and the sense of ownership. Frith and Metzinger point out, first, that the situation captured by the narrative involves a changing status of the sense of agency. I had a sense of control over my actions when in fact I made the wrong choice and acted on it. This sense of agency does not apply to my regret, however, or at least I seem unable to avoid my regret about that action. Adjustments in my sense of agency are reflected in my narrative when I say to myself or to someone else that I regret my action. In contrast, the sense of ownership pertains to both my action and my regret: "while the sense of agency is represented as something we possessed in the past, the state of regret itself does not itself involve a sense of agency. While the phenomenology of ownership is crisp and distinct (I identify with my regret, it is an integral part of myself), regret itself is not an action. It is a kind of inner pain that simply appears in us" (Frith and Metzinger 2016, 202). As they also make clear, my regret is not just a characteristic that I can narrate, it is something that takes over my narration: "The phenomenology of regret can be described as a loss of control over our personal narrative, and in this sense it is also a threat to our integrity. It is a threat to the integrity of our autobiographical self-model, because, on the personal level of description, we become aware of an irrevocable damage to our life narrative" (2016, 202). The emergence of an inner pain reflects the affective aspect of the self-pattern: "Because it is an emotional and frequently also an embodied experience, perhaps with heart wrenching qualities, it is not something we can distance ourselves from—another important way in which regret involves a loss of control" (2016, 202).

The narrative is doing some work in tying together some of the other factors in the self-pattern, and forming a "transtemporal identity" of the subject across time. The relation between action and regret, despite variations in my sense of agency, means that I am the same person who acted in the past, the person who continues to be responsible for my actions. Frith and Metzinger suggest that this is a fictional unity: "a transtemporal, fictional 'self'" constituted by the narrative (2016, 202). Yet the action and affective states—the pain and the regret—are real—real factors that specify a real self-pattern.

We can also acknowledge how an intersubjective or social dimension relates to both agency and affect, since, as the narrative may reveal, others are affected (e.g., frustrated) by my actions. How I relate to those others partially shapes who I am. In Frith and Metzinger's terms, the "important point is that, for any organism that has acquired the capacity to feel regret and whose behaviour is determined by this very special form of conscious content, the self-model and the group-model have become functionally integrated in a much stronger way" (204). The narrative may in fact reflect my identification with the values and desires of others, which may increase my emotional suffering, something that may derive "from a self-caused frustration of group-preferences" (204). I feel regret because, as one might say, my conscience has been formed by my upbringing. Such normative factors are all pervasive. As they put it, the

> group-model has invaded the organism's self-model to such a degree that the conflict between group and individual interests is now internally modelled in a way that a) includes sanctions by the group (regret is internal self-sanctioning), and b) the dynamic competition between group and individual interests is now taking place not only on the level of overt, bodily actions, but has found a new platform—the self-model of the individual.   (2016, 204–5).

That is, there are dynamical adjustments in the self-pattern in which intersubject-ive/social/normative factors determine my reflective evaluation and my feelings about what I have done. Most likely, these also manifest in my behavior and get reflected again (and perhaps repetitively) in my narrative.

My regret and how I, and others, evaluate my past action can have an effect on my future choice of action. My deliberations and actions relate to normative fac-tors, to "cultural practices, such as moral codes and laws. By generating beliefs about self-control [my narrative] shapes the sense of self and gives rise to con-cepts like responsibility, intentionality, accountability, culpability, and mitigating circumstances" (2016, 205). My action, my regret, my pain, mediated in my nar-rative practice, are here making a loop through normative factors that ultimately feed back to influence my behavior.[4] Frith and Metzinger suggest that "the sense of agency and the idea of voluntary action are acquired through cultural learning. The causal link between the group level and the individual level is constituted by the conscious self-model, in which group preferences are increasingly reflected as social complexity increases" (205). Alternatively, as they point out, further phys-ical and affective changes may lead to anxiety and depression (Roese et al. 2009), delayed sleep onset and insomnia (Schmidt & Van der Linden 2013), and onward to additional changes in self-narrative. As adjustments occur in the self-pattern, they get reflected in the self-narrative.

---

[4] The looping is complex. Somogy Varga (2015, 71) writes: "not only does autobiographical self-reflection involve the co-construction of what is recollected, establishing a link between the [narra-tor's] current view of himself and a set of past experiences, but also this process occurs in a loop-like, dynamic way—what is recollected influences the present self-understanding, yet the recollected material [or at least what I recollect and how I interpret it] is itself influenced and altered on the basis of the present self-understanding." See Dings & Newen (2021) for the role of memory in this process.

The point is that we can move forward on understanding the dynamical relations (between experiential, embodied, affective, social, and normative factors) that constitute a coherent self-pattern as they get reflected in self-narrative. We can map out these relations by looking at instances where some action, event, or intervention causes changes in various factors in the self-pattern that get traced out in self-narrative, including those instances where the pattern becomes disordered, or ordered differently.[5]

4.4 Psychopathology

By exploring the hypothesis that all psychiatric disorders are disorders of the self, we can avoid approaches to psychiatric classifications that insist on exclusive taxonomies of either natural kinds or social constructs. We can opt instead for what Peter Zachar (2002) calls "practical kinds." A practical kind model emphasizes relational criteria and the fact that psychiatric disorders tend to be multifactorial. To the extent that we think of such disorders as self-disorders, each individual case of a particular disorder may show different patterns of dynamical relations among the various factors that constitute a particular self. This is because different factors may involve different weights in different individuals (which can be measured in a dynamical analysis, see Section 3.3). For example, anorexia will present differently in a disciplined person with high degrees of self-control than in an impulsive individual (Zachar 2008, 334). Variations in the amount of social support or different cultural contexts may determine how a disorder develops. But we can still expect to see typical patterns of practical kinds associated with different disorders. Schizophrenia, for example, may affect multiple aspects of experience, cognition, mood, and agency in somewhat typical ways (Nekovarova et al. 2014), while panic disorder will be more aspect limited in its impact (D. P. Murphy 2008). A set of recent studies shows that disorders such as anorexia, schizophrenia, and autism can also involve changes in self-recognition and self-other differentiation, and that, in the case of anorexia, different body postures/positions may affect such recognition processes (Lavenne-Collot et al. 2022; 2023; Keromnes et al. 2018).

More generally, as Sass et al. (2017, 12) suggest, in regard to characterizing the elusive aspects of changes in psychopathology, "[M]utations of worldly experience (like mutations of ipseity or basic self-experience) typically have an overall or holistic character that defies ready operationalization into distinct features or

---

[5] In the therapeutic context, narratives not only help therapists to understand patients' experiences, but can also operate as a therapeutic tool that allows patients to incorporate any new awareness or life adjustment into a continuing narrative (see, e.g., Daly & Gallagher (2019); Hutto & Gallagher 2017; Neimeyer 2004; 2016).

factors." Sass's "bio-pheno-social" model attempts to capture the multifactorial complexity of such disturbances. Thus, "alterations at the level of the lived-body [have] profound implications for both interpersonal and intersubjective dimensions of existence," and in schizophrenia, "environmental/social stressors, including childhood trauma and abuse, social defeat, and cultural dislocation/ alienation" may play some pathogenetic role (Sass et al. 2018, 722; see Van Duppen 2017 for a comprehensive review of the phenomenological literature on this point).

One problem that Sass and his colleagues consider is the problem of overlapping symptoms or pathological functions. Some comparative studies (between schizophrenia, depersonalization disorder and panic disorder) suggest a transdiagnostic overlap on some factors, as measured on the EASE.[6] To address this problem Sass et al. suggest a hierarchical ordering of levels where, for schizophrenia, for example, ipseity is the most basic (primary) factor versus other secondary factors and compensatory responses:

> All this supports a revised self-disorder model which recognizes that schizophrenic self-disorder may well incorporate defensive or other 'secondary' phenomena, some of which may involve forms of depersonalization and derealization that also occur *outside* the schizophrenia-spectrum. It suggests that the EASE items (at least many of them) are somewhat less specific to schizophrenia-spectrum conditions than is sometimes claimed.   (Sass et al. 2018, 723)

Secondary factors may also include active reflective attitudes (e.g., motivating feelings of ambiguity toward the illness or toward accepted norms [see Dings & de Bruin 2022]) which "may, in turn, have implications for the nature and course of the illness itself." Although secondary, "these processes might nevertheless be equally *necessary* for development of a characteristically *schizophrenic* form of illness" (Sass et al. 2018, 724).

The notion of self-pattern, however, provides a slightly different framework where symptom overlap is not necessarily a problem. To see this, consider the overlap of pathological functioning in schizophrenia and autism. Vass, Csukly, and Farkas (2022) argue that there is an overlap specifically in anomalous minimal self-experience, as well as in social difficulties, cognitive deficits, and perceptual anomalies. In agreement with Sass and Parnas (2003) and Raballo (2012), they suggest that "[B]oth disorders can be understood as a disorder of self-organisation...[representing] a pathological transformation that takes place at a deeper level than what is commonly captured by diagnostic symptom dimensions"—that is, a transformation of the minimal self. Moreover, it is this "core

---

[6] The Examination of Anomalous Self-Experience (EASE) is a semi-structured, phenomenologically oriented interview focused on disturbances of ipseity or minimal self-awareness (Parnas et al. 2005).

underlying factor" that leads to a variety of "surface-level symptoms," or what Sass calls "secondary" symptoms, such as perceptual anomalies, social deficits, or psychotic symptoms. If this overlap appears to be a problem of diagnosis, one reason may be that Vass, Csukly, and Farkas have adopted a simplified conception of the self—based on the distinction between minimal and narrative self (Gallagher 2000a)—which only captures two aspects of the self-pattern. We can understand the "secondary" factors, however, as fitting into other processes of the self-pattern. When we consider both the broader pattern, and some of the details about particular factors and how they are related, then the overlap does not prove to be pervasive. Thus, for example, even if schizophrenia and autism seem to overlap in regard to social deficits, it turns out that the social deficits, as well as the phenomenology of anomalous body experiences (the sense of body ownership and sense of agency as aspects of minimal or prereflective self-awareness), are different in these two disorders. As Vass, Csukly, and Farkas (2022) point out, for example, the diametrically different anomalous bodily experiences in schizophrenia and ASD lead to differences in intersubjective experience—roughly, inability to distinguish self from other in schizophrenia; and, in contrast, the inability to relate to others in ASD. These differences map into the self-pattern differently. We can still say that both disorders are disorders of self-organization, involving social issues, but the greater detail provided by the wider concept of self-pattern allows for differentiation.

In this regard, differences (that still may involve some overlap) indicate evidence for shifts or differences in dynamical integration. Rather than positing a hierarchical relation that treats ipseity (prereflective self-awareness) as more basic, and then working outward or upward to more secondary factors, the pattern theory posits a dynamical gestalt. This is still consistent with the bio-*pheno*-social model proviso mentioned above, that disorders "typically have an overall or holistic character that defies ready operationalization into distinct features or factors," specifically because of the strong dynamical relations among processes in the self-pattern. For a particular disorder, the focus would be on the pattern as a whole rather than focusing on specific symptoms that overlap with other illnesses. The supposition here is that there will never be a complete overlap of the more holistic patterns.

Perhaps the alternative worry then would be, as Parnas and Henriksen (2014) express it, that "[t]his gestalt is intrinsically elusive and resists any simple, straightforward attempt to define it." The threefold method, introduced in Chapter 3, relying on concepts of meshed architecture, interventionist causal analysis and dynamical correlation, offers a way to address this worry. The gestalt might, just in the case of schizophrenia, organize itself in precisely the hierarchical fashion described by the bio-*pheno*-social model, or possibly in some non-hierarchical pattern depending on individual differences. And in other pathologies it may organize itself differently with different primary versus secondary arrangements, or perhaps in an arrangement that is not easily characterized in terms of primary and secondary factors.

The suggestion that all psychopathologies involve self-disturbances does not limit the self to ipseity or minimal, prereflective self-awareness, but refers to the self-pattern as a whole. It's to be expected that, even in the case of a primary disturbance of ipseity, this would implicate changes in bodily, behavioral, affective, intersubjective, cognitive, reflective, and/or narrative processes—to some varying degree.

Consider, for example, the complex symptomatology of depersonalization/derealization disorder (DPD), as indicated by the Cambridge Depersonalization Scale (Sierra & Berrios 2000). Although no one symptom is present in every case (Simeon et al. 2008), patients experience one or more of the following symptoms:

1. Ipseity disturbance or self-alienation: patients report feeling detached from themselves, or that the self is missing or unreal.
2. Bodily disturbances: patients report disturbed bodily experiences—a lack of body ownership, a lack of felt existence, disembodiment, abnormal body image (macro- or microsomatognosia).
3. Problems with affectivity: Patients complain that they do not feel emotions, pains, or pleasures.
4. Problems with agency: actions are experienced as automatic and mechanical; patients feel like mere observers of their actions.
5. Problems with cognition: Attention deficits, problems with imagery, abnormal thought experiences. Patients describe experiences of their thoughts having "a life of their own" (Sierra & Berrios 2000, 163); or they feel they have no thoughts. Likewise, they experience impairments in short-term memory, and alienation from their episodic memories.
6. Ecological problems: patients report changes in the way they experience the world—without color, lifeless; objects do not seem real; patients feel separated from the world; objects are experienced as unfamiliar, smaller, flatter, or more spatially distant than usual.
7. Problems with intersubjectivity: familiar people are experienced as unfamiliar; experiences of jamais-vu, or déjà-vu, with respect to persons or places.

These symptoms all involve factors or processes contributing to the constitution of the self-pattern. Mapping the dynamical relations among them, in some cases, requires tracing the trajectory of what Kraepelin (1893) called the natural course of the illness (natürliche Krankheitsvorgänge). Seeing how such aspects of the pattern undergo typical changes, comparatively in different disorders, can help to reveal the particular dynamical relations in the self-pattern.

Here again, looking specifically at the narrative aspect can help. We can learn about pathological changes or transformations of self-patterns from what the patient reports, that is, from her own self-narrative, which may be developed in a phenomenological interview, or using an instrument like the EASE. For example, she may report (or her reports may reflect) the loss of a sense of agency, as in some schizophrenic symptoms, or in addiction, without losing other basic experiential elements that are part of a self-pattern. These are not uniform reports across different disorders. In the case of schizophrenic thought insertion, for example, the experience is of some other, external agent invading one's stream of thought, which may not be the case in DPD. In the case of obsessive compulsive disorder (OCD), the patient knows that she makes herself do what she does, but nonetheless cannot resist. In substance addiction there are instances where there is a conflict between first-order desires and second-order, reflective intentions, where the drug wins out in opposition to what the subject really wants. In some episodes of Bulimia the agent is in prospective control as she plans out and executes the binge, perhaps loses control in the middle of it, and then retrospectively feels that she was completely out of control (see Kendler 2008 for these examples). Differences in how the sense of agency works in these different disorders impinge differently on affective aspects of the self-pattern. Addiction and Bulimia may involve positive hedonic experiences at first, and regret later; but this is not the case in OCD where the subject experiences no pleasure in what she is doing, and is motivated by a type of dissatisfaction or sense of incompleteness.

In other disorders patients may exhibit loss of certain psychological and cognitive abilities, such as the ability to recall earlier events (as in amnesia or Alzheimer's disease [AD]). They, or their caregivers, may report these changes; or these changes may start to dramatically shape the patients' narratives. Along with this they may have undergone character or personality changes. In many cases pathological changes can interfere with the individual's autonomy and positive social engagement. Some other aspects of the self-pattern may persist, however. Patients with AD can still respond to bodily discomforts and environmental disturbances (Clare et al. 2008), and they continue to manifest a range of affective/emotional states, even in advanced stages of AD (Magai et al. 1996; Weiler et al. 2016). In still other cases some degree of self-identity and autonomy may continue to be supported by intersubjective relations and/or extended aspects in the subject's surroundings.

Mapping the changes across different aspects of the self-pattern should reveal a set of underlying dynamics that get disrupted or adjusted as one change impinges on the whole pattern. That is, if the pattern is in fact a dynamical gestalt, then we should expect to find not just isolated symptoms affecting one aspect alone, but readjustments (disruptions or compensatory adjustments) in some set of other aspects. One can see this in multiple factor theories of different disorders. If, for example, in schizophrenia, one's prereflective experience of the sense of agency is disrupted (due to some neurological malfunction), this can lead to complex delusions, which in turn can impinge on affect and social relations, as well as changes in the structure of the patient's narratives and self-concept (Berna et al. 2016; Gallagher 2003). For that reason a narrow approach to understanding delusions, for example, is inadequate. That is, understanding delusion simply as a form of false or fixed belief (as emphasized in multiple editions of the DSM) ignores the fact that a delusion may begin (and continue) as a disrupted experience (in some cases, a disruption of prereflective experiential processes) (Gold & Hohwy 2000; Mundale & Gallagher 2009) that reverberates across a number of self-pattern processes—including affect, behavior, cognition, social relations, and self-narrative, changing not just one's beliefs but also one's sense of reality and way of being-in-the-world (Feyaerts et al. 2021; Gallagher 2009a).

In the case of psychopathology, self-narratives may provide a forensic measure of such changes, a linguistic fingerprint, of different conditions (Gallagher & Cole 2011; also see Section 5.5). Junghaenel, Smyth, and Santner (2008) found a lower frequency of cognitive words (e.g., "cause," "know," "ought") in the narratives of psychiatric patients in general, signaling cognitive change. For patients with schizophrenia, negative emotion narratives tend to be less grammatically clear than positive ones, and positive emotion narratives are more likely to involve other people than negative narratives (Gruber & Kring 2008). It's also the case that schizophrenic patients who narrate emotionally loaded facts (versus neutral facts) show higher degree of dyslogia or wrong or novel words (Caixeta et al. 1999). In schizophrenia self-narratives are less coherent and elaborate than controls, suggesting problems connecting self-experience and memory (Berna et al. 2016; Raffard et al. 2010).[7] Building on a model derived from empirical studies of narrative identity (McLean et al. 2020), Cowan, Mittal, and McAdams (2021) found disruptions of narrative identity in schizophrenia, reflected in disjointed structure, an affective focus on suffering, problems with agency, and detached life stories involving disturbances in the metacognitive dimension of autobiographical reasoning, which would include a reflective, or what de Haan (2020) calls an existential dimension (see Figure 4.1).

Borderline personality disorder (BPD) also involves a disintegrated self-narrative, a form of "self-fragmentation" (Fuchs 2007, 381), where the person's experienced identity changes from one situation to another. Philipp Schmidt (2021) argues that this fragmentation or inconsistency leads to or reflects four kinds of "intertwined" instabilities in BPD. First, it interferes with one's ability to gain distance from the present moment or to reflect on past events or future possibilities, a "severe disturbance in reflective processes" that makes it difficult to keep an orderly perspective on the meaning of present experience (2021, 210). Second, affectivity becomes unstable, characterized by emotion dysregulation and the

---

[7] Lysaker and colleagues, looking at narrative, metacognition, and self-esteem, developed a helpful tool, the Scale to Assess Narrative Development (STAND), which can capture some of these changes. (Lysaker et al. 2002; 2005).

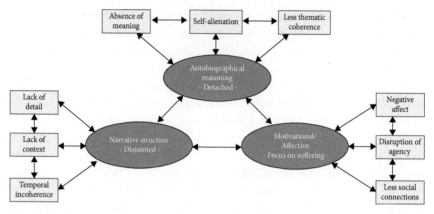

Figure 4.1 Structure of narrative identity in schizophrenia
Source: Based on McLean et al. (2020) and Cowan, Mittal, and McAdams (2021).

experience of intense emotions (anger and pain cycling to dysphoria and reactive apathy), coupled with a lack of "affective self-knowledge" (2021, 212ff.; also see Ratcliffe & Bortolan 2020). A third instability, intertwined with the first two, involves some complex modifications in intersubjective relations, where others are perceived as threats, and as possible targets of manipulation, with some blurring of self-other boundaries (Schmidt 2021, 218ff.).

> Those with BPD diagnoses tend to inhabit a world that is lacking in cohesive, practically meaningful structure, where that structure depends on habitually entrenched, integrated and fairly stable sets of concerns. Moreover, they struggle to relate to other people in ways that are essential to the sustenance of such concerns. So it would be misleading to conceive of emotion dysregulation as something that arises in isolation from one's wider relationship with the social world.
>
> (Ratcliffe & Bortolan 2020, 178)

Finally, BPD involves a diminishment of or alienation from bodily self-experience, which Schmidt suggests is a "concomitant condition of instability in [reflective] identity, affect and the interpersonal" (2021, 224). Reflecting dynamical and holistic relations among these various aspects of the self-pattern, Schmidt emphasizes that these instabilities are "structurally intertwined" and thus "far from being a mere accidental amalgamation of different forms of instabilities" (225).[8]

In depression, the patient may reveal thinking that reflects disorders in mood and affective processing as well as disrupted processes connected to the sense of agency and identity. Depressed patients can experience self-alterations, identity

---

[8] Likewise, Ratcliffe and Bortolan (2020, 180–1) describe an integrated set of effects inextricably linking affect with body, agentive projects, intersubjectivity, and norms, society, and culture.

changes, and they will attempt to integrate these changes into their life by trying to understand the reasons they're feeling this way. They may report feelings of helplessness, desperation, self-loathing, as well as the incapacity to work, to act, to think clearly (Solomon 2001; O'Brien 2004). In the case of major depressive disorder (MDD) patient narratives show that almost all factors in the self-pattern may be affected. In Table 4.1, those aspects listed in the second column are derived from the DSM-5 list of symptoms (ellipses indicate that no symptoms in that category are listed in the DSM-5). Those listed in the third column are from a variety of interviews, vignettes, and patient narratives collated from various sources.[9] Across a collection of such narratives, one finds alterations in what Matthew Ratcliffe (2008) calls existential feelings, mapped out across different components of the self-pattern, including bodily and experiential changes (Fuchs 2005; Fuchs & Schlimme 2009; Paskaleva 2011; Slaby & Stephan 2008). Narrative structures themselves, including temporal and syntactical structures, are sometimes reconfigured in depression. Pennebaker, Mehl, and Niederhoffer (2003) show that increased use of the first-person pronoun in self-narratives predicts both depression and mania. Stirman and Pennebaker (2001), in a study of artists who committed suicide compared to those who did not, found relatively higher frequencies of self-reference words (e.g., I, me, my) as compared to other-reference words (e.g., we, them, they). To define the dynamical connections among these various changes in affect, embodiment, experience, and narrative, one would have to track the etiology and temporal development of specific symptoms and/or that of recovery during treatment where some symptoms may respond quickly while others lag behind or may require different treatments.

One worry may be that the idea of a self-disorder does not differentiate psychopathology from somatic disorders since one could say that many somatic disorders—neurological disabilities, poisonings, drug use, and so forth—can also affect the self-pattern.[10] I think this is correct, but not a problem. Rather, the line between neurological and psychiatric disorders should be rightfully blurred since something that is (or starts) as purely somatic or neurological can lead to psychological and affective and intersubjective problems. I take this to be a virtue of the self-pattern idea—that one should consider all of these aspects when treating patients, because they are all part of who the patient is.

---

[9] Barton et al. (2008); Broome (2005); Flint & Kendler (2014); Wallace (1998); Fuchs (2005); Kelly (2017; 2018); Kirk et al. (2017); Manning (1994); O'Brien (2004); Opel et al. (2014); Radden (2009); Ratcliffe (2014); Solomon (2001); Stanghellini (2017); Stein (2012); Stirman & Pennebaker (2001); Styron (1990); Trigg (2016); Westerbeck & Mutsaers (2008); Wolpert (1999); Wurtzel (1995).

[10] My thanks to one reviewer for pushing me on this issue. Sometimes there are clear differentiations, and sometimes not. On the one hand, there is the idea, stressed in network theory (Borsboom & Cramer 2013), that one important difference may be that in somatic conditions there are identifiable underlying biological dysfunctions (e.g., a tumor), which is not the case with many mental disorders. On the other hand, there are somatic pathological conditions (idiopathic diseases) without clear underlying causes.

Table 4.1 Symptomatology for depression

Elements of self-pattern	DSM-5	Case reports/First-person interviews
Bodily processes	• Significant weight loss or gain, or decrease or increase in appetite nearly every day • Insomnia or hypersomnia	• Lack of appetite • Sleep disturbances • Sleepiness, but sleep is not refreshing
Prereflective experiential processes	• Experiences of fatigue or loss of energy nearly every day	• Fatigue • Feelings of heaviness of body, slow movement • Feeling disembodied or hyper-embodied • Feeling like an automaton—going through the motions [reduced sense of agency] • The world does not open up as a field of possible actions; the sense of "I can" is severely constrained
Affective processes	• Depressed mood most of the day, nearly every day, as indicated by either subjective report (e.g., feels sad, empty, hopeless) or observation made by others (e.g., appears tearful) • Markedly diminished interest or pleasure in all, or almost all, activities most of the day, nearly every day (as indicated by either subjective account or observation) • Feelings of worthlessness or excessive or inappropriate guilt (which may be delusional) nearly every day (not merely self-reproach or guilt about being sick)	• Loss of empathic resonance with others • Loneliness • Self-loathing or low self-esteem • Pervasive sense of dread • Unaccountable fears • Feeling that their experience is absolutely private and absolutely isolating • Despair • Sense of worthlessness or purposelessness • Feeling of being excluded, not understood, underappreciated • Self-alienation ("I would never belong to a club that would have someone like me as a member")
Behavioral / action-related processes	• Psychomotor agitation or retardation nearly every day (observable by others, not merely subjective feelings of restlessness or being slowed down)	• Inability to stop crying • Diminished physical self-care • Self-harm which reduces anxiety

Social / intersubjective processes	...	• Feeling like a burden for others, like a loser • Feeling excluded—feeling of not belonging, profound intersubjective alienation • Concern that others think they are malingerers • Mirror self—negative assessment • Feeling invisible • May have experienced childhood maltreatment
Cognitive / psychological / reflective processes	• Diminished ability to think or concentrate, or indecisiveness, nearly every day (either by subjective account or as observed by others) • Recurrent thoughts of death (not just fear of dying), recurrent suicidal ideation without a specific plan, or a suicide attempt or a specific plan for suicide	• Disordered attention • Excessive rumination • Toxic thought processes • As if "a thick mist in the mind" • Nihilism • Difficulty in imagining a different future • Sense of inevitability • Changed time perception: time experienced as passing very slowly. • The sense of no future opening up—but being swallowed by the present • Diminished reflective perspective on one's life • Difficulty breaking free of the present moment or of thinking about or planning for the future
Narrative processes	...	• Repeatedly re-scripting conversations that were deemed unsatisfactory • Predominance of use of first-person pronouns • Past narratives are couched in terms of loss, failure, and damage • Present narratives hold little or no interest • Future narratives have dried up
Ecological / situated / normative processes	...	• Loss of the sense of personal salience of things (lack of care for loss or damage) • Loss of sense of belonging • Diminished engagement, joy and pride

Source: Based on Daly and Gallagher (2019).

It may also be the case that some mental disorders (e.g., mild cognitive impairment) might not reach the point that we would call a self-disturbance. Hence my frequent mention of things being matters of degree, and changes "above a certain threshold." Even minor changes, however, may involve some degree of decreased coherence or increased rigidity in the pattern, or alterations along one or several processes. More generally, I think the notion of spectrum disorder fits well with the self-pattern idea. Accordingly, one can think of very mild cognitive impairments as still having an effect (but not an extensive effect) on the self-pattern.

4.5 Predictive Processing and Self-patterns

Dan Dennett (1991b, 36), citing Wilfred Sellars and William Wimsatt, notes that the pragmatic character of a pattern will be relative to scale. One should not expect, then, that self-patterns that manifest themselves in the clinic will correlate one-to-one with neural patterns found in the brain. Nonetheless, Tabb and Schaffner (2017, 354) maintain the importance of trying to identify theoretical overlaps in different types of patterns. For them, however, it is also clear that what's useful in the context of clinical diagnosis and treatment, or in the context of everyday being-in-the-world, may not be useful for the geneticist or the neuroscientist. They note that the use of genetic decomposition or cellular pathophysiology may easily result in a different set of taxonomic boundaries among patients than clinical classifiers. This may lead to distinct patterns "that stand in relations of significant tension… [although each may have] value under different perspectives" (2017, 354). Ideally, one would want to find theoretical overlap among diverse decompositions to define a robust psychiatric kind. Practically, however, self-patterns that may be disrupted in psychopathology and that are manifest in the clinical context are more useful in that context than the genetic or neuronal patterns that are more useful in laboratory research. The question is whether some kind of non-reductionist convergence is possible. In this section I'll suggest that a theoretical *détente* between predictive processing accounts focused on the brain (and usually framed in hierarchical terms), and enactive accounts that treat the system as brain-body-environment, may offer such a convergence.

Let me start by offering a caution. A family of computational-predictive models (predictive coding, predictive processing, active inference, and the free energy principle [FEP])[11] have generated a large number of proposals meant to explain

---

[11] Free energy is a measure of the dis-attunement between agent and environment (Bruineberg & Rietveld 2014). The free energy principle is part of a unified brain theory that proposes to account for the diverse empirical data related to action, perception, and learning. Karl Friston explains: "The FEP says that any self-organizing system that is at equilibrium with its environment must minimize its free energy. The principle is essentially a mathematical formulation of how adaptive systems (that is, biological agents like animals and brains) resist a natural tendency to disorder" (2010, 127).

cognition in general, as well as psychiatric disorders, including schizophrenia, psychotic delusions, and depression. Quite often the proposals are concerned with integrating brain processes with biopsychosocial models (e.g., Constant et al. 2022); quite often the analyses involve some conception of the self (e.g., Möller et al. 2021); and quite often they frame the analyses as being in close relation to embodied-enactive approaches. This makes for a great deal of complexity and disagreement, since not only are there a multitude of moving parts (different predictive models, different disorders, different conceptions of the self, different versions of enactivism) but a significant amount of philosophical and technical disagreement about many of these issues, including whether predictive models and enactivism can be friends, given different views about computation, information, representation, and so forth.[12] My aim here is not to settle any of these issues, but to negotiate them pragmatically, while noting the disagreements. Thus, for example, I think that the ongoing debate between predictive models and enactive approaches is not yet ready to be decided, and that theorists on both sides can benefit from continued communication.

To be clear, this section is meant to acknowledge that cognitive neuroscience offers important analyses that can align with and illuminate the wider integration of bodily, affective, social, cultural, and normative factors of the self-pattern and their disruptions in psychopathologial cases.

Studies of depression, for example, suggest that in the depressed subject, abnormal dynamical synchronies exist between the various factors of first–person perspective, bodily/emotional agency, and reflective (narrative-related) agency, as measured by dynamical connections across correlated brain areas (Fingelkurts & Fingelkurts 2017), as well as desynchronization between organism and environment, and individual and society (Fuchs 2001; Lenzo & Gallagher 2021). Patients with MDD

> have abnormal self-related [neural] processing, mostly expressed as increased
> self-focus, excessive self-reflection (rumination) and association of the self with
> negative emotions.... Generally, excessive ruminative self-focus produces such

---

[12] There is ongoing debate about whether the FEP can be seen as consistent with enactivist approaches to cognition and the notion of an autonomous system which produces and sustains its own identity (Thompson & Stapleton 2009, 25). One question is how the FEP relates to the concept of autopoiesis as found in enactivist accounts, and there are significantly different views in play (see Bitbol & Gallagher 2018; Bruineberg, Kiverstein & Rietveld 2016; Clark 2017; Constant, Clark & Friston 2021; Di Paolo, Thompson & Beer 2022; Gallagher & Allen 2018). Some of the issues are highly technical and concern a contrast between the non-equilibrium steady-state features of FEP systems, and the historicity of (the importance of the system's history for) the enactive system (Di Paolo, Thompson & Beer 2022). This entails different conceptions of brain dynamics (hierarchical comparators in PP, versus, for enactive views, dynamical "history-dependence even in the most basic neuroscientific scenario of stimulus processing"). This point has implications for understanding development, plasticity, skill acquisition, and habit formation. Generally speaking, enactivists discount notions of hierarchical processing, and distinctions between top-down and bottom-up, or internal *versus* external, in favor of more gestalt-like relations (Gallagher 2017a; 2023).

feelings as worry, guilt, shame, jealousy, which may lead to insomnia...increased anxiety....Patients with depression showed a higher degree of interoceptive awareness [...and] distorted body self-image.

(Fingelkurts & Fingelkurts 2017, 30)

Drawing on the concept of self-pattern, these researchers suggest that such aspects of selfhood "are not entities that simply modify something that has its own independent existence, but rather together form a dynamic pattern, that as a whole constitutes a complex selfhood" (35). The hypothesis that the dynamical relations among these self-related processes may be reflected in dynamical neural connections offers another way to open such relations to investigation.[13]

This hypothesis has been defended within the framework of predictive processing (PP) and the free energy principle (FEP) by a number of researchers. Limanowski and Blankenburg (2013), for example, argue that the minimal (prereflective) experiential aspects of the bodily self, including the first-person perspective, interoception, and the senses of agency and ownership or mineness, all of which depend on multisensory integration, can be "mapped onto a hier-archical generative model furnished by the FEP and may constitute the basis for higher-level, cognitive forms of self-referral" (1; also see Fotopoulou 2012). Beyond minimal experiential aspects of the self, multisensory integration on the PP model can also explicate connections to affective factors (Seth 2013), and inform self-recognition tasks, which typically involve recognition of the self-as-object, as in, for example, mirror self-recognition (Apps & Tsakiris 2014). As Apps and Tzakiris point out, this approach can explain how self-specific neural processing may arise in any multisensory processing, without positing specialized circuits or parts of the brain that are self-specific (important for avoiding the problems outlined in Section 4.1). Indeed, PP accounts suggest that although self-recognition may involve the specific congruency of predictions driven by efference (motor) processes and incoming sensory input (e.g., Brown et al. 2013; Frith 1992; Friston et al. 2010), the FEP framework "provides flexibility, with fewer constraints on what types of information can drive self-recognition" (Apps & Tsakiris 2014, 8). In this respect, the claim is that predictive models provide the resources to explain all of the various factors that contribute to the self-pattern. As Apps and Tsakiris, focusing just on the complex integration involved in the sense of body-ownership, note: "This is particularly important, given the evidence to suggest that the continuity of the self may be underpinned by many different types of informa-tion, the integration of which leads to a coherent sense of one's body" (2014, 9).[14]

---

[13] A fuller account of the relations that exist between neuronal processes and aspects of the self-pattern would return us to the different time scales involved and their non-linear dynamical relations (see Section 2.5).

[14] This may be one way to address a worry raised by Beni (2016, 3731), namely that it can be partic-ularly difficult to account for the relation of the very different kinds of aspects of the self-pattern, across different dimensions, since "the dynamically constituted self-pattern is not woven around a

Predictive models conceive of a system such as the brain or the organism as perceiving or coping with the world by predicting what it will encounter, and then minimizing prediction errors generated in the processing of sensory input. The uncertainty of experience is measured in terms of the quantity of prediction errors (equivalent to free energy) in the system. The system reduces free energy (minimizes prediction errors, minimizes the dis-attunement between organism and environment) either by revising its predictions ("perceptual inference") or by taking action to change its environment to match its predictions ("active inference"), or both. Although internalist descriptions of PP conceive of the brain as hypothesizing a "hierarchical generative model" of the world (Hohwy 2013), other, more enactive descriptions emphasize active, embodied engagement (active inference) with the aim of maintaining organism–environment attunement.

In general, as Apps and Tsakiris suggest, "the notion that there is a 'self' is the most parsimonious and accurate explanation for sensory inputs. In mathematical terms, this parsimonious accuracy is exactly the quantity that is optimised when minimising free energy or prediction error" (2014, 7). Accordingly, it makes sense to look at various PP accounts of the different processes that make up the self-pattern. Although the primary focus of such analysis may be (or may start) with the brain, it's possible to outline a more enactivist version that takes the system to be brain-body-environment (see, e.g., Miller & Clark 2017). Thus, we can find PP accounts of the prereflective experiential elements of the self-pattern using a model that "successfully predict[s] or match[es] the sensory consequences of our own movement, our intentions in action, and our sensory input" (Limanowski & Blankenburg 2013, 3, citing Hohwy). The embodied system predicts and integrates both exteroceptive and interoceptive multisensory variations in a probabilistic way as we perceive and move and experience ourselves moving. The integrated sensory experience is not *about* the self (as if the self were an intentional object); it's about the world and at the same time (in an ecological fashion) it registers bodily states and self-movement. This cross-modal, self-correcting interoceptive, proprioceptive, efferent/afferent, and exteroceptive integration generates prereflective self-experience manifested phenomenologically in a body-centered spatial frame of reference:

Following this logic, higher-level multisensory areas must predict input in multiple sensory modalities, which according to Apps and Tsakiris [2014] implies 'a high level representation [or model] (of self) that elaborates descending predictions to multiple unimodal systems'.   (Limanowski & Blankenburg 2013, 3)

---

central self that has its own independent existence." This implies that one acknowledges the diversity of elements that enter into the self-pattern, and at the same time allows for the possibility that for any individual some degree of integration will be reflected in neurobiological processes and in processes that characterize organism–environment coupling. More generally, a process ontology, where different factors are just different types of processes running on different time scales, can provide a way to conceive of integration.

As Apps and Tsakiris (2014) and Limanowski and Blankenburg (2013) agree, this system is dynamic and plastic so that basic factors such as the experience of self-location (location of one's body) and the sense of ownership can be manipulated through experimental variances in stimulation, as in the rubber hand illusion (RHI) or whole-body displacement (Blanke 2012; Botvinick & Cohen 1998; Lenggenhager et al. 2007). In the RHI, for example, the subject experiences a rubber hand as incorporated into his own body. Experiential aspects of the self-pattern result from the self-specifying integration of (1) sensory input (e.g., the combination of visual and tactile input in the case of the RHI—the tactile stimulation of the subject's real but hidden hand, plus the visual of the rubber hand undergoing simultaneous tactile stimulation) and (2) priors (e.g., the habitual predictions associated with the subject's body image), which drive the illusion of ownership of the rubber body part. The illusory model (which generates the experience of the felt touch and the observed touch as at the same location) "is selected [by the brain] because it more successfully explains the incoming prediction error in favor of a unified self" (Limanowski & Blankenburg 2013).[15] This model minimizes prediction error (free energy); it can be further refined toward a more veridical model by active inference, that is, by moving my hand. Getting a veridical model of my body and its relation to the environment, or something close to a veridical model (reducing free energy in the system), is important for survival; the self exists "iff (sic) [*sic*] I am a veridical model of my environment" (Limanowski & Blankenburg 2013, 4, quoting Friston 2011).

This last thought, that the organism (the bodily self), rather than "having" a model, *is* itself the model of the environment, is, as I understand it, Friston's way of emphasizing the strong connectivity between organism and environment. In this respect, who we are, even in a very basic embodied way, is shaped by the environment, our interactions with, and our actions in the environment. In terms of the self-pattern, this suggests a dynamical integration between the embodied and experiential aspects of the self-pattern and the ecological and normative aspects (understanding the environment to be social/cultural as well as physical).[16] Evidence for the close connection (which could be modeled as a dynamical causality) between bodily (interoceptive) processes and prereflective experiential processes can also be found in (1) the fact that during the rubber hand illusion the temperature of one's real hand drops as the sense of ownership shifts to the rubber hand (Moseley et al. 2008). This is "interpreted as evidence for top-down

---

[15] For some reservations about internalist PP accounts of perceptual illusions, and why more embodied accounts are important, see Gallagher, Hutto, and Hipólito (2022).

[16] Apps and Tsakiris (2014) note the influence of culturally shaped priors on predictive processing. "There is also evidence of more long-term contextual influences on self-recognition related priors, highlighted by the role that cultural and societal effects have on self-other decision-making. For instance, self-other face recognition has been shown to be different across cultures" (14). Also see Jarvis and Kirmayer (2021) and Constant et al. (2022) for the psychiatric context.

regulations of autonomic control and interoceptive prediction error minimization during the RHI" (Limanowski & Blankenburg 2013, 4). And (2) the idea that self-awareness emerges "from interaction of interoceptive predictions and prediction errors" (Limanowski & Blankenburg 2013, 5, citing Critchley & Seth 2012). Furthermore, Seth (2013) and colleagues (Seth, Suzuki and Critchley 2011; Suzuki et al. 2013) suggest that interoceptive (e.g., autonomic) and efferent or motor control signals give rise to "emotional feeling states." In turn, as Deane, Miller, and Wilkinson (2020) propose, such affective states perform a scorekeeping function that keeps track of one's own adaptive behaviors: "we quite literally feel how well adapted we are to a situation, and those feelings move us [as a form of active inference] in ways that are intended to improve that fit. This has the consequence that our sense of being a self [especially our bodily processes] and affect are mechanistically intertwined." Or in other terms, in this model, bodily processes (not just brain processes), prereflective experience, affect, and ecological aspects are all dynamically intertwined.

Limanowski and Blankenburg (2013) provide further analysis from this perspective to explain how the sense of agency and sense of mineness emerge as part of the experiential aspect of the self-pattern, and how predictive processing also helps to explicate intersubjective self-other relations (see Chapter 6). Here, then, we would find ways to connect embodied, experiential, affective, and intersubjective aspects of the self-pattern. The point I want to highlight here is that PP approaches to understanding various system functions (including the brain in its relation to body and environment) potentially allow for the mapping of dynamical relations among many of the factors and processes of the self-pattern in a way that is reflected in neural processes, although not necessarily in an isomorphic way.

PP suggests that these dynamical relations are *hierarchically* arranged. This would be one way, but not the only way, however, to understand how embodied, experiential, and affective processes of the self-pattern relate to more complex (cognitive, reflective, intersubjective, and narrative) processes. On a more embodied-enactive approach, we may want to give up the hierarchical (bottom-up, top-down) vocabulary (as I suggested in Chapter 2). Thinking of the self-pattern in terms of a gestalt formation, instead of hierarchical organization, would emphasize the reciprocal or dynamical loops that exist within the brain, and between brain, body, and environment. For example, as Miller and Clark (2018, 2563) point out, focusing on reciprocal connections between brain areas that include sub-cortical, body-related areas, "the basal ganglia is connected to the cortex by at least five separate circuits, some of which form closed loops with cortex via the thalamus. This allows information flowing from cortical areas to basal ganglia to return again to the same cortical area." Parvizi describes this as a rich looping relationship which means that "in reality, there is no cortex versus basal ganglia divide. One does not exist without the other, and there is only an inter-linked network of corticostriatal loops" (Parvizi 2009, 356). We find similar reciprocal links in hypothalamus and brainstem connections with cortex (Arnsten & Li 2005). But the very same thing can be said of the intertwinement of brain and body. Indeed, the neural connections suggest a rich reciprocal attunement, an "entanglement" between cortex and body (Miller & Clark 2018; Lewis & Todd 2007), that includes both affective and motor aspects. This entanglement even extends to the immune system, disturbances of which, as Bhat et al. (2021) point out, are implicated in a number of psychopathologies. They propose a model, based on active inference and FEP, that integrates the immune system with other bodily and self-related processes, such that if one set of processes is faced with a threat, other processes within the larger brain-body system, are primed to respond. Accordingly, they suggest that immune insults, even early in life, may be linked to psychiatric disorders decades later (citing the work of Guma, Plitman & Chakravarty 2019).

Predictive processing accounts also suggest explanations of the failures of self-related experience found in psychopathologies. Seth (2013), for example, reviews research on PP deficits in psychiatric disorders affecting self-experience. Comparator models of disturbances in selfhood, or the sense of agency, for example, in schizophrenic delusions of control (Frith 1992; 2011; Frith & Gallagher 2002; Gallagher 2000a; 2004a), foreshadow such predictive models of explanation. On predictive models, delusions and hallucinations may arise from the dominance of priors generating predictions that suppress anomalous extero-ceptive prediction errors (Corlett 2018; Fletcher & Frith 2009; Sterzer et al. 2018). "This view has been finessed in terms of abnormal encoding of the relative preci-sion of priors and sensory evidence to account for a broad range of psychotic symptoms" (Seth 2013, 571). Seth thus proposes PP explanations (especially involving interoceptive processing related to selfhood) for alexithymia, psychosis and anxiety, disorders of body image and body ownership, depersonalization and derealization (also see Ciaunica et al. 2021; Gerrans 2020; Paulus, Feinstein & Khalsa 2019). Others have proposed PP accounts of PTSD (Linson & Friston 2019), depression (Barrett, Quigley & Hamilton 2016; Fabry 2020; Seth & Friston 2016), psychosis (Sterzer et al. 2018), and OCD (Downey 2020).

4.6 Conclusion

In response to skepticism about how the elements of a self-pattern are dynamically related to each other, such that they constitute a relatively coherent, if not strictly unified pattern, I have suggested three ways in which we can discover or investigate such dynamical relations. First, a self-pattern is reflectively reiterated in its narrative component. Various processes and dynamical relations of the self-pattern are reflected in self-narratives in a way that helps us make sense of these relations. Second, they are revealed in the way that they break down in pathologies. The empirical and clinical exploration of psychiatric or neurological disorders can contribute to an understanding of the precise nature of the dynamical relations, and how they can fail. Third, neuroscientific studies, framed in predictive models and linked enactively to other processes of the self-pattern, can help explicate the dynamical relations among those processes that bridge brain, body, and environment.

These three approaches are clearly complementary and speak of integration. Neuroscientific predictive models constantly make reference to organism and environment, indicating processing that goes beyond just the brain; this view can be enhanced by explications of embodied cognition, phenomenology, and psychopathology. Studies of psychopathology are enlightened not only by neuroscience, but also by clinical work and the analysis of patients' self-narratives. The analysis of such narratives can deepen our understanding of the dynamical relations among different first- and second-person aspects of the self-pattern and reveal the complexities that characterize human existence. It should be clear from reviewing some of the evidence in support of these suggestions that explicating the dynamical relations that constitute a self-pattern is a complex task that requires an interdisciplinary approach, and a method, like the one outlined in Chapter 3, that can cut across different types of analysis.

The aim of these chapters is not just to introduce the notion of a self-pattern, or to clarify its dynamical nature, but to show how it can be productively relevant to understanding psychopathology. The pattern theory allows us to think in a holistic fashion about a plurality of factors—addressing the integration problem, extending analysis to include processes and their dynamical intertwinement in ways that go beyond even the biopsychosocial model. While much of this requires navigating through a number of philosophical and theoretical issues, such analyses have implications for clinical/therapeutic work. The following chapters will continue to explore both the theoretical implications and the practical applications of this framework.

5

Disorder, Dissociation, and Disruption in Self-narrative

Self-narrative, as indicated in Chapter 4, tracks a number of the features or processes in the self-pattern. To get a fuller sense of what narrative encompasses, however, we can pursue the idea that the concept of self-narrative addresses what Paul Ricoeur calls the issue of *ipse* identity, or what Marya Schechtman calls the characterization question. This will provide some insight into how to think about coherence, and its disruption, in the self-pattern.

5.1 Varieties of Identity

We return here to some of the philosophical considerations about identity discussed in Section 1.3, and at the end of Chapter 2. Recall that Ricoeur (1992, 116) makes the distinction between *idem* identity (that which remains the same, persisting across time) and *ipse* identity (that which makes me who I am in relation to another, even as I change over time). These are two different problematics addressing two different questions. As Marya Schechtman (1996) puts it, this is the distinction between the issue of reidentification—what makes a person the same from one time to another?—and the issue of characterization—what makes a person the person she is? Given these questions about identity, how does the notion of a self-pattern answer them. With respect to issues concerning psychopathology, we are especially interested in the question about *ipse* identity, i.e., the issue of characterization.

Schechtman (1996, 67) makes a good case for bodily continuity as the criterion of reidentification, and although this continues to be controversial, I think it's the correct way to think about this question, assuming that the concept of bodily continuity, which clearly involves physical continuity, is not reducible to physical continuity. Rather, we should think of it in terms of the continuity of a unique living body, understood as a bodily existence which fits with one's agentive engagement in the world. This concept operates as the principle of *idem* individuation, a kind of ontological anchor that allows us to say this is the same person from one time or context to another, even when some other aspects of the self-pattern change. The idea may require a more nuanced analysis since bodily

The Self and its Disorders. Shaun Gallagher, Oxford University Press. © Shaun Gallagher 2024.
DOI: 10.1093/oso/9780198873068.003.0006

existence also changes, even as it maintains continuity over time; but for our purposes we need not enter any further into questions about *idem* identity.[1]

To answer the characterization question of *ipse* identity, both Ricoeur and Schechtman point to narrative. I think that this answer gets confounded in reference to a third question which we can call the "self-constitution question." Schechtman clearly distinguishes between the reidentification question and the characterization question, and these questions are answered, respectively, in terms of bodily continuity and narrative. In her discussion of narrative characterization, however, Schechtman drifts into a discussion of the following question: What is it that constitutes a person or self? The shift between these two questions takes place as one turns page 93 of her book, *The Constitution of Selves* (1996). On this page she clearly takes narrative to be addressing the characterization question: What is it that makes a person who he is, even as he changes over time? This is a question about a person's character and identity, and Schechtman's view is that "a person creates his identity by forming an autobiographical narrative—a story of his life" (93). She relates this directly to four concepts that are the concern of personal identity discussions: survival, moral responsibility, self-interested concern, and compensation. Once we turn to page 94, however, she starts to answer a different question—the self-constitution question: What is it that makes some entity a person? Her answer, once more, is narrative. Indeed, she calls her position the "narrative self-constitution view." "At the core of [the self-constitution] view is the assertion that individuals constitute themselves as persons by coming to think of themselves as persisting subjects who have had experience in the past and will continue to have experience in the future, taking certain experiences as theirs" (94). Here, then, are the three questions that Schechtman distinguishes:

(1) *Idem*/reidentification: what makes someone the same person over time?
(2) *Ipse*/characterization: what is it that makes a person who she is, even as she changes over time?
(3) Self-constitution: what makes an individual a person (rather than a non-person)?

Schechtman thinks that the answer to the first question is the body, and that narrative is the answer to the second and third questions. Her answer to the third question, that narrative is definitive of personhood, however, leads to some contentious problems about claims such as "to be a *person* at all one must construct a narrative [in the form of a conventional linear story]" (99), and to a later debate with Galen Strawson (2004) who argues against this sort of view. We can

---

[1] See Halsema (2011, 119–20) for a good discussion of this issue.

circumvent such contentious debates, however, simply by giving a different answer to question (3): namely, a person is constituted by a self-pattern. That answer does not require that every person have a strong self-narrative. Indeed, a particular person may lack narrative capacity, as sometimes happens in disorders involving dysnarrativa (Bruner 2002) or loss of episodic memory (Damasio 1999). We would not say, in such a condition, however, that this individual is not a person, since a significant part of the self-pattern still remains in place. What we can say in regard to the self-constitution question is that narrative may contribute to the constitution of the self-pattern, but is not a necessary condition. More generally, persons are more than just their narratives.

To put this in more positive terms, I suggest that we conceive of the person, and specifically the agentive person, as the systemic whole enacted in the processes and dynamical connections of the self-pattern. As we have said, there is no pre-existing entity, agent, or self that operates as the organizer or driver of the self-pattern; rather, the agent develops as the embodied subject constituted by the self-pattern—an agent, typically and generally speaking, is capable of bodily actions, intersubjective interactions, social engagement, and cultural practices, a person who has affective/emotional experiences, and is capable of cognition, reflection, and narrative. In the self-pattern we can find bodily existence that can account for *idem* identity, as well as narrative capacities that account for *ipse* identity. But in each case, the agentive person is more than just a body or a narrative.

Let's consider further the second question, concerning *ipse* identity. Specifically, if narrative is the answer to this question, as both Ricoeur and Schechtman suggest, what does that tell us about narrative in the context of the self-pattern. Let me note that Ricoeur presents a nuanced view of the distinction (or dialectic) between *ipse* and *idem* questions about identity insofar as they can be seen to overlap with respect to the notion of temporality. The concept of character, as it pertains to personal identity, involves not just persistence over time, but also a kind of ipseic consistency over time.[2] Narrative, he suggests, operates as a kind of mediator between these overlapping aspects, and supports what he calls self-maintenance or self-constancy and the capacity to make a promise (1992, 118–19). In terms of the self-pattern, I think what's true about this is, as suggested in the previous chapter, narrative reflects all the other processes of the self-pattern (including bodily processes), not in a passive way but in a way that in some sense mediates across and loops into their dynamical relations. We should not read this as suggesting that narrative solves the reidentification question. If we pursued that line of thought a third more radical view could be established, one that would

---

[2] Ricoeur describes it as partaking "simultaneously of two orders, that of objectivity and that of existence" (1992, 119n4). Ricoeur, however, in the context of his discussion of personal identity moves away from this overly uniform and permanent characterization of character, turning toward a more Aristotelian notion of an acquired disposition or habit that is not unrelated to social and normative factors, which in turn may motivate us to "place a 'cause' above our own survival" (120).

put Ricoeur's position together with Schechtman's and have narrative doing all the work in answer to all three questions. I don't want to go that way. My focus will be to show how narrative works to answer the question about *ipse* identity by reflecting all other aspects of the self-pattern. The self is more than narrative even in regard to *ipse* identity, since narrative depends on a rich pattern of factors and processes.

5.2 How Narrative Connects

If self-narratives reflect, explicitly in content, or implicitly in form, all of the other processes of the self-pattern, then we should be able to trace the connections between narrative aspects and other elements in the self-pattern. To do this I'll bring together a number of considerations that get worked out in a variety of approaches to the concept of the narrative self. Even approaches that make narra-tive central to conceptions of self are unable to avoid pointing to the other factors beyond narrative that support the concept of a self-pattern.

As a first point of connection we should consider our corporeal anchoring in the world. This is reflected in narrative insofar as narrative is primarily about *action*, and action is something accomplished bodily. Ricoeur, in his analysis of narrative and personal identity, makes this clear. The linkage between body and world, between action and context, is part of what narrative reflects. It tracks that linkage in a way that bestows on action the status of genuine action (i.e., as more than mere movement or behavior)—action, especially as it is tied to a practice. Action is never just bodily movement or "basic action" (as defined in action theory); it's a complex embodied performance situated in circumstances that define its meaning (Gallagher 2020a). Precisely in this respect, the *intersubjective, ecological,* and *normative* features of the self-pattern are not isolated realms separated from embodied action. "Practices are based on actions in which an agent takes into account, as a matter of principle, the actions of others" (Ricoeur 1992, 155). Actions are often interactions that involve other agents. Moreover, anything that might count as an individual practice is always derived from the practices of others:

> In our experience the life history of each of us is caught up in the histories of others. Whole sections of my life are part of the life history of others—of my parents, my friends, my companions in work and in leisure. What we said above about practices and about the relations of apprenticeship, cooperation, and com-petition that they include confirms this entanglement of the history of each per-son in the histories of numerous others.   (1992, 161)

A practice, according to Ricoeur, may be a set of actions within a context that constitute a profession or a game—farming or chess playing are his examples.

With respect to chess, "shifting the position of a pawn on the chessboard is in itself simply a gesture, but taken in the context of the practice of the game of chess, this gesture has the meaning of a move in a chess game" (1992, 154). Something similar might be said of a chess piece, for example, the rook. That is, what makes a rook a rook are the rules of chess and the use to which it is put in the context of a game (Haugeland 1998). But in the case of a human agent it is more than norms and the ecological context of action that makes the action *my* action. It is also what we might call the internal relations among the elements of the self-pattern that make the action *my* action. This typically includes my ability to give a narrative account of that action.

Narrative competency is not simply the ability to comprehend and produce stories. It includes the reflective capacity to make reports on one's experiences and actions. It includes not just abilities for understanding narratives, but also capacities for narrative understandings, which allow us to frame our understanding of self and others in a narrative way, and thence to form/produce self-narratives and narratives about things, events, and other people. We can also distinguish between this narrative *framing*, as an implicit process or practice of seeing/understanding events in a narrative framework, and narrative *production*, which is the explicit construction of stories or narrative reports. When Jerome Bruner (1990) describes how we come to know our world and construct our representation of reality through the use of narrative, and when he suggests that "we organize our experience and our memory of human happenings mainly in the form of narrative – stories, excuses, myths, reasons for doing or not doing, and so on" (4)—he is describing narrative framing.

We make sense out of our own actions and the actions of others by placing them in a narrative framework. This is not a new theory of sense-making. It has its roots in hermeneutical traditions. Dilthey, for instance, recognized that it is not sufficient to focus on grasping the mental states of others in order to understand their actions:

> It is necessary to distinguish the state of mind which produced the action by which it is expressed from the circumstances of life by which it is conditioned.... [In some cases] action separates itself from the background of the context of life and, unless accompanied by an explanation of how circumstances, purposes, means and context of life are linked together in it, allows no comprehensive account of the inner life from which it arose.   (Dilthey 1988, 153)

Dilthey rightly emphasizes context. We can grasp the other's life, as well as our own, in its worldly/situational contexts, and that is best captured in a narrative form. Narrative recounts actions, and their reasons, as they figure against a larger history and set of projects. Ricoeur (1992) is close to the mark: I encounter the other person, not abstracted from their circumstances, but in the middle of something that has a beginning and that is going somewhere, and is part of a shared world. I see other people in the framework of a story about some action or practice in which either I have or do not have a part to play. I see their actions and my own actions, or possible actions, in what Bruner (1986) calls the "landscape of action," which is constituted by their embodied actions and the rich worldly contexts within which they act—contexts that operate as scaffolds for the meaning and significance of actions and expressive movements. The landscape of action relates directly to what Rietveld and Kiverstein (2014) call the "landscape of affordances," which includes my ecological possibilities for interacting with others.

Our experience of others transforms our self-experience (the experience of our own possible actions), and narrative has a role to play in this. It is not just that the form of narrative is appropriate for understanding the actions of others because, "we live out narratives in our lives and because we understand our own lives in terms of narratives that we live out" (McIntyre 1981, 212); rather, it begins by going the other way: because we frame our understanding of the actions of others in narratives that follow their action trajectories, the form of narrative is appropriate for reflectively understanding ourselves.

This starts when we are young children. Since we develop in social contexts and normally acquire the capacity for narrative in those contexts, then the development of self-narrative obviously involves others. Katherine Nelson (2003) points out that "with respect to the child's own experience, which is forecast and rehearsed with him or her by parents," competency for self-narrative starts to emerge in two-year-olds. Self-narrative requires building on our experiences of others and their narratives, so "children of 2–4 years often 'appropriate' someone else's story as their own" (Nelson 2003). In addition, carving out one's own character within a set of narratives requires a reflective awareness of having a point of view that is different from others. By the time infants are two or three years of age, and well practiced in understanding immediate environments and events as other people understand them, the acquisition of language, plus the capacity to recognize their own image in the mirror, feed a developing conceptual understanding of themselves that is essential to the onset of autobiographical memory.

> By 18–24 months of age infants have a concept of themselves that is sufficiently viable to serve as a referent around which personally experienced events can be organized in memory.... The self at 18–24 months of age achieves whatever "critical mass" is necessary to serve as an organizer and regulator of experience.... This achievement in self-awareness (recognition) is followed shortly by the onset of autobiographical memory.   (Howe 2000, 91–2)

Autobiographical memory is one aspect that shapes narrative competency—an ability to see things in a narrative framework. Along with a growing linguistic competency, a developing conceptual sense of self, and the interactions associated with pragmatically and socially contextualized secondary intersubjectivity, auto- biographical memory helps to kick-start narrative abilities during the second year of life. Two-year-olds may start this process by working more from a set of short behavioral scripts than from full-fledged narratives; initially their autobiograph- ical memories have to be elicited by questions and prompts (Howe 2000; Nelson 2003). From two to four years, children fine-tune their narrative abilities via fur- ther development of language ability, autobiographical memory, and a more stable self-concept.

When children listen to stories, or play-act (and the same continues in adult- hood when we are exposed to parables, plays, myths, novels, our favorite rap music, films, and other media) they become familiar with characters in a range of ordinary or extraordinary situations, and the sorts of actions appropriate to such characters, all of which helps to shape their normative expectations about others, about themselves, and about which actions are suited to particular situations but also which reasons for acting are acceptable and which are not (Gallagher & Hutto 2008; Guajardo & Watson 2002). Narratives help to build out our norma- tive understanding of what we can expect from others in certain situations, but also what others can expect from us, which in turn shapes our self-identity. Along the same line, narratives are part of the structure that shapes social and cultural institutions (Tollefsen & Gallagher 2017), as well as our folk psychological prac- tices (Hutto 2007) all of which, in turn, inform our intersubjective interactions. Through them we learn the norms associated with social roles that pervade our everyday world and our social practices, in homes, schools, playgrounds, shops, restaurants, and so on.

To summarize:

(1) Narrative is primarily about actions, which are often intersubjective inter- actions, and often involve social-cultural practices;
(2) Actions and interactions are embodied;
(3) Because our bodies are always in-the-world, our actions are always situated;
(4) Action-situations involve ecological, worldly processes, but especially other people and social practices constrained in a normative fashion;
(5) Narrative reflects such structures and allows us to frame our understand- ing of both our own actions and those of others in ways that recursively shape those actions and our own experiences;
(6) The development of narrative competency and self-narrative begins at a young age reflecting and contributing to the development of our linguistic and cognitive abilities, fostering the development of episodic- autobiographical memory and self-concept.

5.3 Narrative Identity: Fiction or Reality

Someone might object: this is all well and good, but this kind of narrative identity, this making of coherency, or some degree of coherency, in the self-pattern is still only a kind of construction; it has no real depth and may be a kind of fiction, as suggested by thinkers like Hume (1739) or Dennett (1991a). One response to this concerns the role of affect. If narrative hits on every aspect of the self-pattern— bodily, experiential, behavioral/action-related, intersubjective, psychological-cognitive, reflective, ecological, and normative, Schechtman (1996, 97) makes it clear that affect is also an important part of this mix of elements: "We expect a person's beliefs, desires, values, emotions, actions, and experiences to hang together in a way that makes what she says, does, and feels psychologically intelligible." Schechtman introduces the idea that affect is something like the glue that keeps these various elements meshed together, and she does this through her interpretation of John Locke's classic account of personal identity. In contrast to interpretations that emphasize the role of memory, that is, psychological continuity, as the basis for personal identity, Schechtman emphasizes that Locke

> stresses the *affective* side of consciousness. He paints a picture of consciousness as the faculty whereby we experience pleasure and pain, happiness, and misery. He tells us, for instance, that "*Self* is that conscious thinking thing…which is sensible, or conscious of Pleasure and Pain, capable of Happiness or Misery, and so is concern'd for it *self* as far as that consciousness extends," thus emphasizing the definition of identity in terms of sameness of consciousness precisely because it is in consciousness that we experience the affect that underlies self-interested concern, compensation, and justice of punishment.   (Schechtman 1996, 108–9)

Affectivity, part of what William James called the "warmth and intimacy" of bodily experience (together with interoception and proprioception), is what makes one's body one's own, providing for a sense of body-ownership. On the same basis of affectivity, we own our past and present actions. Affect, in this regard, operates as a glue that binds narrative identity to bodily existence and action. Schechtman makes it clear that affect does not always work in a conscious way. The affective associations connected with past actions condition our current actions, sometimes even if we do not have explicit memories of those past actions. More generally, Schechtman points out, the affective dimensions that are part of the way we have been raised, may contribute to our feelings of worthiness and self-esteem: "It is no great revelation that a person who feels loved and valued by a stable family in childhood is more likely to grow up feeling worthy, entitled, and secure than a person who is made to feel worthless and incompetent" (111). Importantly, this general orientation toward the world will affect a person's interactions with others, her choice of action, and her specific dispositions in various situations. All of this, in turn, is reflected in one's narrative, since these affective experiences

> give us a "script"—a sense of self, an idea of who we are and what kind of story we are living.... This, then, is how Locke's insight can be used to yield a helpful understanding of what is involved in having a narrative self-conception.... To have a narrative self-conception ... is thus to experience the events in one's life as interpreted through one's sense of one's own life story, and to feel the affect that follows upon doing so.   (Schechtman 1996, 111–12)

I interpret Ricoeur to be offering a similar conception of the relation between self-narrative and affect (a relation that makes self-narrative personal). Ricoeur makes it clear that there is an unusual causal relation between narrative and the events narrated, which involve "action dynamics" (Ricoeur 1992, 144). It's possible, he suggests, to give a causal, impersonal account of a series of events or actions. A narrative, on its own, does not necessarily add extra causal forces to the series of events. At the same time, however, a narrative can transform the meaning of an event; it can have an affective effect. Narrative provides extended context, and for that reason, the event narrated can take on a certain personal (and this means "affective") significance that it otherwise would not have. More specifically, "by entering into the movement of a narrative which relates a character to a plot, the event loses its impersonal neutrality. By the same token, the narrative status conferred upon the event averts the drift of the notion of event which would make it difficult, if not impossible, to take the agent into account in the description of the action" (142n1).

Ricoeur uses the example of the promise, but we can go back the example of regret (discussed in Chapter 4) to see the same dynamics, and the importance of affect. Regret involves a form of narratival self-knowledge in which I, as the narrator, can give an account, and evaluate my past action. Sometime in the past I made the wrong choice. Now I come to regret that choice, and this manifests itself in my self-narrative. Specifically, what gets reflected in my narrative are changes or adjustments in my self-pattern. Recall that Frith and Metzinger (2016) show how this works in regard to the minimal experiential aspects of the self-pattern, which include the sense of agency (which changes between the action and the regret) and the sense of ownership (which remains the same). They also point out that the regret can take over my self-narrative. Despite the change in the sense of agency, my self-narrative connects my action and my subsequent emotion, which means that I am the same person who acted in the past, and who continues to be responsible for my actions.

It's at this point that Frith and Metzinger suggest that this is a fictional unity: "a transtemporal, fictional 'self' constituted by the narrative" (Frith & Metzinger

2016, 203n6). Again, however, I think that one should say that this is a very real unity or coherence because the action and the affective states—the pain and the regret—are real, as they have real effects on my self-narrative and self-pattern, which in turn may influence my present and future behavior, or have an effect on my intention formation and future choice of action, which then again will be reflected in my ongoing self-narrative. My action, my regret, my pain, mediated in my narrative practice, are here making a loop through normative factors that ultimately feeds back to influence my behavior.[3] Narrative traces the threads of the very real processes of the self-pattern that are already woven together— actions, affective feelings, cognitive processes that are embedded in social and cultural practices.

Self-narrative plays a double role in the self-pattern. It is not only reflective of the other processes of the self-pattern, it is itself an active component of the self-pattern. In other words, narrative is not a one-way disinterested reflective format-ting of the self-pattern (as if operating as an external observer). If it is affected by and shaped by all those other factors, and affected when those other processes become discordant, narrative practices can also contribute to reshaping those processes and their dynamical connections. This is why narrative therapy can work.

Ricoeur understands the "emplotment" or plot process involved in narrative identity "in dynamic terms [as] the competition between a demand for concordance and the admission of discordances which, up to the close of the story, threaten this identity" (1992, 141). Concordance, for Ricoeur, is a "principle of order (141) that effects a 'synthesis of heterogeneity'; an 'unstable structure of discordant concordance'" (142). In this respect narrative has the resources to deal with just the kinds of dynamics involved in dynamic patterns. One can think here of Scott Kelso's analysis where dynamic patterns involve a dialectic of coherence/dissipation. The self-pattern is necessarily heterogeneous, and emerges from heterogeneity, since it integrates very diverse phenomena. The integration, however, brings some kind of coherence.

One question is how heterogeneous elements can be coherently integrated in a form of *ipse* identity, and the answer is, as Ricoeur proposes, via narrative:

By this I am attempting to account for the diverse mediations performed by the plot: between the manifold of events and the temporal unity of the story

---

[3] The looping is not only complex, as Varga (2015, 71) points out, but pervasive throughout our lives. Normative factors, closely tied to culturally defined familial practices shape our lives very early and are made more complex by other institutions. As Gadamer put it: "Long before we understand ourselves through the process of self-examination, we understand ourselves in a self-evident way in the family, society, and state in which we live....The self-awareness of the individual is only a flickering in the closed circuits of historical life" (Gadamer 2004, p. 278). Narrative, perhaps, allows for a more elongated self-awareness.

recounted; between the disparate components of the action—intentions, causes, and chance occurrences—and the sequence of the story.   (1992, 141)

In a self-narrative "the character preserves throughout the story an identity correlative to that of the story itself" (143). If the self is, in effect, a self-pattern, it can be more or less discordant, especially since a self-narrative is not just about a character *simpliciter*; the character is connected to his actions, which are always contextualized, along with the various processes that contribute to the self-pattern. Through narrative, the character is situated in a set of "action dynamics" (Ricoeur 1992, 144). Furthermore, part of the context involves others who are not just action observers, but interactors and evaluators; this introduces a normative structure in which agents are "raised to the rank of persons [with a moral status] and of [responsible] initiators of action" (145).

If narrative plays a constitutive role in self-identity, it does so only to the extent that it contributes to a self-pattern, which is always something more than a character in a narrative. Even if narrative reflects a degree of cohesiveness in the self-pattern, and contributes to the *ipse* identity of the person, the "narrative unity of life" (MacIntyre) is never the totality of a life. Our narrative is always incomplete, and not always as unified as we might think. Ricoeur calls it the "narrative incompleteness of life" due, in part, to our entanglement with others' life histories (1992, 161), and to the extent that one is never the sole narrator of one's story.

5.4 Dissociation and Narrative Distance

To gain some further perspective on how it is possible that self-narrative not only reflects the structure and dynamics of the self-pattern, but may contribute to them, or in some cases of psychopathology, may disrupt them, we should consider how, within the structure of narrative, a specific kind of dissociation can arise. Here the concept of narrative distance is relevant. This concept goes back to Aristotle's *Poetics,* and it has been used in narrative theory to indicate how far removed the narrator is from the narrated events (Lothe 2000; Andringa 1996). There are, in fact, a number of different kinds of narrative distance: perspectival distance, evaluative/affective distance, temporal distance, and hermeneutical distance:

- *Perspectival distance.* For example, there is less distance between the narrator and the narrated events if the narration is done in the first-person versus third-person perspective. One would expect less narrative distance in autobiographical narratives where the narrator is using the first-person pronoun.
- *Evaluative/affective distance.* Narrative distance measured in terms of the extent and the valence of the narrator's evaluation of the events, or how the

narrator feels about the events. This affective or emotional valence reflects how pleasurable or painful the narrated experience was for the narrator, or how the narrator is currently feeling about the event. The phenomenon of regret, as we saw in Chapter 4, is a good example of this.

- *Temporal distance.* A third kind of narrative distance can be characterized as the distance between the time when the narrator narrates and the time represented by the narrated events. This has to do with both content and structure. With respect to content, if my narrative of events is based on episodic memory, then the limitations imposed by my memory may introduce important discrepancies between what I narrate and what actually happened—a difference between narrated events and historical events. With respect to structure, one ought to consider both internal and external time frames. The internal time frame reflects the serial order within the narrative. One can think of this in terms of McTaggart's (1908) notion of the B-series, cast in terms of earlier and later. Plot depends on this, as Ricoeur (1992) explains in terms of configurations of *discordance* (where a novel event is introduced) and *concordance* (where an event is integrated with the plot). In contrast, the external time frame refers to the temporal perspective of past versus present versus future (McTaggart's A-series). Specifically, from the narrator's viewpoint, events are either past, future, or present relative to the narrator's own present time. The narrator has a temporal perspective on the events that are narrated, with greater temporal distance between events in the distant past compared to events in the near past, for example. In self-narrative, then, the narrating self has a temporal perspective on the narrated self.

- *Hermeneutic distance.* These various kinds of differences—in perspective, valuation/emotion, and temporality—are factors that can introduce limitations and biases into the recounting of events (see Goldie 2011). Narrative distance is unavoidable, and this means that all narrative practice involves interpretation, the veracity of which is measurable in degree, but is never 100 percent, due to factors such as the narrator's interest and affective state, the intended audience, and of course the ever present sheer impossibility of any narrative description conveying everything in a given scene or event. Every narrative involves selection.[4]

Narrative distance, along any of these variables, is not necessarily a weakness. It is not only in descriptive power and relative eloquence that good biography, like good fiction, resides, but also in the selection of events and of the pertinent,

[4] Beyond questions about narrative distance, the hermeneutical complexity concerning autobiographical narrative, and especially important limitations concerning self-narratives of people with psychiatric disorders, are well described by Varga (2015, Ch. 3).

signal aspects of them, for example, how strongly one feels about them. It is also the case that the different types of distance can modulate each other in the construction of the narrative. One past event, for example, might have a greater temporal distance compared to another more recent event, but if the first event has more of an emotional valence than the second, it may feel closer and stronger. Traumatic events in the past may feel as if they are still present.

In autobiographical (or self-)narrative one may, specifically, ask about the distance between the self who narrates and the self who is narrated. Within the context of autobiographical accounts, narrative composes a relation between both the *narrating self* (the narrator) who in the act of narration, "here and now," is telling the story and is being affected by it, and the *narrated self*, the object (the protagonist) of the narrative. When the narrator says, for example, "I had a great time in college," the "I" points in two directions. It points to the person who is telling the story, the narrator, and signifies that the narrator means to say something about herself; but it also points to the person or character who the narrator *was* at some point in the past. The narrator thus expresses an identity between herself as-subject and the person she is talking about, although there is always some degree of dissociation or narrative distance involved. We might think of this as a non-pathological psychological dissociation. That is, in a first-person autobiographical narrative, the person who the narrator is today is not necessarily identical to the person she was. In narrative theory, *ipse* identity is a concept that allows for a difference between *I*, the narrator, and the narrated *me* at an earlier (or later) time, despite numerical (*idem*) identity. A person might say, "I did this in college, but I certainly wouldn't engage in that activity today. I've changed quite a bit."

Furthermore, it's also quite possible that the narrator isn't correct when she says, "I had a great time in college." To some extent this will depend on the veracity or selectivity of her memory (perhaps she can only remember the few good things that happened). It will also depend on certain hermeneutical biases generated, for example, by the kind of things she is interested in reporting, or by the kind of effect that she would like her narrative to have, or the kind of audience she is addressing, and whether her narrative aims for truthfulness; she may want to appear as someone who had a great time, even if she did not.

It seems possible to regard narrative distance and its various aspects as reflecting two different kinds of processes involved in narrative practice. Both the perspectival and temporal aspects may be considered functions of the structural features of narrative, which depend, in turn, on the language or the particular narrative stance taken by the narrator. In contrast, the evaluative/affective and hermeneutical aspects seem to reflect something closer to psychological factors that involve the narrator's experiences, and her interpretation of them in general, and how she wants to portray herself. In an analysis of narrative, however, these different aspects may not be clearly distinguished, as I'll now try to make clear.

Together with colleagues, I conducted an experiment to investigate the dynamics of *ipse* identity in self-narrative (Bedwell et al. 2011). We asked subjects (university students) to orally give four short autobiographical narratives: (a) about an event that actually happened to them during high school; (b) about an event that actually happened to them involving their family; (c) a fictional or made-up story where they recount their experience of an event in high school that did not actually happen to them; and (d) a fictional or made-up story where they recount their experience of an event involving their family that did not actually happen to them. We gathered 176 short, oral, autobiographical narratives in this way, half of which were intentionally fictional or deceptive, and half non-deceptive. Our aim was to test a hypothesis: that there would be an increase of narrative distance in intentionally deceptive autobiographical narratives compared to non-deceptive autobiographical narratives. If so, it raises questions as to why narrative distance might increase and what kind of narrative distance is involved.

The oral narratives were transcribed and we did a comparative analysis using the software program Coh-Metrix. Coh-Metrix automatically computes several linguistic indices, of cohesion within a text, for example, word-level indices like familiarity, syntactic analysis, referential and semantic cohesion indices, and situation model indices (Graesser et al. 2004; 2007; McNamara et al. 2005). We identified seven linguistic variables that showed a statistically significant effect for deception versus non-deception and no statistically significant interaction with story type (family versus high school):

1. *Flesch Kincaid Grade Level*: a traditional formula for calculating the grade level (0–12) of textbooks. The higher the number, the harder it is to read the text. Deceptive stories had a lower Flesch Kincaid Grade Level than the non-deceptive stories.
2. *Number of sentences*: Deceptive stories contained more sentences than the non-deceptive stories. Since there was no significant difference in the number of words used between the deceptive and non-deceptive conditions, deceptive studies contained, on average, more, but shorter, sentences.
3. *Sentence Syntax Similarity*: comparison of syntactic tree structures of sentences. Coh-metrix returns the proportion of nodes in the two tree structures that are intersecting nodes. This is an indication of how similar sentences are in structural complexity. Deceptive stories had greater sentence syntax similarity than the non-deceptive stories.
4. *Explicit action words (intentional content)*: The number of actions involved estimated by counting the number of main verbs that imply intentional or goal-driven action. Examples: "put," "skip," "eat," "cut," "give," and "play." Deceptive stories contained a greater amount of action words/intentional content than the non-deceptive stories.

5. *Log min in sentence for content words*: Returns the log word frequency value for the rarest word in each sentence and computes the mean across sentences. Scores range from 0 to 6. Lower values relate to the general use of relatively rare words. Non-deceptive stories had a lower value than the deceptive stories, indicating more use of relatively rare words in the truthful stories.

6. *Stem Overlap*: a form of referential cohesion, in which a noun in one sentence has the same or a similar morphological root as a word in another sentence. Non-deceptive stories contained a greater degree of stem overlap than the deceptive stories.

7. *Anaphor Reference*: An anaphor is a word (usually a pronoun) that substitutes for a previously mentioned noun to avoid repetition. Coh-metrix calculates the proportion of anaphor references that refer back to its constituent within five sentences. Anaphor reference is another aspect of referential cohesion. Deceptive stories contained fewer anaphor references than the non-deceptive stories.

Generally, the intentionally deceptive narratives (versus non-deceptive narratives) showed:

- *less referential coherence* (measured by Anaphor Reference and Stem Overlap)
- *less complexity* (lower Flesch Kincaid Grade Level, higher number of simple short sentences) with *similar syntax* (Sentence Syntax Similarity) and *less rare words* (Log Min. in Sentence for Content Words)
- *significantly higher number of action words,* that is, more descriptions of actions, than in the non-deceptive narratives.

As I indicated above, there are at least two possible interpretations of narrative distance that we can use to understand these results. On the first interpretation, narrative distance may signify a psychological dissociation. If we take descriptions of actions to involve a more impersonal perspective than a description in terms of experience or feelings, then the higher number of action words (i.e., descriptions of self in terms of actions and external events) in deceptive narratives reflects a greater narrative distance (a higher degree of impersonality) between the narrator and the narrated self. One way to think of this is to consider the person described in the deceptive narrative as more like another person (not me, not the true me). That is, if in fact I am lying about myself or about what I have done in the past, then in some sense I am describing someone who is not the present me, implying a greater distance between the narrator and the narrated. In that case I (the narrator) am giving a description of someone (myself—the narrated self) as another, and from the outside.

The easiest way to run a first-person description of someone else is not in terms of the other's mental states but in terms of their actions, as anyone who compares pulp fiction with, say, Proust or Henry James will know. So, in describing others, actions become the main focus (Genette 1983). The prediction, then, is that my narrations about people other than myself will reflect a higher number of action words. That is, they will offer a description more in terms of actions and external events than in terms of the other's motives or reasons for acting. A study by Krackow (2010) makes a related point. Krackow compared narratives of *remembered* childhood events to *imagined* childhood events and found a higher number of mental state terms in the remembered events. Accordingly, the fact that deceptive self-narratives reflect a higher number of action words suggests that the narrating self is distancing (dissociating) herself from the narrated self.

Bruner's (1986) distinction between the landscape of action (LoA) and the landscape of consciousness (LoC) can be informative here. LoA narratives describe what happens in terms of a series of actions or external events. LoC narratives describe "what those involved in the action know, think, or feel, or do not know, think, or feel" (Bruner 1986, 14). An example of LoA: "I walked to the store to get some candy." An example of LoC: "I *decided* to walk to the store because I *wanted* to get some candy." Feldman et al. (1990) show, in a study of narrative comprehension in adults, that people easily understand the gist of a story cast solely in the less complex LoA, and it is clearly possible to represent the major events in a drama without always being able to decipher or explain, with full clarity or perhaps at all, the *reasons* why a protagonist will have acted. The main idea, however, is that if in the case of deceptive autobiographical narrative I am describing myself as if I were another, and from the outside, then, we would expect the narrative to be framed more in the LoA (more action words) than in LoC (more mental state words). That turns out to be the case in our elicited deceptive narratives.

This, however, is not the only interpretation available. A second interpretation can be given in terms, not of psychological dissociation, but simply in terms of narrative reflecting certain cognitive-linguistic requirements related to less syntactical complexity in the deceptive narratives, which is also something we found. Less referential coherence, for example, may reflect the fact that the participants are constructing the deceptive narratives on a more ad hoc basis (they were given only four minutes to construct their narratives) than narratives based on memory of their own activities, which they may have described before. Despite the similarity in the total number of words in deceptive and non-deceptive narratives, the reduced complexity in the deceptive narratives is consistent with previous research showing less detailed information delivered (Vrij 2001; Vrij & Heaven 1999) and shorter sentences with simpler syntax for deceptive communication (Miller & Stiff 1993).

But if deceptive narratives themselves are less complex, generating them may still be *more* cognitively complex than generating non-deceptive narratives.

As Bedwell et al. point out, deceivers must use additional cognitive resources to maintain a coherent and consistent version of a false story. There's a difference in cognitive complexity between generating autobiographical narratives on the basis of imagination (as in deceptive narratives) than on the basis of memory (as in non-deceptive narratives), presuming for the sake of argument that memories are fairly truthful. In the case of memory, where I have a direct memory of my experience of the past event, I do not require an extra step of identifying who the subject is. I know that it was I who experienced X. In the case of imagining myself doing something, however, the structure involves: (1) imagining someone doing X; (2) knowing that I did not do X; but (3) nonetheless identifying that someone as myself. In other words, pretense enters into the deceit as an extra cognitive step.

So the cognitive complexity involved in generating a false narrative does not automatically translate into complex narratives. The fact that a deceptive narrative may be expressed with a higher syntactical simplicity than a non-deceptive narrative may be viewed as a compensatory effect—a way of balancing out the cognitive complexity. In other words, in order to be able to do all the cognitive work involved in deception, the narrator may keep the story as simple as possible. Likewise, if, as in non-deceptive narrative, the cognitive work is not as complex, the narrator may have more resources available to enhance the story or embellish the details (Kronsted et al. 2023).

This same reasoning, however, may explain the higher number of action words in the deceptive narratives. Generating LoA narratives requires less cognitive work than LoC narratives, which may help to balance out the higher cognitive demands of deception. This can be seen in the developmental literature. As children gain narrative competency, they begin with narratives that are dominated by actions, and only gradually learn to add intentional language (Hutto, 2008; Nelson, 2009). In addition, to explain one's reasons for acting may be easier than to explain the motives or reasons of another person. Describing another person's motives, emotions, intentions, and so forth, in narrative form seems more complex than describing their actions.

My interest here is not in deceptive narratives, but in the different interpretations that may be possible in regard to narrative distance. Narrative distance is not pathological dissociation, but we can ask whether similar dynamics are at work, or whether they fail to work in the self-narratives of people with different psychiatric disorders. A key question is whether pathological dissociation, as reflected in self-narratives, follows structural lines that lead to the same or to different interpretational strategies, where we need to understand that either the narrator treats the narrated self as if it were someone other (which may be a genuine psychological dissociation), or simply operates with a less complex cognitive/syntactic strategy as compensatory in regard to cognitive load (resulting in something that looks like psychological dissociation, but may simply be compensatory for a cognitive deficit that may accompany a psychiatric disorder). I'll return to difficulties in distinguishing between genuine psychological dissociations versus compensatory processes in the next section.

5.5 Narratives and Psychopathological Disorders

Much of interpersonal expression is ephemeral; body language and prosody may be potent communication channels but without video or film they are lost as moments pass. In contrast, recorded oral language and written language can endure. Within medicine there is a tradition of recording and examining narrative accounts of patients with psychiatric and neurological conditions. Scientists from Weir Mitchell to Alexander Luria and Oliver Sacks were able to find extraordinarily rich narratives of brain damage, autism, aphasia, blindness, and so forth. Yet rarely are the accounts that are taken from the patients themselves (in interviews, for example) questioned in regard to their narrative structure, despite the fact that certain conditions may of themselves affect the range of narrative possible to a given patient, and may constrain the very shape of the narrative. Simplifying for the moment, if we distinguish the various elements which make up an expressive narrative it would include expressed contents (experiences, thoughts, feelings), narrative structure, and the linguistic and embodied expressive channels or mechanisms of communication. In the analysis of narratives of neurological patients the latter set of factors tends to be the focus while content and structure are presumed to be fairly well intact. For example, in cases of aphasia one sees curtailment of language (and gesture) but we might presume that the patient's experience and feelings are largely intact, even if in some respect they may be affected by the person's condition. The generative problem is with expressive channels. Alternatively, in adult-onset blindness linguistic skills may be unaffected, but there are likely radical changes in what the patient has to say and narrative content changes dramatically.

In other cases, however, there can be differences in narrative structure, related to narrative style and vocabulary. Someone with high-functioning ASD may use language differently from individuals who are not autistic, reflecting in part the landscape of their experience. In depression one might see a profound change in mood with no overt change in linguistic skills, although the person's use of language and of various words may change, and we may find compensatory adjustments that address cognitive difficulties. In other conditions an alteration in one's experience of one's body, through neurological loss, or trauma, may not only change thoughts and feelings but may affect communication and alter the person's use of narrative. In fact, some conditions motivate us to ask if these two sides—the experiential and the expressive—are so interlinked as a continuum that a simple binary consideration has little utility.

Here I return to the question raised in Chapter 4: Can narratives provide a forensic measure, a linguistic fingerprint, of psychopathology? In other words, in the narratives of individuals with psychopathological conditions, do narratives reflect disorders in the self-pattern in a veridical fashion, or might the narratives themselves be considered disordered, in ways that complicate this question? This question, or more precisely, this strategy, as indicated in Chapter 4, has been pursued in a number of studies that have examined the self-narratives of people with psychopathological conditions. Such studies found lower frequencies of cognitive terms in the narratives of psychiatric patients in general (Junghaenel, Smyth & Santner 2008), and specifically in patients diagnosed with schizophrenia, less grammatical clarity in reference to negative emotions, and more social reference in narratives about positive emotions (Gruber & Kring 2008); higher degree of dyslogia or wrong or novel words in emotional (versus neutral) narratives (Caixeta et al. 1999); and less coherent and elaborate self-narratives connecting self and memory (Berna et al. 2016; Raffard et al. 2010). In cases of major depressive disorder (MDD), compared to non-depressed patients, self-narratives reflect reconfigured temporal and syntactical structures (Lenzo & Gallagher 2021); increased frequencies of self-reference words (Pennebaker, Mehl & Niederhoffer 2003; Stirman & Pennebaker 2001); impaired memory for positive emotional events (Werner-Seidler & Moulds 2011); overly generalized reports on past events (Mackinger et al. 2000); and alterations in affect (Ratcliffe 2008) and bodily experience (Fuchs 2005; Fuchs & Schlimme 2009; Paskaleva 2011; Slaby & Stephan 2008). Different types of amnesia involve different patterns in first-person pronoun use in self-narratives. Although patients with transient global amnesia consistently use first-person pronouns, patients with functional amnesia tend to use general pronouns in their self-narratives, which may reflect a link to experiences of depersonalization (Becquet et al. 2021).

Thus, a variety of data can be collected from the analysis of self-narratives of patients with psychiatric disorders. Accurate interpretation of such data, however, is not always easy. Interpretation of narrative, in terms of its semantic and syntactic structures, is constrained both by psychopathological theory and hermeneutical-narrative theory. Consider, for example, three different views on the nature of schizophrenia and how they impinge on one's interpretation of schizophrenic narratives.

First, on one view, in schizophrenia a disruption in the sense of agency may be the result of problems with certain introspective practices. The problems are directly related to what Graham and Stephens call "our proclivity for constructing self-referential narratives." They suggest that, normally, an agent's experience of agency for her actions or thoughts depends on her sense that the actions or thoughts fit well with her own self-narrative, or on "whether she finds [their] occurrence explicable in terms of her theory or story of her own underlying intentional states" (Graham & Stephens 1994, 102). In contrast, for the schizophrenic who suffers from delusions of control or thought insertion, "what is critical is that the subject find her thoughts inexplicable in terms of beliefs about her intentional states" (1994, 105).

A second view takes a bottom-up approach and points to impairments in self-temporalization at the level of prereflective ipseity as disruptive to a sense of agency, which then gets reflected in narrative (Bovet & Parnas 1993). Disorders of temporal experience are clearly present in self-narratives of patients with schizophrenia. Consider the following bits of narrative:

> [...] there....In the middle of time I was coming from the past toward myself....Before there was a before and after. Yet it isn't there now.
> (Cited by Minkowski 1970, 286)
>
> I get all mixed up so that I don't know myself. I feel like more than one person when this happens. I'm falling apart into bits.   (Cited by Sass 1995, 70)
>
> Then I, through this combination of myself projecting into the other person, and the other person in itself, am monitored to react as expected...and that happens so rapidly that I, even if I had wanted to, am unable to stop myself.
> (Cited by Sass 1999, 334)

Consistent with this phenomenological view, Phillips (2003) suggests that in schizophrenia, self-narratives become impoverished and fragmented, or overly focused on the present, on what is happening to the subject now—and they are often specifically about the experience of their condition.

A third view is represented by Lysaker and Lysaker (2002) who suggest that narrative structure derives from an internal self-dialogue: "The self is inherently 'dialogical,' or the product of ongoing conversations both within the individual and between the individual and others" (210). In some cases of schizophrenia, they suggest, narrative becomes monological, or the self-dialogue becomes distorted.

Here, then, are three approaches to understanding narratives in cases of schizophrenia:

1. We control our narratives; the narrative reflects a complex (meta-)cognitive mistake, for example, about agency (Graham and Stephens).
2. Some factor other than narrative (e.g., affect or prereflective ipseity) is disrupted and is simply reflected in narrative (Bovet and Parnas).
3. Something in the linguistic-narrative-dialogical practice itself goes wrong (Lysaker and Lysaker).

In (1) and (2), narrative might operate as a neutral vehicle that expresses disturbances in some other processes, or may itself become disordered because of these disturbances. In (3), it seems, narrative is complicit in the disturbance, that is, the narrative is itself pathological, and not just reflective of the pathology. One might think that it should be easy to distinguish between neutral or complicit narratives; or that it would be easy to distinguish between (2) and (3)—a distinction that might parallel a distinction between the prereflective experiential processes of the self-pattern (an awareness of one's present embodied situation, or one's ipseity), and narrative processes that involve a temporally extended sense of (narrative) self. The fact that these two elements in the self-pattern are dynamically related, however, doesn't make this an easy distinction.

Accordingly, if one followed the general research strategy of identifying features of narrative structure that might be shifted around or disrupted as the result of living with a given condition, one would still have to work out how to distinguish between these alternative interpretations. The strategy of searching for the fingerprints of pathology in narrative, may not, on its own, distinguish between these possible interpretations. Deciding which is most appropriate may depend on how one views the relation between elements of the self-pattern as they are reflected in the narrative itself.

This may also involve the concept of narrative distance discussed in the previous section, and the distinction between genuine psychological dissociation and compensatory processes. Consider the following self-narrative by a schizophrenic patient:

> I get all mixed up so that I don't know myself. I feel like more than one person when this happens. I'm falling apart into bits...I'm frightened to say a word in case everything goes fleeting from me so that there's nothing in my mind....My head's full of thoughts, fears, hates, jealousies. My head can't grip them; I can't hold on to them. I'm behind the bridge of my nose—I mean, my consciousness is there. They're splitting open my head, oh, that's schizophrenic, isn't it? I don't know whether I have these thoughts or not.   (Cited in Sass 1995, 70)

Are narratives like this reflecting a real psychological dissociation that touches on ipseity ("I feel like more than one person...")—the Bovet-Parnas interpretation? Or might it reflect a cognitive/linguistic difficulty ("I'm frightened to say a word in case everything goes fleeting from me...")—in this case a compensatory strategy related to cognitive workload or a problem in dialogical structure—the Lysaker-Lysaker interpretation? Or might the patient's narrative suggest that the expression of what is being felt may lead of itself to a dissolution of the self-pattern, which is closer again to the Bovet-Parnas interpretation? Or is this either-or view too simplistic? Might we say that both issues—disruptions in both ipseity and dialogical structure—are involved? To distinguish these we may have to look to extra-narrative indications that concern other aspects of the self-pattern.

This brings us back to the question of whether narrative itself can be neutral or complicit. Can one distinguish disordered narrative, involving language with exceptional structures, for example, in verb use, in syntax, from narrative that simply reflects disruptions in other aspects of the self-pattern and the experience of living with unusual conditions. It is certainly imaginable that someone with, say, depression, may have a perfectly normal use of language, and so use narrative to express their pathological condition—a condition that can have significant impact on other aspects of the self-pattern, which then gets reflected in narrative content. Alternatively, someone with a pure dysphasia may have profound changes in use of language, isolated from psychological problems. In more complex and severe psychoses, like schizophrenia, the relations between narrative structure and content, and between expression and experience, are far more complex (see, for example, the discussion of "clang" below).

5.6 Self-narrative in Schizophrenia

Generation of a self-narrative depends on the proper functioning of a variety of cognitive capacities, including:

(1) a capacity for temporal integration of events;
(2) a capacity for first-person self-reference;
(3) a capacity for encoding and retrieving episodic-autobiographical memories;
(4) a capacity for engaging in reflective metacognition.

Neuropsychological research suggests that in schizophrenia, beginning at the prodromal stage (Hartmann et al. 1984), processes involved in each of these capacities are frequently disrupted. It should not be surprising then, that, as a result, schizophrenic narratives are problematic, both in structure and content. Indeed, if any one of these capacities fails we would expect that failure to be reflected in the subject's self-narrative. If, in schizophrenia it's possible that all of them fail, then the situation is far more complex. Let's take each in turn.

5.6.1 Temporal Integration

I already indicated that narrative involves a twofold temporal structure. First, a time frame that is internal to the narrative itself, a serial order (B-series) in which one event follows another. This internal time frame allows for the composition of narrative structure. I mentioned Ricoeur's notions of concordance and discordance in this regard, related to configurations of plot structures of narrative. The second, external time frame (the A-series, past-present-future) defines the narrator's temporal relation to the events of the narrative. Even if this relation is left unspecified ("Once upon a time…") it is usually open to a specification that these events happened in the past, or will happen in the future, relative to the narrator's present. Of course, it is possible that if the events never happened and never will happen (as in the case of fictional events) we might think of them precisely as not having a specifiable place in time relative to the narrator. This cannot be the case with respect to *self*-narrative, however. Even if the event in question never did happen (e.g., an event falsely remembered), or never will happen (e.g., a planned event that never comes to be actualized) in self-narrative it is still set in a temporal relation to the narrator.

The external time frame is perspectival in a way that the internal time frame is not. The external time frame is defined relative to the narrator who defines the present. From the perspective of the narrator telling the story, the events of the story, which internally maintain their serial relations (x happens before y), may be more or less remotely past (or future). In self-narrative it is always the case that the narrator (oneself) is related to the events in the narrative in a perspectival way. The events recounted in the narrative are part of the narrator's immediate or remote past, or are projected to be part of the narrator's future, or are happening to the narrator in the present. Someone incapable of maintaining a normal perspectival frame of reference is unable to generate a self-narrative properly specified in its temporal framework.

There is a large body of evidence indicating that some schizophrenic subjects have problems pertaining to temporal experience in ways that interfere with both internal and external temporal frameworks. Future time-perspective is curtailed in schizophrenia. Minkowski, for example, describes schizophrenia as involving "acts without concern for tomorrow." He quotes a patient: "There is an absolute fixity around me. I have even less mobility for the future than I have for the present and the past. There is a kind of routine in me which does not allow me to envisage the future. The creative power in me is abolished. I see the future as a repetition of the past" (Minkowski 1970, 277). Lysaker's patient C produces monological and rigid narratives with sustained delusions (Lysaker, Wickett & Davis 2005). He interprets all events in a delusional manner, that is, believing that he was the subject of persecution by a former high-school teacher. The narrative is fixed and absolute; any challenge to it is perceived as further persecution organized by the teacher, and this simply becomes part of the narrative. In this regard new events in C's self-narrative are dominated by events (veridical or not) that are past. His self-narrative is nicely characterized by the same terms expressed by Minkowski's patient: absolute fixity and the lack of motivation that would enable him to envisage a future that would be different from the past, reflecting problems with temporal structure specifically in regard to the external, perspectival A-series.

Schizophrenics also experience difficulties in indexing events in time, and these difficulties are positively correlated to symptoms of auditory hallucinations, feelings of being influenced, and problems that involve distinguishing between self and non-self. Some schizophrenic narratives are characterized by a temporal derailing, by constant tangents, the loss of goal, the loosening of associations or the compression of a temporally extended story to a single gesture (see Cowan, Mittal & McAdams 2021).

Self-narratives of some schizophrenic patients reflect more general problems in the proper sequencing of events (in the B-series), and self-placement in appropriate temporal frameworks. For example, one patient reports:

> I felt as if I had been put back, as if something of the past had returned, so to speak, toward me...so that not only time repeated itself again but all that had happened for me during that time as well...In the middle of all this something happened which did not seem to belong there. Suddenly it was not only 11:00 again, but a time which has passed a long time before was there...In the middle of time I was coming from the past toward myself...Before there was a before and after. Yet it isn't there now...[When someone visits and then leaves] it could very well have happened yesterday. I can no longer arrange it, in order to know where it belongs.   (Cited by Minkowski, 1970, 284–6)

Schizophrenics have difficulty planning and initiating action, problems with temporal organization, and experienced continuity. Bovet and Parnas (1993, 584) describe these problems in general terms as involving an "impairment of self-temporalization."

Impairment of self-temporalization manifests itself not only across these internal and external frames, but also in short-term integration. Capabilities related to temporal integration and the linear ordering of events within a temporal framework are essential to the formation of the narrative perspective and to the sequential order that characterizes narrative. Working memory involves the temporal integration of experience over very short periods of time, and its proper functioning is a necessary condition for capabilities that are directly relevant to the formation of self-narrative, namely, capabilities that involve minimal self-reference and episodic-autobiographical memory.

Studies of spatial ordering (Keefe et al. 1997), temporal ordering (Dreher et al. 2001), and verbal (Wexler et al. 1998) tasks in schizophrenics show marked deficits of working memory (Goldman-Rakic 1994). Difficulties with the processing of working memory sometimes manifest themselves as "formal thought disorders"—a breakdown of the temporal organization of reasoning and speech, relatively slow speeds of cognitive processing (Fuster 1999) and "cognitive dysmetria" (Andreasen et al. 1998). Problems that some schizophrenics have in keeping track of recent actions (Mlakar, Jensterle & Frith 1994), affecting the sense of agency, may involve their inability to anticipate or sequence their own actions in working memory (Gallagher 2000b). They also perform poorly on delayed response tasks (Fleming et al. 1997). Disorganized cognition includes perspectival shifts that disrupt the subject's ability to block out alternative perspectives (Sass 1995, 144), an ability that is necessary for unconfused action and clear communication.

Related to working memory, problems with the intrinsic temporal (retentional-protentional) structure of experience,[5] for example, can result in narrative disruptions known as clang associations. In the case of clang associations, schizophrenic subjects can lose their way and get ensnared in a current (present) aspect of language or the narrative itself; subjects are captured by semantically non-relevant aspects of the story and they go off on extreme digressions. Clang associations are usually explained in terms of rhyming words—"whip," "tip," "lip"—where patients are more likely to connect words because of similarity of sound, rather than by meaning. This is something often seen in clinical interviews. Susan Duncan (2005) shows that it also occurs in gesture, where a particular iconic gesture will lead the patient into digression—and she appeals to problems with protention (loss of a sense of where the narrative is going) to explain this.

As a result of disturbances in temporal integration, the semantic continuity of experience often breaks down in schizophrenia (Pöppel 1994). The same problems involving temporal integration are linked to action-related neurological dysfunctions involved in voluntary movement in individuals with schizophrenia (Singh et al. 1992), as well as the failure of intermodal sensory integration in schizophrenic experience (Parnas et al. 1996). It is not surprising, then, that problems with temporal integration and intermodal binding are reflected in the narratives of schizophrenics. One patient reports: "[S]ometimes everything is so fragmented, when it should be so unified. A bird in the garden chirps, for example. I heard the bird, and I know that he chirps; but that it is a bird and that he chirps, these two things are separated from each other" (cited by Minkowski 1970, 285).

5.6.2 First-person Self-reference

To begin to form a self-narrative one must be able to refer to oneself by using the first-person pronoun. In turn, the development of the ability to use the first-person pronoun depends on a primitive embodied sense of differentiation between self and non-self. This experiential differentiation is certainly in place in early infancy. It's implicit in proprioceptive and kinaesthetic experience, and it relates to being able to recognize the difference between being moved and moving oneself, and in this way relates to the senses of ownership and agency. This sense of differentiation is the basis for a related experiential process—the prereflective self-awareness that is referenced when one says "I." It is this experiential

---

[5] For more detail about the phenomenological concept of the retentional-protentional structure of intrinsic temporality, see below, Section 9.4.

"I" which is extended and enhanced in self-narrative. Without the basic sense of differentiation between self and non-self I would not be able to refer to myself with any specification, and self-narrative would have no starting point.

Certain forms of self-awareness cannot be mistaken, and as a result, specific uses of the first-person pronoun in self-reference are immune to error through misidentification (IEM) (Shoemaker 1968). For example, if I say, "I think it is going to rain," I may be entirely wrong about the rain, but I cannot be wrong about the "I." I cannot say "I" and mean to identify someone else by that word. If I say "I see that John is at his desk," I can be wrong about it being a desk; I can be wrong about it being John; and I can even be wrong about my cognitive act (it may be hallucination rather than visual perception). It would be nonsensical, however, to ask me, "Are you sure that you are the one who sees that John is at his desk?" Wittgenstein indicates that this use of the first-person pronoun, which is IEM, is a use "as-subject."[6] There are some uses of the first-person pronoun, however, that may involve misidentification. For example, surrounded by several other people, I may look in a mirror and exclaim "I'm sunburned." In this case I may be wrong if I mis-perceive someone else's image as my own. This is what Wittgenstein calls use of the first-person pronoun "as-object," and such uses are not IEM.

Importantly, it can be argued that even in cases where I do objectively misidentify myself (e.g., if, when practicing my archery, I mistakenly claim that I am the one who hit the target, when in fact it is somebody else who hit the target), I am not mistaken in my subjective self-reference. This is the idea of guaranteed self-reference (Strawson 1994). When I say "I," I am referring to myself, even though I may be wrong about who hit the target. Indeed, I can objectively misidentify myself in this respect only because I have correctly self-referred. In such cases, my mistake about who hit the target when I did not hit the target is a mistake only because I correctly referred to myself in saying "I."

In whatever way we parse this out, we can agree with Shoemaker (1968) that IEM holds for cases of self-reference because they are cases in which there is no need for identification, and thus no chance of misidentification. In other words, we are immune to error in this regard, not because we are so proficient, or so infallible at judging who we are, but because this kind of self-awareness doesn't involve a judgment at all. This makes the capacity to use the first-person pronoun an extremely secure anchor for self-narratives.

For the construction of self-narrative, not only the use of the first-person pronoun, but also the experience of agency for one's actions, are essential. Ricoeur (1992) makes it clear that in narrative a character is either (or alternatively) an agent or a sufferer. In self-narrative the construal of the character (the narrated self)

---

[6] For one possible, although ambiguous exception to this principle see Gallagher (2015).

as agent or sufferer depends on the ability of the narrator to self-attribute action. This means that even if other elements in prereflective experiential processes of the self-pattern (e.g., first-person perspective, sense of ownership) are intact, a lack of a sense of agency may still be disruptive to self-narrative.

In schizophrenic symptoms of thought insertion, delusions of control, and auditory hallucinations, various aspects of self-awareness are disrupted. Specifically, such experiences may involve a lack of a sense of agency. John Campbell (1999) goes so far as to suggest that in the case of schizophrenia the lack of a sense of agency represents a failure of IEM. That is, phenomena like thought insertion, where the patient claims that it is not his thought, seem to involve errors of self-identification. The patient who suffers from thought insertion is not in error about the thought content, but rather is wrong about whose thought it is. Here is an example, patient K, an eighteen-year-old male (from Sandsten, Zahavi & Parnas 2022, 5):

> The way I believe everyone else experiences thoughts, is that when they think, it is like having your own voice in your head, but without the sound. It is just like that, but it is not me who is doing the thinking. So, it is a foreign body, which is not coming from the outside, but is within as a slightly different voice. And the voices are foreign, so I am not in control of them whatsoever.

One can argue, however, that certain aspects of prereflective self-awareness and self-reference remain intact even in cases of thought insertion, delusions of control, and auditory hallucinations (Gallagher 2000b). That is, on at least one interpretation, patients who suffer from these symptoms wrongly attribute their experiences to someone else only with respect to agency (i.e., they claim that someone else caused the action), but they correctly self-attribute these experiences in terms of ownership (i.e., they acknowledge that they themselves are the ones who undergo the experience)—indeed, that is why they are complaining. Understood in this way, they correctly, and with IEM still intact, use the first-person pronoun to formulate their complaints.

Accordingly, a patient may be seemingly lost in a confusion of self and other, but she is nonetheless able to use the first-person pronoun properly and consistently. For example, a woman with schizophrenic symptoms describes what she experiences when she is in a conversation: "[T]hen I, through this combination of myself projecting into the other person, and the other person in itself, am monitored to react as expected…and that happens so rapidly that I, even if I had wanted to, am unable to stop myself. And after that, I am left by myself and very lonely" (quoted in Sass 1998, 334). Another patient with schizophrenia spoke of "no longer [being] able to distinguish how much of myself is in me and how much is already in others. I am a conglomeration, a monstrosity, modeled anew each day" (Freeman et al. 2013, 54). In such cases, nonetheless, when the patient uses the first-person pronoun, she is not referring to someone else; she is referring to and is not misidentifying herself. The disruption in the sense of agency, however, can still derail the self-narrative.

Just here, however, the notion of narrative distance has some importance. Some studies suggest that in schizophrenic self-narratives, although the narrator correctly uses the first-person pronoun to identify himself *as narrator*, the narrator will sometimes use a third-person pronoun to designate himself as a character in the narrative (Bernal 2001). The difference (and the narrative distance) represented by different pronouns may signify precisely a failure of the subject to treat himself as agent of his own narrated actions. Again, this would not be a violation of IEM since it involves, at most, a failure of objective identification; but it would be a disruption of narrative self-identity.

5.6.3 Episodic-autobiographical Memory

Both the capacity for temporal integration and the capacity for first-person self-reference seem necessary for the proper working of episodic-autobiographical memory. These capacities are related to two aspects normally understood to define autobiographical memory: the recollection of the specific time in the past when an event took place, and self-attribution, the specification that the past event involved the person who is remembering it. It is possible, however, that someone who is able to self-attribute actions (e.g., when they are occurring) and is also able to specify the proper time frames for events (e.g., in following a set of instructions) still may not be able to acquire memories, or to recollect autobiographical events.

There is a long philosophical tradition, starting with Locke (1690), which holds that just such memories form the basis of personal identity. It seems clear that narrative identity is primarily constituted in narratives that recount past autobiographical events. If there is any degree of unity to my life, as Ricoeur (1992) suggests, it is the product of an interpretation of my past actions and of events in the past that happened to me (all of which constitute my life history). If I am unable to form memories of my life history, or am unable to access such memories, then I have nothing to interpret, nothing to narrate that would be sufficient for the formation of self-identity.

The importance of episodic memory for the construction of narrative is also recognized in neuropsychology. Maguire, Frith, and Morris (1999) point out that the successful use of stories to convey and acquire information depends on two factors: that the story makes sense, and that the person who hears the story has access to prior knowledge. The coherence of the story depends on these factors. In the construction of self-narrative, autobiographical memory provides the prior knowledge out of which the coherent narrative is formed.

It is quite common, in philosophy and neuropsychology, to discuss episodic memory in terms like "encoding" and "retrieval" and thus to conceive of memory on the metaphor of information storage. Some psychologists and philosophers, however, going back at least as far as Frederic Bartlett (1932), propose that memory is not simply a matter of reproduction or retrieval of stored information, but a reconstructive process (Barclay & DeCooke 1988; Schechtman 1996). In this sense the narrative (and self-narrative) process is not simply something that depends on the proper functioning of episodic (and autobiographical) memory, but in fact contributes to the functioning of that memory. Just to the extent that the current contextual and semantic requirements of narrative construction motivate the recollection of a certain event, that recollection will be shaped, interpreted, and reconstructed in the light of those requirements. For this reason a variety of issues involved in a discussion of memory are also relevant to our discussion of metacognition in the next section.

Impairment of episodic-autobiographical memory is a cognitive deficit commonly found in schizophrenia. Schizophrenics do not have problems with all types of memory, but they do have a focused deficit in the type of remembering that involves mental re-living of their own actions and experiences (Danion et al. 1999). PET studies show that schizophrenic patients, relative to controls, have reduced hippocampal activation during verbal episodic memory retrieval (Heckers et al. 1998). The same researchers also found evidence for hippocampal hyperactivity in the schizophrenic patients they tested, something associated with abnormal thought processes, hallucinations, and delusions (also see Goldman-Rakic 1994; Frith et al. 1995; Dolan & Fletcher 1997).

It seems clear that if schizophrenic patients have problems in either the encoding or the retrieval of memories, they will also have trouble in constructing a viable self-narrative. This is not just a question of whether they can remember their own story. Rather, the episodic–autobiographical memory system delivers content for the construction of self-narrative. If autobiographical content is confused, if it is dramatically incomplete, inaccessible, or entirely fleeting, this will be reflected in one's self-narrative. The explicit and self-conscious formation of a life story depends on the material provided by memory. Lacking such material, there are at least two possible responses. The first can be seen in some cases of transient global amnesia. A patient may feel completely disoriented and ask such things as "Where am I?" "What day is today?" or "Where are we going?" Here we have questions, but no narrative. A second possible response results in a narrative, but one that is confabulated or extremely enhanced by metacognition that has become hyperreflexive.

5.6.4 Reflective Metacognition

The process of interpretation that ordinarily shapes episodic-autobiographical memories into a narrative structure depends on the capacity for reflective metacognition. A life event is not always meaningful in itself; rather, it depends on a narrative structure that lends it context and sees in it a significance that may go beyond the event itself. As Merlin Donald (2006) puts it, metacognition provides the "cognitive governance" that allows for disambiguating and differentiating events within the narrative. To form a self-narrative, to be a self-interpreting animal, one needs to do more than simply remember life events. One needs to consider them reflectively, deliberate on their meaning and decide how they fit together semantically. Metacognition allows for that reflective process of interpretation. It also enhances the product delivered by autobiographical memory. As Ricoeur points out, narrative identity "must be seen as an unstable mixture of fabulation and actual experience" (1992, 162). It is possible, for the sake of a unified or coherent meaning, to construe certain events in a way that they did not in fact happen. To some degree, and for the sake of creating a coherency to life, it is normal to adjust, or sometimes to confabulate and to enhance one's story. Self-deception is not unusual; false memories are frequent. Whether in any particular case metacognition contributes to this process, or limits it, it is clearly essential for the interpretive process that produces the self-narrative.

Cowan, Mittal, and McAdams (2021) found disruptions of narrative identity in schizophrenia, reflected not only in disjointed structure, but also in detached life stories, which involves disturbances in the metacognitive dimension of autobiographical reasoning. Chris Frith (1992), likewise, suggests that metacognition is problematic in schizophrenia. Specifically he contends that there is a disruption of self-monitoring in both motor and cognitive domains. Self-monitoring can include introspective metarepresentation, a second-order reflective consciousness, a form of introspection that is disturbed in the schizophrenic. We note, however, that it is possible for metarepresentation to go wrong in at least two ways. First, as Frith emphasizes, it can fail in a way such that the schizophrenic is left without the ability to monitor his or her own experience. Second, however, as Louis Sass (2000) suggests, metarepresentation and a certain degree of over-monitoring of experience can be generated in hyperreflexive experience, when processes that are ordinarily tacit (processes that I normally do not have to monitor explicitly or consciously) come to the subject's attention. Neurological dysfunctions (in prefrontal cortex, premotor cortex, supplementary motor area, hippocampus, and so forth), as well as affective and intersubjective processes, can lead a subject to attend to what is ordinarily tacit in experience, leading to problems that may involve the sense of agency or sense of ownership, or working memory (and the retentional-protentional aspects of experience).

Either kind of metacognitive disturbance holds consequences for the schizophrenic self-narrative. It is possible that the disruption of metacognition can be selectively Frithian and Sassian in succession. Either a failure of self-monitoring, or a hyperreflexive shift, where the subject begins to focus on normally implicit aspects of experience, could motivate the schizophrenic to introspect explicitly about what is absent from or odd about his or her experience. In turn, this reflection can lead to a further, compensatory hyperreflection that may entail a failure to monitor other normally monitored aspects. A schizophrenic may have great difficulties with attention, not because of a complete lack of attention, but because she is attending in a high degree to certain aspects of her experience that are not usually the focus of attention. The failure of self-monitoring may be that there is too much of it going on. This possibility is not unrelated to what Sass calls a central paradox of schizophrenic experience: "a strange oscillation, or even coexistence, between two opposite experiences of the self: between the loss or fragmentation of self and its apotheosis in moments of solipsistic grandeur" (Sass 1998, 317). The failure of self-monitoring to which Frith attributes thought insertion and symptoms of influence may lead to first-person narrative claims like "I didn't want to do this, that machine made me." Failures of self-attribution that may involve a disruption in the sense of agency and a lack of self-monitoring are not sufficient, however, to explain why the subject attributes agency for the action to someone or something else. If in some respect there is a shrinking of the self ("these are not my actions") there is at the same time an expansion of the narrative that accounts for the self—an expansion that includes other people or things.

It is possible that schizophrenic hyperreflexive experience is motivated by precisely the kind of failures reviewed above. If there is a failure in my sense of agency, and I experience thought insertion, for example, or if there is some experienced lack of temporal integration, it seems likely that certain aspects of my experience, which are usually tacit or implicit, would begin to manifest themselves in an explicit way. That would motivate an introspective search for explanations to account for such experience. Indeed, as Bruner and Kalmar (1998) suggest, the driving force for the formation of narrative in the mode of metacognition is "trouble," or a sense of jeopardy.

Based on experiments with split-brain patients, Michael Gazzaniga (1995; 1998) suggests that a specific left-hemisphere mechanism, which he calls the "interpreter," is responsible for the neurological process involved in generating narratives that compensate for missing or distorted information. The interpreter mechanism weaves together autobiographical fact and newly devised fiction to produce a self-narrative that maintains the sense of a continuous self. In agreement with Dennett's characterization of the narrative self, Gazzaniga contends that we have a propensity to enhance our personal narratives with elements that smooth over discontinuities and discrepancies in self-constitution (Gazzaniga & Gallagher 1998). The greater the discontinuities and discrepancies, as in schizophrenia, the more one's personal narratives involve deliberations, abstractions, withdrawals, and confabulations that may include attribution of agency for one's actions to some other agent.[7]

---

[7] In some cases there are ongoing auditory hallucinations or quasi-hallucinations experienced as running commentary and/or arguing voices—a heard voice commenting on the patient's ongoing actions or thoughts; or hallucinatory voices discussing the patient in the third person.

The self-narratives of some schizophrenic patients can break down across all four capacities required for narrative competency: *temporal structure* (internal temporal disruptions and disorganization), *ipseity* (incoherent sense of self), *autobiographical memory* (impoverished content), and *metacognition*. We can see this in some of the narratives collected by James Phillips (2003). For example, he describes a patient with schizophrenia, Mr. B, as providing impoverished and fragmented self-narratives characterized as involving disordered and incomplete thoughts, interruptions of ongoing narrative "with statements about how it all started," a lack of a coherent sense of self, a minimal sense of future (also see Lysaker et al. 2005). With respect to metacognition, Mr. B appears to have problems with over-monitoring rather than a Frithian failure of monitoring, at least in regard to interrupting and sending the narrative back to "how it all started." In effect, this kind of narrative demonstrates problems with all four cognitive capacities related to the formation of self-narrative (Table 5.1).

Such disruptions of narrative competency both reflect and contribute to the broader disruptions in the patient's self-pattern. Although schizophrenics are able to use the first-person pronoun in a way that anchors their self-narrative to themselves, they sometimes have problems with self-attribution and the sense of agency for their actions. They attribute such actions to other agents as causes, and this is reflected in the content of their self-narratives. Structural problems in the self-narrative are apparent when schizophrenics cannot maintain the serial order or temporal perspective for life events. Essential structures of the narrative process having to do with sequential plot and perspectival time frames are disrupted in important ways. Even if such temporal frameworks remain intact, however, problems with autobiographical memory may deprive the subject of the proper or adequate content with which to fill such frames. The lack of structure and/or content may motivate the overactivation of a reflective metacognition that is ordinarily at work in the explicit construction of narrative. It is not the case that in schizophrenia metacognition simply ceases. Indeed, it may become hyperreflexive and lead to the confabulation of unusual self-narratives. Failures in some or in all of these areas help to explain the problems that schizophrenic subjects have in constructing a self-narrative.

5.7 Narrative as a Forensic Tool: The Case of Borderline Personality Disorder

Borderline personality disorder (BPD) is another complex disorder that presents a challenge for any psychiatric analysis that seeks an integrative explanation. BPD involves a disintegrated self-narrative, a form of "self-fragmentation" (Fuchs 2007, 381) or "identity diffusion" (Baptista et al. 2020, 5; Kernberg 1985; Jørgensen 2006; Jørgensen et al. 2012) where the person's experienced identity changes from

Table 5.1 Correlations among phenomenological aspects, cognitive problems, neurological dysfunctions, and narrative effects in schizophrenia

Self-narrative in schizophrenia	Phenomenology	Cognitive problems	Neurological dysfunction	Narrative effects
Temporal structure	Curtailed future perspective; derailed temporal order; impairment of self-temporalization	Dysfunction of working memory; slowed cognitive processing; breakdown of semantic binding	Prefrontal dysfunction	Lack of internal concordance; lack of temporal perspective as narrator; fragmented self-narrative
Minimal self-reference	Lack of sense of self-agency; thought insertion, delusions of control, and auditory hallucinations	Dysfunction of *forward* comparator and preaction processes; 'who' system	Abnormal pre-movement brain potentials in SMA, premotor, and prefrontal cortices	Misattribution of agency; objective misidentification
Autobiographical memory	Difficulties remembering past personal events; incomplete and fleeting memories	Encoding and retrieval problems	Reduced hippocampal activation during retrieval; hyperactivation of prefrontal areas	Impoverished content; incoherent contexts
Metacognition	Focus on normally tacit dimensions; attention problems; introverted reflection	Hyperreflection; problems with self-monitoring	Overactivation of left-hemisphere "interpreter"	Confabulated narratives; "sick" narratives

Source: Gallagher (2003).

one situation to another. The fragmented self-narrative does not stand simply on its own as the primary explanation, even if at some times narrative distance between narrator and narrated self appears to be absolute, a complete "rupture in narrative processes" (Schmidt & Fuchs 2020, 2). Rather, self-narrative clearly reflects disorders of the self-pattern, as specified by Philipp Schmidt (2021), who argues that BPD involves four kinds of "intertwined" instabilities pertaining to reflective capacity, affectivity, intersubjectivity, and bodily self-experience.

First, the fragmentation interferes with one's ability to gain distance from the present moment or to reflect on past events or future possibilities, a "severe disturbance in reflective processes" that makes it difficult to keep an orderly perspective on the meaning of present experience (Schmidt 2021, 210). This is a disruption to the temporal structure of reflective self-narrative generating an experience of discontinuity. Second, affectivity, in this situation, becomes unstable, characterized by emotion dysregulation and the experience of intense emotions (anger and pain cycling to dysphoria and reactive apathy), coupled with a lack of "affective self-knowledge" (Schmidt 2021, 212ff.; also see Ratcliffe & Bortolan 2020). A third instability, intertwined with the first two, involves some complex modifications in intersubjective relations, where others are perceived as threats, and as possible targets of manipulation, with some blurring of self–other boundaries (Schmidt 2021, 218ff.; also see Bilek et al. 2017 for how these dynamics manifest in lower cross-brain connectivity):

> Those with BPD diagnoses tend to inhabit a world that is lacking in cohesive, practically meaningful structure, where that structure depends on habitually entrenched, integrated and fairly stable sets of concerns. Moreover, they struggle to relate to other people in ways that are essential to the sustenance of such concerns. So it would be misleading to conceive of emotion dysregulation as something that arises in isolation from one's wider relationship with the social world.
> (Ratcliffe & Bortolan 2020, 178)

Finally, BPD involves a diminishment of or alienation from bodily self-experience, or "disrupted body experiences" which blur the boundaries between self and non-self (Baptista et al. 2020, 7, 10), and which Schmidt suggests is a "concomitant condition of instability in [reflective] identity, affect and the interpersonal" (2021, 224). Reflecting dynamical and holistic relations among these various aspects of the self-pattern, Schmidt emphasizes that these instabilities are "structurally intertwined" and thus "far from being a mere accidental amalgamation of different forms of instabilities" (225).[8]

Baptista et al. (2020) hypothesize that all of the disruptions found in BPD derive from a disturbed complex experience of agency. One would need to do

---

[8] Likewise, Ratcliffe and Bortolan (2020, 180–1) describe an integrated set of effects inextricably linking affect with body, agentive projects, intersubjectivity, and norms, society, and culture.

further empirical interventions to show whether this is the right way to think of the dynamics of the self-pattern in this case, but the review by Baptista et al. provides evidence that at the very least there are correlations between disturbed sense of agency and the other processes that are disrupted in the self-pattern in BPD. There is also evidence that the lack of the sense of agency in BPD is accompanied by a lack of narrative coherence (Adler et al. 2012). These disturbed processes also correlate to ecological disruptions—including environmental, economic, and early social factors (e.g., household instability, physical violence, sexual abuse) during development. These researchers suggest that to gain a full understanding of BPD, one needs to take an interdisciplinary approach that brings together studies in evolutionary biology, social cognition and psychopathology, and life history.

Two points follow from such attempts to map the variety of hypothetical links between disruptions in bodily processes, affect, self-narrative, intersubjectivity, the sense of agency, ecological factors, long-term development, and life history in BPD. First, the concept of a self-pattern can helpfully show how these disparate factors might in fact link up, providing a broadly integrative approach which goes beyond simply trying to piece together multiple disciplines and methodologies that tend to address these factors separately. The interventionist and dynamical systems approach outlined in Chapter 3 may provide the methodological tools for empirical studies in this area. Second, given the importance of the ecological-developmental aspects of life history, the examination of self-narratives may offer an important forensic tool for diagnosis and therapy.

Importantly, there is a more central point that finds clarification here. Although we may be able to treat the self-narrative as a forensic tool, as we have indicated before, as part of the self-pattern it is also more than that. Here we can specify the significance of it being more than a reflection of disorders in the self-pattern. The specific kind of disruption in self-narrative associated with BPD is something that the subject suffers. As Schmidt and Fuchs (2020, 1) put it, individuals with BPD "suffer from recurrent feelings of emptiness, a lack of self-feeling, and painful incoherence, especially regarding their own desires, how they see and feel about others, their life goals, or the roles to which they commit themselves." Such disturbances in narrative processes involve a painful form of self-experience.

This leads to a stronger claim, namely, that a disruption of self-narrative is not simply a sign or symptom of the disorder, it is a constitutive part of BPD. More generally, a disruption in self-narrative, or a disruption in any of the processes that constitute the self-pattern, is not simply a sign of a particular psychopathology that underpins such phenomena, it *is* the psychopathology, or part of what constitutes the disorder. In this regard, we can reject both the kind of strict naturalism that would claim a disorder to be a natural kind (some essential thing that exists independently of the subject's experience or self-pattern), and the loose relativism that would hold it to be a mere socially constructed interpretation.

6

Phenomenological Anchors

Mapping Experiences of Agency and Ownership

In Chapter 5, I proposed a way to think of the agentive person as the systemic whole enacted in the processes and dynamical connections of the self-pattern, an embodied agent capable of bodily actions, intersubjective interactions, social engagement, and cultural practices, a person who has affective/emotional experiences, and is capable of cognition, reflection, and narrative. As Scott Kelso puts it, "The emergence of [a] self is a disorder-order transition in the coordination dynamics" (Kelso 2020). What emerges is clearly an agent that is more than just a body or a narrative. In this chapter I want to explore some of the complex elements in the phenomenology of the self-pattern—the experiences of agency and ownership.[1] Our awareness of our own agency is phenomenologically complex, involving various kinds of intentions and experiences, for example, prereflective experiential aspects tied to sensory-motor processing, as well as reflective orders of intention formation and retrospective judgment. I intend to map out how the experience of agency is interwoven with the experience of ownership and other elements of the self-pattern. The way that various complex contributory elements manifest themselves in such experiences demonstrates a variety of dynamical connections. Such connections can break down in psychiatric disorders, and we can find instances of a missing or reduced sense of agency in such cases. As part of this analysis I also want to highlight the importance of how experiences of agency and ownership relate to social and intersubjective processes. Embodied action happens in a world that is physical and social and often reflects perceptual and affective valences. The effects of a variety of forces and affordances that are both physical and social contribute to the complex dynamics of the experiences of agency and ownership.

---

[1] Not only complex, but philosophically controversial. As we'll see in the following sections, there is no unanimous agreement about the sense of agency or the sense of ownership—how they manifest or fail to manifest in psychopathology, for example, or even whether there are such experiences. Although I'll be endorsing a phenomenological view, supported by a growing number of neuroscientific studies, I'll discuss, or at least note, dissenting views.

The Self and its Disorders. Shaun Gallagher, Oxford University Press. © Shaun Gallagher 2024.
DOI: 10.1093/oso/9780198873068.003.0007

6.1 Complexities in the Phenomenology of Bodily Movement

In a variety of studies over the past twenty years, experiences of agency and ownership have been shown to be phenomenologically complex, involving different factors, from a basic sense of agency connected with sensory-motor processing (e.g., Farrer et al. 2003; Tsakiris & Haggard 2005; Tsakiris, Bosbach & Gallagher 2007), to the more complex cognitive accomplishments of intention formation and retrospective judgment (e.g., Gallagher 2012a; Pacherie 2006; 2007a; Stephens & Graham 2000; Synofzik, Vosgerau & Newen 2008).

The prereflective sense of agency (SA) and sense of ownership (SO) can be distinguished in the experiential aspects of the self-pattern. The SO for movement is the sense that I am the one who is undergoing the movement—that it is *my* movement or *my* body moving, whether the movement is voluntary or involuntary. When I engage in intentional action, SA is the experience that I am the one who is causing or generating the action (Gallagher 2000a; 2000b). SA is missing in the case of involuntary movement, but I still have SO for such movement. If I am physically pushed, for example, I still have the sense that I am the one moving, even if I did not cause the movement. These experiences are prereflective, which means that they do not depend on the subject taking an introspective reflective attitude. Nor do they require that the subject engage in an explicit perceptual monitoring of bodily movements. Just as, in most everyday situations, I do not attend to the details of my own bodily movements as I am engaged in action, neither my SA nor SO is something that I attend to, or something of which I am explicitly aware. As such, SA and SO are phenomenologically recessive. Indeed, this recessiveness motivates some abstract philosophical puzzlement, as nicely expressed by Wittgenstein: "[W]hen 'I raise my arm', my arm goes up. And the problem arises: what is left over if I subtract the fact that my arm goes up from the fact that I raise my arm?" (1953, §621). Despite the "thin and elusive" character in the phenomenology of volition, Frith and Haggard nonetheless suggest an answer: "we have a vivid sense of agency—the experience of controlling the world through our actions" (2018, 405).

The case of involuntary movement provides a good clue about the (neuro) physiological processes that correlate with these self-experiences. In the case of an initial involuntary movement, I experience the movement as my own (SO), but do not experience self-agency for it. My SO correlates with reafferent sensory feedback (visual and proprioceptive/kinaesthetic information that tells me that I'm moving). In both involuntary and voluntary movement SO is generated by this sensory feedback. The contrast between voluntary and involuntary movement registers the presence (in the case of the former) or absence (in the case of the latter) of initial motor commands (efferent signals). This suggests that in the case of voluntary movement efferent signals may play some role in generating the prereflective SA (Tsakiris & Haggard 2005).

Sensory suppression experiments (Tsakiris & Haggard 2003) suggest that SA arises at an early efferent stage in the initiation of action, that is, in processes anterior to actual bodily movement. Experiments with subjects who lack proprioception but still experience a sense of effort reinforce this conclusion (Lafargue et al. 2003; see Gallagher & Cole 1995; Marcel 2003). Tsakiris, Longo, and Haggard (2010) found independent activations in midline cortical structures correlated with SO, but absent for SA; and activation in the pre-SMA linked to SA, but absent for SO. Although this finding supports an "independence" model, where SA and SO are understood to be two "qualitatively different experiences, triggered by different inputs, and recruiting distinct brain networks" (Tsakiris, Longo & Haggard 2010, 2740), there is behavioral and phenomenological, and further neurological evidence for a more integrative model where SA and SO are strongly related (e.g., Caspar, Cleeremans & Haggard 2015). In this respect, an intervention on SA may have an effect on SO, and vice versa, and this supports the idea that the phenomenology of most of our everyday actions does not always reflect a clear experiential distinction between agency and ownership. Their integration in the minimal experiential aspect of the self-pattern is relatively tight (see Liesner, Hinz & Kunde [2021] for review).

As I continue my action, efferent signals and motor control processes, including afferent feedback from my movement, contribute to an ongoing, albeit phenomenologically recessive SA. I have an experience of *what* I am doing, framed in terms of my intentional goal, rather than of any details of *how* I am doing it, for example, what muscles I am using. My goal or intention, what I am trying to accomplish, constrains my body-schematic (motor control) processes and the motor intentionality that keeps me attuned to the world. In this respect SA includes a basic sense of what I am accomplishing in the world. A number of experiments help to distinguish between the purely motor control aspects of SA and the intentional aspects, that is, the most immediate and perceptually based sense that I am having an effect on my immediate environment (Farrer & Frith 2002). In this respect, SA already has a prereflective complexity.

6.2 Deflating the Senses of Ownership and Agency

Let me head off one worry about understanding the phenomenology of SA and SO as dimensions of prereflective experience. Several philosophers have lined up to criticize the notion of a prereflective sense of self, including the idea that there is a prereflective SA or SO (e.g., Bermúdez 2011; 2017; Dainton 2008; 2016; Di Francesco, Marraffa & Paternoster 2016; Grünbaum 2010; see Gallagher 2017b for a response). Generally speaking, these critics take the phenomenological conception of prereflective experience to be inflationary.

Barry Dainton (2008), for example, in his discussion of what he terms the "isolation thesis," that is, the idea that there could be just one isolated bodily sensation (for example, a pain), takes issue with the phenomenological concept of prereflective self-awareness. He contends that, typically, in contrast to the isolation thesis, when I experience some sensation, I experience it "against the backdrop of various other forms of consciousness: a range of bodily experience, tactile sensations, visual and auditory experience, intentional or willed bodily movements, conscious thinking...[etc.]" (2008, 239–40). This recessive backdrop of experience, to which we are not attending when we attend to the pain, he calls the "phenomenal background." This background consists of two regions—a worldly region where I experience, for example, in exteroception, the sights and sounds around me, and an "inner" region, an elusive set of bodily experiences, thoughts, memories, and so on. He suggests that this inner aspect of the phenomenal background contributes to (and perhaps constitutes) "the feeling of what it is typically like to be me (or you)" (240). This inner background may be relatively stable, as Dainton suggests, but it does not consist of a particular kind of sensation or feeling. Specifically, he argues, it does not consist of a prereflective self-awareness or sense of mineness or ownership.

> I can see no reason to take this stability as indicative of a single special type of experience, something over and above the changing stream of thought, perception, volition, emotion, memory, bodily sensation, and so on.   (240)

He argues that if we subtract all of these various experiences, there would be nothing of experience left; therefore, there is nothing over and above just these experiences—no extra or additional experience that we would identify as the experience of mineness. Rather, he suggests, the "ambient sense of self" is something like the product of all of these experiences. This phenomenal background is always something of which we are co-conscious, but always something precisely in the background, and of which we are not explicitly aware. It's this ubiquitous presence of the phenomenal background, this ambient sense of self, that makes it impossible to imagine an "ownerless" isolated pain sensation.

Although Dainton takes this argument to be an objection to the phenomenological claim that there is a particular form of self-awareness, of the "nonreflexive" variety, that is always implicit in experience (Gallagher & Zahavi 2020; 2021), his account seems to be an expression of the very same phenomenon. Dainton denies anything like an additional experience of mineness, over and above the phenomenal background he describes. Two things follow from his analysis. "First, we can account for the phenomenology of mineness without positing any primitive 'ownership' quality" (243). And second, "our sense of self is not the product of a single simple form of experience, but rather the joint product of several different sorts of (quite ordinary) experiences" (243). Dainton, then, does not deny that there is a sense of mineness (SO), but just that it is a separate or additional quality, added to the phenomenal background.

It's difficult to see how this would count against the phenomenological concept of SO, since the phenomenologists, including Zahavi and myself, describe the sense of mineness as an *intrinsic* aspect of experience, not as something extra that is added, or an additional quality that one experiences in addition to experiencing pain, or bodily sensations, or thinking, and so forth. As Zahavi puts it, "Whether a certain experience is experienced as mine or not, however, depends not on something apart from the experience, but precisely on the givenness of the experience" (2005, 124). That is, SO and SA are features that are instrinsic to the structure of our experiences:

> Experience happens for the experiencing subject in an immediate way and as part of this immediacy, it is implicitly marked as my experience…[P]rereflec-tive self-consciousness is prereflective in the sense that (1) it is an awareness we have before we do any reflecting on our experience; (2) it is an implicit and first-order awareness…The mineness in question is not a quality like being scarlet, sour or soft. It doesn't refer to a specific experiential content, to a specific what; nor does it refer to the diachronic or synchronic sum of such content, or to some other relation that might obtain between the contents in question. Rather, it refers to the distinct givenness or the how it feels of experience…That prereflec-tive self-awareness is implicit, then, means that I am not confronted with a the-matic or explicit awareness of the experience as belonging to myself. Rather we are dealing with a non-observational self-acquaintance.
>
> (Gallagher & Zahavi 2020)

Michael Martin (1995), focusing on the sense of body-ownership, understands the SO for bodily sensations to depend on a sense of one's spatial boundaries. According to Martin, "when one feels a sensation, one thereby feels as if some-thing is occurring within one's body" (267). This is not a matter of explicit judg-ment, as if I were experiencing a free-floating sensation and then judging its spatial location as falling within my body boundaries. Rather, according to Martin, the experience of location is an intrinsic feature of the sensation itself. This experience depends on the SO for one's body as a whole; that is, the SO for a particular body part depends on it being a part of that whole body (1995, 277–8). In this regard, SO is not a quality in addition to other qualities of bodily experi-ence, but "already inherent within them" (278). This can be viewed as consistent with the phenomenological view where SO is an intrinsic aspect of

proprioceptive and kinaesthetic experiences of bodily position sense and movement, and other bodily sensations.[2]

Similar to Dainton, and in contrast to Martin (1995, 267), José Louis Bermúdez
(2011; 2017), rejects the idea that SO is a "special phenomenological relation,"
and denies that there is a positive first-order (non-observational) phenomenology of ownership or feeling of "mineness." He thus offers a deflationary account,
in contrast to what he calls "inflationary" phenomenological conceptions:

> On a deflationary conception of ownership the sense of ownership consists, first,
> in certain facts about the phenomenology of bodily sensations and, second, in
> certain fairly obvious judgments about the body (which we can term judgments
> of ownership).   (Bermúdez 2011, 162)

According to this deflationary view an explicit experience of ownership only
comes about when we turn our reflective attention to our bodily experience and
attribute that experience to ourselves. His claim that there is a phenomenology of
ownership such that "[w]hen we experience our bodies we experience them as
our own…" (Bermúdez 2015, 38) means that there is a *second-order* phenomenology of ownership derived from the judgment of ownership. A second-order,
reflective experience of ownership results only as a product of this judgment, but
it is not something that is there to begin with. "There are facts about the phenomenology of bodily awareness (about position sense, movement sense, and interoception) and there are judgments of ownership, but there is no additional feeling
of ownership" (Bermúdez 2011, 166). Accordingly, he regards the prereflective
SO as a philosophical fiction. Although one does experience a sense of body
boundedness and connectedness, one does not experience, in addition, SO as a
separate and independent feeling.

The response to Bermúdez has to be the same as the response to Dainton. On
the phenomenological view, to say that SO is an intrinsic aspect of proprioceptive
and kinaesthetic experiences is to agree that it is not an additional or independent
feeling, but rather, a sense "already inherent within" the phenomenology of bodily
sensations, an intrinsic aspect that is prereflectively there without having to make
a reflective judgment about ownership. Isn't this just the deflationary account that
Bermúdez is looking for—one that does not posit an additional feeling, or "perfectly determinate 'quale' associated with the feeling of myness" (Bermúdez 2011,
165), independent of proprioceptive and kinaesthetic sensations, or, for that matter, the necessity of a reflective judgement? Indeed, this is what Jerome Dokic

---

[2] Frederique de Vignemont (2017) considers cases in which there is no SO for a bodily limb
although sensations may register on that limb. In such cases, for example, somatoparaphrenia and
deafferentation, it is important to note that proprioception/kinaesthesia is missing (Gallagher & Cole
1995; Vallar & Ronchi 2009). This means that for a more precise characterization of SO in terms of
body boundaries, one should define such boundaries as proprioceptive.

(2003) endorses in an account that Bermúdez identifies as deflationary. "Bodily experience gives us a *sense of ownership*... The very idea of *feeling* a pain in a limb which does not seem to be ours is difficult to frame, perhaps unintelligible" (Dokic 2003, 325). This just is a prereflective experiential SO, an intrinsic aspect of experience that makes first-person bodily (proprioceptive, kinaesthetic) aware-ness itself (i.e., prior to any judgment) a form of self-consciousness. It's what puts the "proprio" in proprioception (Gallagher & Trigg 2016).

Parallel to such critiques about SO, Thor Grünbaum (2015) offers a detailed critique of the notion of the sense of agency (SA), drawing a similar conclusion, namely that there is no separate and distinct prereflective SA that acts as the basis for a judgment about agency. "One can accept that there are conscious mental states or processes that are proprietary to action, such as practical deliberation, practical decision-making and intending, without accepting that there is a special phenomenal feeling associated with motor control" (2015, 3314). Grünbaum's analysis is focused on accounts of SA that make it the experiential product of comparator mechanisms involved in motor control. Although he doesn't deny the possibility that a comparator mechanism may be involved in motor control, he challenges the idea that such subpersonal mechanisms can generate a distinct experience of agency.[3]

Grünbaum also sees a problem in the way the concept of SA is used in experi-mental designs. Experiments attempting to understand problems with SA in schizophrenia (he cites Daprati et al. 1997),[4] or, using a similar experimental paradigm, to identify the neural correlates of SA (e.g., Farrer & Frith 2002) involve asking subjects to distinguish between actions they cause in contrast to actions caused by someone else. In Farrer and Frith, for example, for each trial the subject performs a hand movement to control a joystick, which in turn controls movement on a computer screen. According to Grünbaum, if SA is generated by motor control processes, the motor processes involved in the hand movement should generate SA for each action, and that should remain constant across all trials. Yet subjects who are moving the joystick seemingly fail to experience self-agency in those cases where movement on the computer screen is caused by

---

[3] Grünbaum interprets the claim that SA is generated by such subpersonal processes to mean that SA is intention-free. That is, on such accounts, SA would be generated even if the agent had not for-mulated a prior, personal intention to act in a certain way. Reaching for my beer as I watch the football game, however, does not require that I consciously deliberate and form a plan to do so, although it still counts as an intentional action and certainly involves a motor intention and a present intention (or intention-in-action) (see Pacherie 2006; 2007a). Indeed, comparator models include the idea that there is a functional element in the system that correlates with intention. The comparator process just is the comparison of this intentional element with efference copy or sensory input from the movement to facilitate motor control (e.g., Frith 1992). In this respect it's not clear that SA should be character-ized as intention-free.

[4] Daprati et al. (1997) show that subjects mistook the actions of the other person as their own in about 30% of the cases; schizophrenic subjects with a history of delusions of control and/or hallucin-ations misjudged 50–77% of the cases.

someone else. Grünbaum thinks there is a confusion here about SA. I think he's right, but it's a confusion that leads to a better explanation.

Farrer and Frith, despite endorsing the idea that SA is generated in motor control processes, argue that SA varies depending on whether subjects felt they were in control of what was happening on the computer screen. What this suggests, however, is that the prereflective SA is more complex than an experience generated by motor control processes. Specifically, SA involves at least two aspects—one having to do with the control of bodily movement in action, and one having to do with the intentional aspect of the action, that is, my awareness of what the action accomplishes in the world. As this and other experiments (see e.g., Haggard 2005; Kalckert & Ehrsson 2012; Moore, Wegner & Haggard 2009) show, this depends on a sensory-motor integration ("cue integration" or an integration of perceptual, proprioceptive, and efferent processes, reflected in the activation of integration areas which Farrer and Frith [2002, 602] identify as the anterior insula).[5] Indeed, such integration processes suggest that in action contexts there is a complex meshing of motor control and intentional aspect, as well as a meshing of SO and SA in their shared proprioceptive dynamics (Gallagher 2005; 2012b).[6]

Grünbaum may be right about comparator mechanisms; there are in fact good reasons to question whether comparator models offer the best explanation of SA. Still, SA may be generated in processes that integrate motor control and perceptual monitoring of what our actions are accomplishing in the world. One alternative to the comparator model is Peter Langland-Hassan's (2008) explanation in terms of filtering models (also see Friston 2011; Synofzik, Vosgerau & Newen 2008; Bu-Omer et al. 2021). Although Langland-Hassan (2008) also raises worries about the positive phenomenology of SA, similar to Dainton's worries about SO, he concludes that the phenomenology of agency is "one that is embedded in all first order sensory and proprioceptive phenomenology as diachronic, action-sensitive patterns of information; it does not stand apart from them as an inscrutable emotion" (392).

Despite concerns raised about prereflective SO and SA, in the end the critics reinforce the point I want to take from the phenomenological account, and from what we can learn from neuroscientific experiments, namely, that SA and SO are

---

[5] The idea that the intentional aspect of action (i.e., what the agent accomplishes in the world) contributes to SA, and in some cases dominates over motor control processes, is clearly demonstrated in experiments that intervene on the interactions between agent and the physical environment (the use of tools and artifacts). Di Plinio et al. (2019) used intentional binding as an implicit measure of SA (Haggard, Clark & Kalogeras 2002; Moore & Obhi 2012; Dewey & Knoblich 2014; see Figure 6.1) and showed a decrease in SA, approaching psychosis-like experiences, in some cases when interactions with instruments were automated. In schizophrenia SA fails for the most part due to noisier and less reliable motor processes; subjects then compensate by a greater weighting of external cues (Synofzik et al. 2010; Voss et al. 2010).

[6] See Meyer & Hunnius (2021) for an interesting study of SA in early infancy and the importance of temporality in the dynamics of sensorimotor processes. For more on the dynamical processes involved in SA, see Gallagher (2020a, §2.3).

dynamically integrated with the experiential aspects of bodily existence. This is an integration, not of added features, but of intrinsic relations. As I'll argue in the following sections, this kind of dynamical integration also extends to other factors of the self-pattern, including reflective, psychological/cognitive, and narrative factors.

6.3 Reflective Judgments and Narratives about Agency

For some theorists the experience of agency is closely tied to self-narrative. Graham and Stephens (1994; Stephens & Graham 2000) understand the experience of agency to depend on whether the subject experiences her actions and thoughts as consistent with her self-understanding or self-narrative. In discussing the schizophrenic symptom of thought insertion, their focus is on having a particular thought or belief. We can conceive of thinking itself to be a kind of action, and accordingly, I take this account to extend to delusions of control, which involve bodily movement, as well. For Graham and Stephens, agency is understood in terms of "our proclivity for constructing self-referential narratives" which allow us to explain our behavior retrospectively: "such explanations amount to a sort of theory of the person's agency or intentional psychology" (1994, 101; Stephens & Graham 2000, 161):

> [W]hether I take myself to be the agent of a mental episode depends upon whether I take the occurrence of this episode to be explicable in terms of my underlying intentional states.   (1994, 93)

To the extent that someone perceives her action or introspects her thought as not being consistent with her self-narrative, she does not experience agency for it. Whether this explains thought insertion or delusions of control, there does seem to be a connection between the experience (the sense and/or the attribution) of self-agency and self-narrative.

Graham and Stephens are not alone. Bortolotti and Broome (2009), also addressing the question of thought insertion, hold a related view, although they consider the problem to be one of ownership rather than agency. Bortolotti and Broome, however, clarify the more general theoretical background concerning the link between agency and/or ownership, and narrative.[7] Narrative allows for the possibility of giving reasons, and, on their view, thought insertion involves a

---

[7] Bortolotti (2010) makes a clearer distinction between authorship and ownership, and seemingly associates authorship with agency (or at least control). "A subject can gain control over her attitudes by deliberation, when she forms an attitude on the basis of reasons that are regarded by the subject as her best reasons for endorsing its content; or justification, when she defends the content of her attitude on the basis of reasons that she takes to be her best reasons. In these circumstances, the subject

"failure to ascribe to oneself and give reasons for a first-personally accessed and reported thought" (2009, 18):

> Subjects with thought insertion do not have any difficulty in satisfying the intro-spection condition [they are able to introspect the thought], but they do not feel entitled to the thought they can introspect and struggle in making it an integral part of their own self narrative and self image.   (2009, 18)

Despite their interpretation of the issue in terms of ownership, their conclusion comes out of a tradition of equating agency with authorship, where authorship means something like authoring one's own narrative. "There is a sense in which people are the authors of a story that they recognize as a story about themselves. The implications of these self narratives have been related to metaphysical ques-tions about the nature of the self" (2009, 4). Bortolotti and Broome cite David Velleman (2005; 2007) who emphasizes the prospective function of narrative, and its importance in the formation of self-identity and the autonomous formation of intention.

Richard Moran also connects this notion of authorship with deliberation and intention formation, which depend on reasoning and being able to give reasons for believing something or for acting in some way. "Thus a person able to exercise this capacity is in a position to declare what his belief is by reflection on the reasons in favor of that belief, rather than by examination of the psychological evidence. In this way [...] avowal [or endorsement] can be seen as an expression of genuine self-knowledge" (Moran 2004, 425). The important point here is that for someone to be considered an author or agent of a particular propositional attitude or a particular action, she is "expected to be in a position to offer some justification," to be able to give reasons for believing something or acting in some way, and thereby to endorse the belief or action. If a thought or action does not fit with one's reasoned narrative, if one cannot give any reasons for having that thought, or doing that action, then one is not the author of it—and since author-ship is equated with agency, one is not the agent. Or for Bertolotti and Broome, one is not the owner of the thought. Thought insertion, on this view, is a failure of endorsement (2009, 15), and ultimately, perhaps, a failure of narrative.

More generally, and outside of the debate about schizophrenic symptoms, this same connection between narrative authorship and agency can be found in Schechtman's view which emphasizes the idea that narrative constitutes the self. Narrative in this sense is what makes us agentive selves:

can ascribe an attitude to herself on the basis of an act of authorship" (210–11). The sense of agency for an action seemingly derives from the reflective act of authoring a justification for the action.

At a general level, we can see that a person needs a narrative self-conception in order to be an agent at all... The kind of psychological organization that makes an individual a person on the narrative self-constitution view is precisely the kind required for being an agent.   (1996, 159)

Again, the idea is that a particular action needs to fit into a person's self-narrative in the right way for that person to be an agent with respect to it. Intelligibility thus becomes the criterion for agency:

The more an action seems to stem from a coherent and stable pattern of values, desires, goals, and character traits, the more it seems under a person's control. When a person's action is anomalous or inexplicable in terms of the rest of her experience and psyche, it seems less likely that the impetus for it comes from her...   (159)

Reflective or narrative attribution may seem an overly intellectualized way of thinking about agency, emphasizing the semantic content of thought and narrative, and downplaying the processual action-specific experiential aspects of agency—the idea that I have an experience of agency implicit in action or in the process of thinking. Nonetheless, it points to the relevant role of reflection and narrative, and makes it clear that narrative involves a reflection on action, and also that it is structured in a way that reflects action and agency.

Regarding the relation between action and narrative, it's important to get clear on the order of things. For example, there are some theorists who argue for a strong integration of action and narrative. Thus, Bruner writes: "Narrative structure is even inherent in the praxis of social interaction before it achieves linguistic expression" (1990, 77; also see e.g., Halliday 1978). In some therapeutic settings, one finds a similar claim about "body narrative," not in the sense of a narrative about a body (as in e.g., Charon 2006; Ling & Liu 2008; Scholz 2000) but in the sense of the body generating narrative through its movement. These are considered "nonverbal narratives... the body telling its stories on its own nonlinear and nonverbal terms... [C]onscious body movements generate a fluid, nonverbal narration of self and identity no less important than the verbal stories we may tell" (Caldwell 2014, 89). In the therapeutic practice the aim is to restore the feeling of self-authorship. Elsewhere I've argued that although we can enact a narrative through bodily movement, much in the way that an actor can act out a scene, this does not mean that action itself has a narrative structure or that narrative is inherent in action (see Gallagher 2020a; Gallagher & Hutto 2019, in contrast to Erskine 2014; Delafield-Butt & Trevarthen 2015). Action is different from narrative. One difference is that narratives involve a reflective process that introduces a distinction between the reflecting and that which is reflected (see the discussion of narrative distance in Section 5.4). Furthermore, all of the bodily processes involved in actions and interactions—movement, gesture, intonation, affect, and so on—if *evidenced* in a reflective narrative, are not fully expressed in the narrative. The attempt to express them all in narrative would issue in a narrative longer than, yet still not as detailed as the action itself. Moreover, because the temporal structure of narrative is quite linear, it is difficult to represent the full richness of the contemporaneous situation in narrative. Narrative is selective so that some things always have to be left unsaid, while other things have to be repeated. For example, to narrate in any detail actions that happen simultaneously, one has to narrative them successively.

The structure of embodied activity itself is not essentially or already narrative in nature. Rather, we should say that embodied activity is structured in a way that naturally lends itself to narration. Accordingly, it is no accident that what counts as a faithful narrative about such activity should replicate or approximate that structure. On this view, embodied actions have a pre-narrative, albeit narrative-ready structure (Kerby 1993; Hutto 2006). Richard Menary captures this precisely: "[o]ur embodied experiences are ready to be exploited in a narrative of those experiences. Narrative arises from a sequence of bodily experiences, perceptions and actions in a quite natural manner" (2008, 75). Action does have a structure, but it is not at all clear that it has a narrative structure. To put things in the right order, we should say that the structure of narrative derives from and reflects the structure of action, rather than vice versa. As Ricoeur puts it, it is not "that practices as such contain ready-made narrative scenarios, but their organization gives them a prenarrative quality..." (1992, 157).

Granted this, we also have to say that the dynamics that operate between narrative and agency are not one-way. There is a reciprocal relation between narrative and action. Narratives do not simply report sequences of events or actions. As Catriona MacKenzie rightly suggests, when narratives explain the connections between actions they recount, "they give shape and coherence to our lives, or at least to the various sequences that make up our lives..." (2007, 268–9), and they inform future actions, providing motivational, normative, and intentional connections in the "space of reasons." This is what the authorship idea is trying to get at. This is what Ian Hacking (1995a) calls a "looping effect." Our actions, in some cases, come to be guided by narratives, which prospectively can enter into intention formation through reflective practices. In addition, more implicitly, narratives, to the extent that they reflect norms and customs as well as personal experiences, may start to inform our behaviors without our being aware of it. My actions, my affordances, what I can do, what my possibilities are, are shaped by the effects of my own narrative and my normative understanding of what is possible.

It is in this sense that narrative not only reflects, but contributes to, by being part of, the self-pattern. This is why, as we've seen, disturbances in narrative processes can involve a painful form of self-experience, as in individuals with BPD

Table 6.1 Prereflective and reflective aspects of the experience of agency and ownership

Experience	Pre-reflective (Gallagher 2000)	Reflective (Stephens & Graham 2000)
Agency (authorship)	*Sense of agency*—as I act or think, the prereflective *experience* that I am the cause/initiator of my action or thinking, and have some control over it	*Attribution of agency*—the reflective (retrospective) attribution or *judgment* that an action or a thought was caused by me.
Ownership (subjectivity, my-ness or mineness)	*Sense of ownership*—the pre-reflective *experience* that I am moving (or keeping still) or thinking—that the movement, action, or thinking is mine.	*Attribution of subjectivity*—the reflective (retrospective) realization or *judgment* that I am the one who moved or had a specific thought.

Note: Terminology varies from one theorist to another. Sometimes a distinction is made between agency and authorship, and sometimes these are treated as equivalent terms. Likewise, SO is sometimes equated with a sense of subjectivity (a sense that I am living through an experience), and sometimes with a feeling of mineness (this is my experience).

Source: From Gallagher (2020a, 50).

(Section 5.7). When things go well, however, my self-narrative can add coherence to the self-pattern to the extent that it pulls together my actions, my sense of agency, my reflective abilities, the affordances offered by the environment, the normative forces that constrain my life, and my intersubjective relations.

In addition to prereflective experiences of agency and ownership, then, one can reflectively (and retrospectively) attribute agency and ownership to oneself based on a judgment about one's first-order experience or action (Synofzik, Vosgerau & Newen 2008; see Table 6.1). What sort of criterion does one use to make a judgment about one's agency? The most straight-forward possibility is that one simply uses a phenomenological criterion. That is, I judge that I am the agent of a certain act if I prereflectively experience SA while engaged in that action. Alternatively, as Graham and Stephens suggest, one might use a criterion of consistency between one's actions and one's beliefs, desires, or self-narrative:

> Whether I count something as my action thus depends upon whether I take myself to have beliefs and desires of the sort that would rationalize its occurrence in me. If my theory of myself ascribes to me the relevant intentional states, I unproblematically regard this episode as my action. If not, then I must either revise my picture of my intentional states or refuse to acknowledge the episode as my doing.   (Graham & Stephens 1994, 93, 102)

Although it is possible that I can be engaged in action while on automatic pilot, which may still involve a prereflective SA for that action, it is also possible that my prereflective SA for my current engagement in a particular action may coincide temporally with an ongoing reflection about what I am doing or how I am doing it. My reflection may be of different sorts and different degrees. It may be finely attuned to detailed particulars about the action or action context. For example, in various types of athletic performance, one may need to attend and act strategic-ally to take into account the precise situation (the layout of the field, the position of other players, the speed of the ball, and so forth). This would not entail a heavy introspective type of reflection, but it may involve something more than just per-ceptual monitoring or being aware *that* one is doing something (see Christensen, Sutton & McIlwain 2016).

Graham and Stephens describe a heavier type of reflection where I might be considering whether I ought to be doing what I'm doing, or what the implications of my action are. They link it to "our proclivity for constructing self-referential narratives" (1994, 101). Do my intentions and actions and their consequences line up with the type of person I think I am? Do they fit my self-conception or self-narrative? This type of reflection may happen after the fact, *retrospectively*. I may engage in some action spontaneously and then consider whether I should have done that, a process that may lead to regret. If my action had been spontan-eous, then the SA that I had during that action would be supporting my memory of what I had done, confirming that I had indeed acted in that way, thereby informing my reflective process. It is also possible to reflect *prospectively*, prior to action, either for pragmatic (strategic or planning) purposes or for purposes closer to moral reasoning and intention formation. In that case, engaging in an action after reflecting on it is likely to strengthen my prereflective SA for that action, reinforcing my sense of control, for example.

For example, if I deliberate and create an action plan or prior intention to do something (for example, buy a new car next week), when the time comes and I put that intention into action, the fact that I had planned it out and am not acting in a completely spontaneous way should increase my sense of control over my action. If, in contrast, I found myself in the car dealership, as a result of a spon-taneous desire for a red Mustang convertible that I spotted on the lot, I might in fact feel a little out of control, and this feeling of lack of control (or decreased SA) may be reinforced when I start to evaluate my action in terms of my self-narrative or in terms of a violation of my long-term intention to reduce my dependency on fossil fuels. In this respect, either the presence or the absence of deliberative reflection or the judgment or attribution of agency that I make about my action, may in fact have an effect on my ongoing SA for the action.

On this view we can identify several different contributories to a complex experience of agency distributed across multiple elements in the self-pattern.

- Prereflective SA based on proprioceptive/kinaesthetic and efferent motor-control processes that generate a first-order experience linked to bodily movement in and toward an environment (*bodily* and *experiential processes*)

- Prereflective perceptual monitoring of the effect of my action on the world in terms of specific intentional or means-ends relations in specific situations (*behavioral, ecological,* and *experiential aspects of SA*)
- Formation of prior intentions, often involving a prospective reflective deliberation or planning that precedes some actions, and retrospective attributions or judgments of agency that follow action (*cognitive, reflective,* and *narrative processes*)

It's easy to see that these various processes occur across different time scales (from elementary to integrative to narrative), and that they line up respectively with distinctions made between motoric, present, and distal intentions as discussed in action theory.[8] We can add to this the reflective long-term sense of one's capacity for action over time, which Elisabeth Pacherie identifies as related to self-narrative "where one's past actions and projected future actions are given a general coherence and unified through a set of overarching goals, motivations, projects and general lines of conduct" (2007a, 6).

6.4 Intersubjective and Social Constraints

Everything that we have said so far about the experience of agency and ownership, however, is still too narrow in the scope of what should be included in such an analysis. Experiences of agency and ownership are fully embodied and situated (Buhrmann & Di Paolo 2017). We've already seen that they are embodied since they involve bodily action, and proprioceptive and kinaesthetic processes. Autonomic and vestibular processes are also involved, as are affective and emotional aspects. Christensen et al. (2019), for example, have shown that fear and anger can reduce an implicit measure (intentional binding) for SA. That experiences of agency and ownership are situated means they can be modulated—increased or decreased—by physical and spatial features of environments as well as social factors that include, not only other people, but also normative, social, and institutional practices that may constrain or enhance personal agency.

Both practically and normatively the presence of others has an effect on what my possibilities for action are, and the way that I perceive the world in action contexts. This effect even manifests itself in prereflective behavior. For example, when another agent sitting next to me engages in what seems an independent task, it can slow my reaction time for my own task—the so-called Social Simon

---

[8] See Pacherie's (2008) distinctions between M(otor)-intentions, P(roximate)-intentions, and D(istal)-intentions, or Searle's (1983) distinction between prior intentions and intentions-in-action.

Effect (Sebanz et al. 2003; see Sebanz et al. 2006).[9] Things may get even more complex since the nature of one's interpersonal relationship with the other can affect the results. A cooperative relationship with a co-actor can strengthen the effect; a competitive relationship can abolish or significantly decrease the effect (Dolk et al. 2011). Cultural factors may also modulate the effect. It increases among members of a collectivistic religion (Dolk et al. 2014), and when there is perceived similarity between co-agents (Müller et al. 2011), as well as when the subject takes the other to be acting as an intentional agent (rather than a non-intentional robot) (Stenzel et al. 2012).

Although such Simon Effects occur even if one is not interacting with the other person, in cases where there is interaction the effects are greater (Takahama et al. 2005). In one study, for example, experimenters observed co-actors in a coordin-ated joint action that required synchronous delivery of objects to a target loca-tion. One agent was constrained by an obstacle, requiring more movement than the other agent. Across a number of experiments the agent without constraint nonetheless moved as if an obstacle were obstructing her way suggesting that unconstrained agents were affected by their co-actor's task constraint and adjusted accordingly (Schmitz et al. 2017).

Such effects, although they happen in non-conscious ways, can have an effect on one's prereflective sense of agency. They may also become much more expli-citly self-conscious. Consider the effects on performance when an individual becomes overly self-conscious in front of others. Likewise, the influence of other people often shapes prospective and retrospective processes of intention forma-tion and action evaluation. My deliberations to act in a certain way, for example, may be influenced by what my friends consider to be an appropriate choice. Peer pressure, social referencing, which may be implicit or explicit, or our habitual behavior when in the presence of others may detract from or increase our feeling of agency. We located these intersubjective and culturally normative variables on the horizontal axis in the meshed architecture model. In typical behavior they get integrated into prereflective and reflective factors and become part of the dynam-ical gestalt of the self-pattern. In this regard, one's experience of agency will be a matter of degree; it can be enhanced or reduced by physical, social, economic, and cultural factors that work their way into and through our own practices, but

---

[9] The Simon Effect is found in a traditional stimulus-response task. Participants respond to differ-ent color stimuli, pressing a button to their left with their left hand for blue and a button to their right with their right hand for red. They are asked to ignore the location of the color (which may be dis-played either in their right or left visual field). An incongruence (mismatch) of right versus left between the color location and hand used to respond results in increased reaction times (Simon 1969). When a subject is asked to respond to just one color with one hand there is no conflict and no effect on reaction time. In the Social Simon Effect the subject has exactly the same task (one hand-one color) but is seated next to another person who is responding to a different color. Each agent acts like one of the hands in the original experiment and reaction times increase (Sebanz et al. 2006). The presence of the other agent seemingly has an effect on my action even in this very simple task.

also, in pathological cases, for example, by loss of motor control or disruptions in prereflective action-consciousness.

Considerations about the experience of agency hold important implications in regard to therapeutic settings. Interactions between patient and psychiatrist may be such that they rob the patient of a sense of agency if, for example, the psychiatrist fails to respond or to show interest in the patient's reports on their experience. Houlders, Bortolotti, and Broome (2021) describe cases of patient–psychiatrist conversations or clinical encounters where patients' reports are discounted or entirely ignored, and the indifference of the psychiatrist is problematic (something that might be considered a form of epistemic or hermeneutical injustice):

> Some of the evidence on clinical encounters gathered by using conversation analysis offers a good insight into exchanges that have the potential to adversely affect people's sense of agency. In exchanges between a psychiatrist and users with psychotic symptoms, for instance, users actively describe their experiences but often the doctor provides no response and avoids direct questions that users might have about their experiences. This suggests to the users—and to a neutral observer—that there is no engagement: the psychiatrist does not explain or discuss the relevant experiences despite these being important to the users and users seeking to know more about them.   (Houlders et al. 2021, 7700)

Houlders et al. also suggest that to the extent that the patient's report, their self-narrative, typically tends to reinforce their sense of agency, ignoring or discounting that narrative in such situations leads to a diminishment in that sense and may have a deleterious effect on both diagnosis and therapeutic results. Given the importance of others in the co-constitution of self-narrative, the psychiatrist has an opportunity to bolster the patient's sense of agency and to promote a better outcome.

6.5 Disordered Experiences of Agency and Ownership in the Self-pattern

The conceptual articulation of the different aspects of the experience of agency suggests that the loss or disruption of this experience in different pathologies may be varied. In schizophrenic delusions of control motor control processes may be disrupted. In other cases the attribution of self-agency may be disrupted due to problems with reflective cognition. In cases of narcotic addition, for example, an addict may feel that something other than himself is compelling him to use drugs despite his reflective attempt to resist (Frankfurt 1988; see Grünbaum 2010, for discussion). Disruptions in the experience of agency in various pathologies—including schizophrenia, anarchic hand syndrome, obsessive-compulsive behavior, narcotic addiction, and so on—may in fact involve different sorts of selective loss and very different experiences. In the following sections I'll focus on symptoms of schizophrenia and of agoraphobic anxiety.

6.5.1 Schizophrenia

We noted that in typical cases of involuntary movement, efferent signals and SA may be absent but SO for the movement is maintained because of the presence of afferent sensory feedback signaling me that this is *my* body that is moving. In such cases, then, my experience is that I am moving, although I did not initiate the movement. The same logic may explain some aspects of schizophrenic delusions of control. At least on one interpretation, if there are neurological problems, for example, with efference copy in forward motor control processes, this may result in a loss of SA for the action (Frith 1992; Gallagher 2000a). Consider the following report by a patient suffering from delusions of control:

> They inserted a computer in my brain. It makes me turn to the left or right. It's just as if I were being steered around, by whom or what I don't know.
>
> (Cited in Frith et al. 2000, 358)

The patient expresses no question about who is being turned or steered (he has an intact SO—it is he who is moving); but his experience is of something (or someone) else controlling his movement (he has no sense of self-agency for that movement).

Typically, when explaining the forward model, reference is made to an action intention. The efferent signal is compared to the specific intention or goal of the action to verify that the motoric components of the action are on track. With respect to the schizophrenic symptom of thought insertion, however, it's not clear that motor control processes or anything like an intention to think, are involved in the thinking process, and accordingly, it's not clear that thought insertion can be explained in the same way as delusions that involve bodily movement (Gallagher 2004a; Frith 2004). First, there is no reason to think that a subpersonal comparator or efference copy would be involved in monitoring thought processes if thinking is conscious and one is able to consciously track one's thinking. It may be possible, however, to appeal to a disruption of neurobiological processes that are more distributed than the specialized processes of motor control or comparator mechanisms to explain delusions of control and thought insertion—that is, to more general processes that affect not just SA for motor action, but also for cognitive processes, resulting in delusional symptoms (Daprati et al. 1997; Singh et al. 1992). Second, to posit an intention to think for every thought would lead to an infinite regress if the intention itself is conceived of as a form of thinking. In any case, it's not clear that we monitor our every thought, or that we have a sense of agency for every thought or thinking process (Gallagher 2004a; López-Silva 2021; Proust 2009). Indeed, the phenomenon of unbidden thoughts (Frankfurt 1988), that is, thoughts that passively enter one's stream of consciousness, and that are not initiated under our agentive control (in contrast to the kind of thinking involved in methodically solving a problem) suggests that things are more complex. Furthermore, even with respect to delusions of control, the absence of efference copy in forward motor control processes (which may explain a lack of SA) does not explain the full phenomenon, since the anomalous delusional experience also feels alien and there is usually an attribution of agency to another person or object.

Accordingly, Billon and Kriegel (2014) suggest that rather than there being "something missing" (e.g., SA), delusions of control and thought insertion really involve "something added"—namely an experience of alienation, reflected in the subject's claim that someone or something else is making his movements or thoughts. One possible explanation for the alien feeling is that a disruption in the integration of proprioceptive, perceptual, and efference processes in the anterior insula (Farrer & Frith 2002), or bodily processes more generally (Fotia et al. 2022), or in mechanisms that allows for the proper discrimination between self and non-self (Georgieff & Jeannerod 1998), may generate a sense of alien control in one's prereflective experience.

According to phenomenological approaches to schizophrenia, delusions of control are considered disorders of prereflective self-experiences—or what Sass, Parnas, and Zahavi (2011; Sass & Parnas 2003) call *ipseity-disturbance*. Ipseity "refers to the most basic sense of selfhood or self-presence: a crucial sense of self-sameness, fundamental (thus nearly indescribable) sense of existing as a vital and self-identical *subject* of experience or *agent* of action" (Sass 2014, 6). Sass, for example, argues that in cases of ipseity disturbance in schizophrenia, first-person experience is disrupted in two ways. First, the patient engages in "hyper-reflexivity," marked by an amplified self-consciousness of processes and phenomena that would normally remain tacit (2014, 6). Second, the subject experiences a "diminished self-affection," such that he undergoes a diminished "sense of existing as a subject of awareness or agent of action" (2014, 6), accompanied by a feeling of alienation. According to this model, an initial heightened self-awareness (hyper-reflexivity, directed, for example, toward one's bodily processes) leads to a diminished self-awareness and alien feeling, similar to the way in which if you stare at the back of your hand long enough it starts to feel as if you are staring at something that is not you.[10] The ipseity-disturbance model is grounded in a

---

[10] As Dylan Trigg (in Gallagher & Trigg 2016) points out, it may be that in delusions of control the person experiences what Merleau-Ponty has called the impersonal aspects that accompany our personal life: "if I wanted to express perceptual experience with precision, I would have to say that one perceives in me, and not that I perceive. Every sensation includes a seed of dream or depersonalization, as we experience through this sort of stupor into which it puts us when we truly live at the level

broader distinction between a minimal or prereflective sense of self-experience and a reflective, more conceptual self-consciousness that may involve self-narrative. On this model, the disturbance at stake in schizophrenia is a disturbance in the prereflective experiential aspect of the self-pattern rather than in aspects of self-narrative.

In contrast, as we saw above (in Section 6.3), Graham and Stephens (1994; Stephens & Graham 2000) propose a more cognitive view: in cases of schizophrenic delusions of control or thought insertion, they contend the problem is with reflective and narrative processes. The subject fails to attribute agency to his actions or thoughts because they seem radically inconsistent with his self-narrative. Pacherie (2007b, 211) calls this the narrative explanation. In such cases the important change is in the reflective judgment of agency. According to Graham and Stephens, there is no change in the attribution of ownership; the subject does not deny that the action is being carried out by his own bodily movement, or that the thought is occurring as part of his own experience. Indeed, that is precisely his complaint—that this action or thought involves his body or his thinking, but does not seem consistent with his beliefs or self-conceptions. This rationalist account may be more consistent with the view that a delusion is "a false belief based on incorrect inference" (as it has been defined in various editions of the DSM). This account, however, doesn't provide a full explanation since it's not clear why an inconsistency between action and narrative would prevent an attribution of self-agency rather than, for example, promote a sense that one has made a mistake or was simply inconsistent in one's actions, or, again, why it would motivate a misattribution of agency to someone else. Furthermore, it doesn't address a puzzle raised by Bayne and Pacherie (2004, 8): "We are also puzzled by the question of how a top-down [i.e., cognitivist or rationalist] account of delusions could explain the damage to the autonomic system that one finds in the Capgras and Cotard delusions. Is this caused by the delusional belief? That seems unlikely." Even if one can point to an organic malfunction that correlates with delusions, for example, the correlation between problems in judgment of agency in schizophrenia and a deficit in cortical activation in the default mode and central-executive networks (Spaniel et al. 2016), the etiology is not clear. Furthermore, even if we could specify that cognitive or narrative capabilities are in some way undermined by organic damage (see e.g., Armstrong 2020), it is not clear why the subject's delusions would be selectively about certain topics and not others—that is, why the subject is not delusional about everything he believes, or why some actions or thoughts are considered alien, but not others. I've called this the problem of specificity (Gallagher 2004a; 2009a), and Pacherie, Green, and

---

of sensation" (Merleau-Ponty 2012, 249/223). We typically do not live within our sensation, however, we are typically perceivers and agents living in the world. In schizophrenia, this natural attitude can be disrupted.

Bayne (2006, 575) suggest that it remains unsolved. This also seems a problem for empiricist accounts that would explain the loss of SA solely in terms of a faulty comparator. It makes more sense to explain the specificity of delusions as dependent on dynamic alterations in the way certain social and cultural factors are incorporated into the self-pattern. Indeed, delusions are often based on concepts found in popular culture—robots, brain implants, aliens from outer space, zombies, and so forth (Gallagher 2009a).

One starts to see here that any explanation of delusions of control and thought insertion needs to take into account not just a disorder in one exclusive factor of the self-pattern—whether that be conceived in terms of neurobiology, phenomenal ipseity, reflective or narrative capacities, or social-cultural factors. Rather, the account should look to disruptions in multiple processes and the dynamical connections among these various processes in the self-pattern. Moreover, it is important to understand the developmental picture. Henriksen, Parnas, and Zahavi (2019, 6) point out that a phenomenon like thought insertion arises from an already altered experiential history, specific to schizophrenia:

[S]uch psychotic phenomena are often the outcome of a profound sense of self-alienation that already exists prior to the onset of psychosis. The self-alienation in question is fundamentally speaking a pervasively *felt distance* between the experiencer and his experiences. When reaching its full potentiation in psychosis, this felt distance becomes unbridgeable, as it were, allowing some of the patient's own thoughts to appear so strange and unfamiliar that they no longer are recognized as his own thoughts.

Despite a great deal of empirical evidence in support of the idea that the experience of agency is the thing at stake in delusions of control and thought insertion (see, e.g., Graham et al. 2014; Hur et al. 2014; Jeannerod 2009; Kozáková et al. 2020; Prikken et al. 2017; Krugwasser et al. 2021), not everyone agrees. The disagreements return us to the different views of the senses of agency and ownership discussed in Sections 6.2 and 6.3. Bortolotti and Broome (2009), who focus on the symptom of thought insertion,[11] for example, deny that such delusions involve problems with the experience of agency. Their proposal is that such delusions involve problems with the experience of ownership, and specifically, attributions of ownership. This requires, they suggest, a "more demanding notion of ownership" that involves a self-ascription or endorsement condition according to which a subject acknowledges an action or thought as her own and ascribes it to herself on the basis of introspection, or on the basis of her reasons for acting or thinking

---

[11] They limit this analysis to thought insertion and do not think it necessarily applies to delusions of control. I agree that there are important differences in explanatory requirements for delusions of control and thought insertion (Gallagher 2004a).

in that way. That there may be a problem with the attribution of ownership in such cases, however, does not rule out the possibility that the primary problem is still a problem with the experience of agency. If we ask why the subject reflectively disowns the action or the thought, two answers still seem possible. Either (1) the thought doesn't fit with her self-narrative (as suggested by Graham and Stephens), and therefore is not endorsed by the subject since she is not able to provide reasons for it (as suggested by Bortolotti and Broome), or, (2) the action or thought actually feels or is experienced as alien—a first-order experience that may have initially motivated the second-order reflection. Moreover, this first-order feeling of alienation may result from, or may result in, a modulation or displacement of SA for that action or thought. So, even if Bortolotti and Broome are right that the person's second-order, retrospective report indicates a problem with the attribution of ownership, this problem may be due to a first-order, experiential problem with SA and/or feeling of alienation (see Humpston 2018 for a critical view on this solution).

Alexander Billon (2013), who also thinks that thought insertion involves problems with the attribution of ownership, provides a different argument against the involvement of SA. He argues that the subject doesn't actually have a first-order experience of the thought. Rather, the inserted thought is generated and inserted by a second-order reflection. Such thoughts lack first-order (prereflective) phenomenality and therefore there can't be a first-order SA or SO for the thought.

Billon offers a clarifying analogy. The inserted thought is akin to a sentence uttered by someone else, or a sentence in a text that one is reading. I may have reflective access to the thought in a way that is akin to my perceptual awareness of a sentence on the page or of the sentence you just uttered. There may be something it is like to have that reflective access, or to perceive the sentence, but the sentence itself does not have a thought-like phenomenal character. I come upon a certain intentional content, a certain thought-meaning that seems independent of any process of thinking that would bestow on it a phenomenal feeling such that it would feel like I was the one thinking it. In that case it's a thought that I seemingly did not think—something that did not get generated in my thinking process. It's not clear, however, that this totally eliminates the involvement of the experience of agency; if what's missing in the case of the sentence, and in the case of the inserted thought, just is the sense that I am the one generating the thought in a process of thinking, then what's missing is precisely the sense of self-agency—the prereflective SA which just is the sense that I am the generator of the thought or action. If there is no SA for the thought, then my reflective discovery of the thought in my stream of experience is a surprise. This assumes, however, that there usually is SA for one's thinking; otherwise one would be surprised more often and would constantly be experiencing inserted thoughts.

The analyses of Bortolotti, Broome, and Billion highlight the complexity and ambiguity involved in these issues—that is, the complexity and ambiguity that is sometimes intrinsic to the actual relations that exist within the experiences of agency and ownership. It's possible that SA and SO are closely related in prereflective experience (consistent with the *ipseity-disturbance* model); and it's also possible that there are reciprocal relations between SA/SO and reflective judgments and narratives about agency and ownership. We should think here of dynamical relations within the self-pattern, and modulations that cross time scales in a reciprocal, albeit non-linear fashion. If, for example, SA is disrupted by neural or extra-neural factors, then reflective attributions of agency and ownership may be affected such that I am led to judge an action or thought as not mine or as not under my control.[12]

6.5.2 Experiences of Agency and Ownership in Other Disorders

Experimental measures of the experience of agency are generally of two types: implicit measures using intentional binding (Haggard, Clark & Kalogeras 2002; Moore & Obhi 2012) or sensory attenuation (Kühn et al. 2011), and explicit measures using rating scales and questionnaires, which may also capture SO (Marotta et al. 2017; Sato & Yasuda 2005; Yamaguchi et al. 2020). In the case of voluntary action, in contrast to involuntary movement, for example, perceived times of action onset and its perceived worldly effect are temporally compressed, that is, shifted toward each other (Figure 6.1). Sensory attenuation, associated with a measurably reduced N1 component in electrophysiological ERP studies (Hughes, Desantis & Waszak 2013), may rely on a close match between sensory feedback predictions generated by forward models and actual sensory input; a lack of match would indicate unintended consequences and could elicit more (hyper-reflexive) attention to action processes. These measures putatively correlate with prereflective SA rather than reflective (judgment, attribution) processes (Duerler et al. 2022; Gallagher 2020d; Smigielski et al. 2020). They may also measure different (albeit related) processes, and if such processes can be modulated by changes in ecological and social contexts, this may explain why there is not perfect consistency across all measures (see Dewey & Knoblich 2014; Lafleur, Soulières & d'Arc 2020; Barlas & Obhi 2014).

Variations and different types of disruptions in the experience of agency can be found in different disorders. Not just in schizophrenia, but in non-clinical

---

[12] For variations on how SA and SO relate in schizophrenic thought insertion, see for example, Gennaro (2021); Henriksen, Parnas & Zahavi (2019); López-Silva (2019); Pedrini (2015); Seeger (2015); Sousa & Swiney (2013). Most of these variations assume that there are in fact experiences that we can call senses of ownership and agency. For a very different, Wittgensteinian, expressionist conception of thought insertion, see Feyaerts and Kusters (2022). For a review of evidence concerning variations in SA and SO in regard to body-self-experience in schizophrenia (using body transfer illusions such as the rubber hand illusion) see Baum et al. (2022).

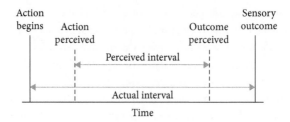

Figure 6.1 Intentional binding: Subjects typically underestimate the actual time interval between action onset and sensory outcome for intentional action
Source: From Gallagher 2020b, with permission.

subjects manifesting schizotypy characteristics, in patients with anosognosia for hemiplegia, in mirror-touch synaesthetes, in anarchic hand syndrome, OCD, addiction, and so on. In the case of schizotypy, for example, a disruption of SA depends less on motor control processes and more on intentional aspects, that is, perceptual cues (Asai & Tanno 2007; Moore, Tang & Cioffi 2020). In contrast, in the case of anosognosia for hemiplegia, a disorder in which patients, following stroke, are unaware of their paralysis or motor deficit, and report that they are able to, or are in fact moving their paralyzed limb, their SA for such illusory movement is based primarily on motor control processes that seemingly fail to register sensory feedback (Berti & Pia 2006), or on a discrepancy between efferent signals and sensory feedback which fails to reach threshold for awareness (Preston & Newport 2014).

In mirror-touch synaesthesia (MTS) a subject feels a tactile experience on her own body when observing another person being touched. In this regard there is evidence that differences in SA are linked to anomalies in SO and self-other differentiation. In vicarious agency experiments (which blur the distinction between self-initiated and other-initiated actions) people with MTS experienced higher SA over the movements that were not their own, suggesting that SO entrains SA via sensory (visual-proprioceptive) feedback (Cioffi, Banissy & Moore 2016).

In the case of anarchic hand syndrome one limb seems to have a will of its own and engages in action that the subject experiences as alien (Della Sala, Marchetti & Spinnler 1991). Subjects have no SA for the action although they can reflectively attribute agency to their own body and they continue to have SO for the limb. This differs from somatoparaphrenia (or alien hand syndrome) where a subject has no SO for the limb, and in many cases attributes the limb to someone else. It also differs from utilization behavior (following frontal lobe damage) where subjects are unable to inhibit acting on environmental cues (for example, if they see a hammer they cannot help but pick it up and use it, even if it is inappropriate to do so), but they continue to have SA for the action and don't experience it as alien (Pacherie 2007b).

When we engage in action our motor system typically attenuates sensory feedback, which not only allows us to pay more attention to environmental features than to features of our own movement, but also allows for a discrimination between self-movement and externally generated movements, which contributes to SA. In the case of OCD a deficiency in anticipatory aspects (predictions generated by forward motor control processes) means that patients fail to attenuate the sensory consequences of their own actions. There is a mismatch between expected and actual outcomes leading to feelings of incompleteness even when actions are properly executed. This involves conflicting modulations in SA (involving a decreased sense of control) and in judgments of agency (Gentsch et al. 2012; Giuliani et al. 2021).

Questions about the experience of agency in addiction can be very complex. Narcotic addiction can lead to a loss of SA. As mentioned above, if an addict withdraws from taking drugs and starts using again, he may feel that he is not the agent and that some force is moving him to take drugs. SA, as measured by intentional binding, may be modulated by changes in neurotransmitter (e.g., dopamine or ketamine) levels (De Pirro et al. 2019). Changes in the experience of agency, however, are not just the result of chemically induced dependency. There is no strong correlation between compulsive drug use, degree of pleasure, or reductions in withdrawal symptoms as measured in placebo studies, and the subjective reports of users. On one view, the experience of agency in addiction is inhibited by reflective evaluations of one's own behavior and the formation of self-narratives that undermine one's belief in agentive control (Snoek, Kennett & Fry 2012; Wiens & Walker 2015). Beyond changes in neurotransmitters or beliefs, however, pathological addiction shows high correlation with the salience of socially situated drug-related behaviors and stimuli (Robinson & Berridge 1993; 2000). Addiction can alter an agent's perception of specific social situations, which may become increasingly hedonically significant to the agent. In this case dynamical relations between social/cultural, affective, and cognitive/narrative factors have an impact on prereflective experiences of agency and ownership.

6.5.3 Agoraphobic Anxiety

This is also clearly the case in a variety of anxiety disorders. The experience of anxiety is in counterpoint to that of schizophrenia. Unlike schizophrenia, which can entail a "severe erosion of minimal self-experience or real confusion of self and other" (Sass 2014, 5), including a disruption in the experience of agency, in some cases of anxiety the boundary between self and other is retained, at least in a patchwork fashion (Gallagher & Trigg 2016). Indeed, it is precisely because this boundary is retained rather than destroyed that anxiety and a loss of control emerges.

In agoraphobia, for example, a disruption in the experience of agency is part of a more pervasive disruption in the self-pattern, involving experiences of the body (heart palpations, trembling of the legs, nausea, alienation), intersubjectivity (social discomfort), social/cultural context (including avoidance of certain environments), and the formation of behavioral habits—a collection of symptoms that pose a threat to the integrity of the self-pattern.

Agoraphobia is often thought of as a spatial disorder (Vidler 2002) involving a reaction to a specific kind of public spatiality. According to Clark (1988), a subject with agoraphobia initially perceives a threat in the environment, which seems more dangerous than it actually is. This is often the case with "either large expanses in which the subject feels 'trapped' in the middle, or narrow spaces flanked on all sides by open space, for example, a bridge. This fits well with the idea that the experience of agency may be affected in some cases by relations that extend to environmental features" (Gallagher & Trigg 2016).

The subject changes his behavior; he habitually avoids places that arouse undesirable sensations, and he becomes more vigilant in anticipating both the onset of anxiety and possible "threats." This way of coping leads to further snowballing effects on the subject's experienced loss of agency (Trigg 2016). The anxiety about space is reflected in bodily sensations so that the perception of threats in the environment transforms into a "misinterpretation" of specific bodily sensations regarded as signals of impending disaster (Clark 1988). This anxiety can also disturb bodily motricity (our capacity for meaningful movement in response to affordances in our surroundings), including the inability to move or the sudden urge to move, which is felt as a loss of control and as if it comes from nowhere:

> If you are very attuned to sensations in your legs, you will notice that they seem to have a mind of their own... The flight impulse is felt keenly in the legs; it feels almost as if your very limbs were demanding that you run.   (Shawn 2008, 119)

Such losses of control include a sense of impending collapse, an anxiety about passing out, and a more generalized anxiety over "losing one's mind" (Barlow 2002, 107).

In the clinical literature, agoraphobia "is intimately tied to a deep sense of the absence of control over one's feelings and actions" (Capps & Ochs 1997, 152; Barlow 2002, xiii). In contrast to the typical experience of spatiality, where the body operates in the mode of a forward-looking *I can*, a trustworthy center of orientation actively engaged with the affordances that surround it, a person with agoraphobia may experience space in the mode of hesitancy, disquiet, and a lack of trust in how he or she will respond to unpredictable or unfamiliar situations. This fits well with Dylan Trigg's (2016) bodily-inhibition model of anxiety which includes a disruption in the experience of agency, leading to a broader destabilization in the self-pattern. The disruption in the experience of agency involves a shift in bodily motricity and the feeling that the body has its own autonomy (Chambless et al. 1986). The subject's hesitant movement in the world frequently involves a connected awareness that anxious sensations and movements originate less from the agent as an integral and unified subject, and more from the body as an autonomous thing.

Loss of control and the experienced alienation from the body also involve a modulation in the sense of ownership. It is not *I* who am running from danger, but rather it is *the* legs that are instructing *me* to run. This presents an impediment to experiencing the body as "one's own." Bodily motricity transforms from an *I can* to an *I cannot*, and the body seems other than self. In this respect the sense of ownership becomes ambiguous since I know that it is I who am undergoing and enduring the anxiety, but it seems uncertain to what extent the body is irreducibly *mine*. Individual body parts can assume an uncanny quality that reflects a broader discordance in the self-pattern during anxiety (Trigg 2014).

The somatic symptoms that emerge relate directly to what Dainton (2008) called the phenomenal background, and the experience of ownership that is intrinsic to it. In this kind of anxiety, there is a restructuring where the phenomenal background comes to the fore in a schizophrenic-like hyperreflexivity (Sass 2014): "becoming short of breath and beginning to breathe rapidly...feeling my heart beat at twice the normal rate...finding my vision growing dark and blurred, feeling my face grow cold, and my legs tremulous, weak, and then extraordinarily stiff" (Shawn 2008, 117). In addition to these changes, there is also a reflective skepticism: "will I get to the end of the road and be the person I was when I started the journey?" These are not just uncomfortable sensations and thoughts, but a more pervasive threat to the subject's self-pattern, in both prereflective and reflective processes.

Although there are parallels between the *ipseity-disturbance* model of schizophrenia and the *bodily-inhibition* model of anxiety, for example, hyperreflexivity in regard to bodily sensations (Trigg 2016), there are also critical differences. Notably, if schizophrenia involves the sustained diminishment of ipseity (Sass & Parnas 2003), in agoraphobic anxiety, diminishment of self-presence is ambiguous and intermittent, punctuated by patchwork moments of bodily integrity, spatial coherence, and self-presence alongside moments of bodily disintegration, spatial incoherence, and self-alienation. Space is divided into safe/familiar versus dangerous/unfamiliar regions. So long as the subject avoids the latter, he can function, building a form of control over his body by controlling externals and avoiding situations where control is threatened.

This ambiguity also manifests itself in the subject's narrative. For one patient, "with the exception of [being unable to cross open spaces without anxiety], he likes to believe he is healthy" (Knapp 1988, 63). Subjects feel "normal" in secure surroundings: "I even pretend to myself that my 'personality' is somehow incompatible with agoraphobia...Agoraphobia *is* at odds with the tone of some of what

I do. I am not wary in every domain" (Shawn 2008, 119–20). Shawn is able to assume the role of a performing pianist, able to face a "hostile audience," courageous enough to posit a "minority view" at a faculty meeting, and tolerant of "good and bad reviews" of his work (120). This "normal" self is defined by a strong sense of being both the originator and controller of bodily movement coupled with a tacit sense that *I* am the one undergoing the movement. The narrative of the subject with agoraphobia is cut up into different regions, similar to the spatiality of his world.

Notably, this patchwork dissection extends to intersubjectivity, too. Other people are not perceived as innocuous bystanders, they are either threatening or supportive. The role of the "trusted person" assumes a defining importance in the subject's ability to navigate space without anxiety. The presence of a trusted person signals a familiarity, constancy, and understanding that is lacking in the subject's otherwise precarious experience of the world (Trigg 2013). More generally, however, other people do not assuage the subject's anxiety; they amplify and reinforce an already existing anxiety. Clinical research suggests that another's gaze is a significant factor in precipitating the onset of anxiety (Davidson 2002). Other people become, in some instances, a critical problem for the person with agoraphobia. Whereas choices of spatial routes and behavioral routines are subject to a degree of control via a set of habitual patterns, control over how another person perceives us seems impossible. In this respect, the spatiality of the home, defined as the safe place par excellence, is predicated on its function of concealing the gaze of the other (Davidson 2003, 84).

One thus sees in agoraphobic anxiety different configurations of self-pattern than in schizophrenia or other disorders. Such differences should inform the art of psychiatric diagnosis understood, perhaps, as a form of pattern recognition across what Kraepelin (1893) called the natural course or development of the illness. Although these conditions may involve some overlap in disruptions in the experiences of agency and ownership, they play out differently, both in the precise dynamics of those experiences, and across other aspects of the self-pattern. Even allowing for the complexity of schizophrenia, which may also involve comorbid experiences of anxiety, there are clear differences, not only where the DSM-5 puts them in regard to agoraphobia—in behaviors where fear is the motivating affect, and in specifications about experienced spatiality—but also in the re-ordering of intersubjective relations and in the experiences of agency. Such differences in self-patterns will also be reflected in the self-narratives of these patients.

7

Autonomy in the Self-pattern

Implications for Deep Brain Stimulation and Affordance-based Therapies

Questions about the nature of self and self-consciousness are closely aligned with questions about the nature of autonomy. These concepts have deep roots in traditional philosophical discussions that concern metaphysics, epistemology, and ethics. They also have direct relevance to practical considerations about therapeutic treatments in medical contexts. In this chapter, with reference to understanding specific side effects of deep brain stimulation (DBS), which is increasingly employed as a therapeutic approach in the treatment of Parkinson's disease (PD), obsessive compulsive disorder (OCD), and major depressive disorder (MDD), I'll argue that the best way to think of autonomy with regard to the self-pattern is to think of it in terms of relational autonomy as it connects to affect, agency, and the notion of affordances.

7.1 DBS: An Altered Sense of Self and Personal Identity

In DBS treatment electrodes are implanted in specific brain areas (different brain areas for different disorders) allowing the modulation of neural activity. The use of DBS has been successful in treating movement disorders like PD and dystonia, and psychiatric disorders like OCD and MDD. In some cases, however, this treatment can also lead to unpredictable changes or adverse effects in the experience of self and personal identity. In a few instances, such changes may be serious enough that it remains unclear whether the patient is the same person (i.e., retains the same *ipse* identity) before and after DBS.[1] The possibility of adverse effects raises some ethical issues. To be clear, however, the results of DBS treatment are mostly positive. Indeed, the point of DBS is to resolve symptoms of serious

---

[1] How extensive the problem of adverse effects is, and how precisely DBS is involved, are still open questions (Gilbert et al. 2021). Moreover, the problems that one finds in extreme cases should not be equated with the lesser degree of personality changes found in typical patients (Bluhm, Cabrera & McKenzie 2020). For example, Eich, Müller, and Schulze-Bonhage (2019) conducted a systematic evaluation of neurostimulating devices, including DBS. They found that DBS patients showed only moderate changes in self-perception, and minor changes in those aspects that involve self-alienation. For a discussion of some of these issues, see Pugh (2020); Zawadzki (2021).

The Self and its Disorders. Shaun Gallagher, Oxford University Press. © Shaun Gallagher 2024.
DOI: 10.1093/oso/9780198873068.003.0008

disorders when other options have not worked. DBS can lead to diminishment of anxiety, improved mood, and many other positive benefits in treating disorders such as OCD and PD (Alonso et al. 2015; de Haan et al. 2015; Greenberg et al. 2006). Setting aside the ethical issues that may be involved with respect to adverse effects, the relevant issue that I want to address concerns just how DBS can change the self-pattern. In this regard we should consider both the adverse and beneficial effects of this kind of treatment.

A review by Schüpbach et al. (2006), for example, listed the following adverse effects reported by patients (overall nineteen out of twenty-nine patients reported at least one of these side effects) subsequent to DBS treatment for PD:

1. Altered body image. Patients had difficulties accepting the presence of a device in their brains—they reported they felt "like a robot" or "like an electronic doll"
2. Feelings of estrangement: patients could no longer "find themselves"; they were "not feeling like themselves anymore"
3. Loss of vitality
4. Feelings of helplessness—patients felt "mentally unable to resume a more normal life style"
5. Loss of meaning in life—feelings of emptiness or meaninglessness.

Agid et al. (2006) noted additional problems concerning retrospective evaluation. For example, patients felt they had been damaged by the consequences of their disorder; or they voiced regret that the disorder took up so much of their life. They also experienced persistent problems concerning prospective attitude. For example, they continued to anticipate the same disabilities as in their prior state. Christen et al. (2012), reviewing treatment of PD by means of stimulation of the subthalamic nucleus (STN) in sixty-six case reports, sixty-nine review papers, and 347 outcome studies published between 1993 and 2009, categorized adverse side effects or sequelae to include effects on behavior, cognition (reasoning, memory), mood (depression, anxiety, apathy), the autonomic system, language, social aspects, and quality of life. Other studies found increased anxiety, panic, fear, hypomania, hyper-sexuality, increased impulsivity, increased anger, forgetfulness, mild aphasia, difficulties concentrating, planning, and organizing, depression, suicidal behavior, impulsivity, worsened verbal fluency, or executive dysfunction, acute olfactory, gustatory, or motor sensations—variations that depend on the disorder treated, symptoms, and the area of the brain stimulated (Appleby et al. 2007; Bronstein et al. 2011; Burdick et al. 2011; de Haan et al. 2015; de Koning et al. 2011; Denys et al. 2010; Gilbert 2013; Goodman & Alterman 2012; Morishita et al. 2014; Müller & Christen 2011; Okun et al. 2007; 2012; Synofzik 2013).

Schüpbach et al. (2006) also report more positive effects: "feelings of new self or new life," feelings of "awakening" or having "a second birth" after treatment.

Both negative and positive changes, however, may complicate the patient's relations with people close to them. Patients may be more easily annoyed by others, more irritable, more aggressive (Agid et al. 2006); some studies report psychosocial maladjustment or no improvement in the social domain for patients (Ooms et al. 2014). Some participants report that they have difficulties in their personal relationships after DBS treatment. Their partners need to accommodate sudden changes in their behavior, or "in being confronted with 'a different person'" (de Haan et al. 2015).

Given the extent and the diversity of post-DBS side effects, researchers have rightly expressed concern for the patient's sense of self (e.g., Baylis 2013; Glannon 2009; Kraemer 2011; Schermer 2009; Witt et al. 2013). One worry is that DBS might negatively affect personal responsibility (Klaming & Haselager 2013; Leentjens et al. 2004), one's sense of autonomy (Gilbert 2015; Schüpbach et al. 2006), or authenticity (Johansson et al. 2011; Kraemer 2011). Since there is a significant degree of uncertainty related to the effects of DBS, De Ridder et al. (2016, 245) raised the question about what patients "have to sacrifice for this beneficial effect," and they suggest "it is important that theoretical models are developed that can help us understand the function of possible neuromodulation targets and make predictions about possible neuromodulation targets." Likewise, Schermer (2009) calls for more theoretical research into what constitutes the self, alongside the empirical research on DBS. Indeed, depending on the degree of uncertainty involved about possible changes in personal identity, at the very least these concerns have implications for clinical practice, informed consent, and policymaking (Mathews 2011). Furthermore, theories that take the self to be in some measure socially constituted, and that take autonomy to be relational, raise important questions about how responsibility gets distributed among patients, physicians, and other players in the context of treatment (Gallagher 2021b). Again, in this chapter I don't pursue these explicitly ethical issues but rather focus on questions about self and autonomy in the context of DBS therapy.

7.2 Deflationary versus Plural Models of the Self

What theoretical conceptions of the self can explain the variety of side effects and symptoms post-DBS? Some theorists have attempted to explain the changes to self-experience and personal identity resulting from DBS by appealing to what we have called "deflationary" conceptions of the self (see Chapter 1). A deflationary conception of self is one that states that the self is just one thing and nothing more. Such conceptions can range from Metzinger's (2004) "self-model," to Dennett's (1991a) notion of an abstract center of narrative gravity. Aligned with such deflationary strategies the following proposals have been made to explain the side effects of DBS:

- DBS leads to changes in self, understood purely in cognitive terms. For example, Synofzik and Schlaepfer (2008) offer an account in terms of the notion of self, understood as the objective "cognitive representational system with special characteristic self-representational capacities." Witt et al. (2013) consider this to be too broad or nonspecific; they propose a model of self, defined as a specific set of core propositional attitudes (beliefs, desires), which have an impact on the identity of the person, a view consistent with Dixon and Gross (2021) who describe a belief-network theory of self where the self is equated with a network of beliefs about oneself.
- DBS leads to changes in self, understood purely in narrative terms. Marya Schechtman (2010), for example, argues that we should understand the reported changes as changes in the patients' narrative identity—DBS disrupts the narrative flow or, in the case of successful treatment of depression, causes the depressed self-narrative to suddenly stop and a new happy one to suddenly start (also see Schermer 2011; Müller, Bittner & Krug 2010). DBS may disrupt an ability to reflectively articulate reasons for any changes that may occur in one's self-narrative (Schechtman 2010).
- DBS leads to changes in self, understood purely in phenomenological terms of alienation and authenticity. Kraemer (2013), for example, focuses on the experience of alienation from one's previous self, and therefore on the absence of authenticity—a feeling of being who one is.
- DBS leads to changes in self, understood primarily in terms of the person's sense of agency. A number of theorists (Brown 2020; Goddard 2017; and Lipsman & Glannon 2013) suggest that DBS affects agency or the sense of agency; in some cases it affects the patient's experience of the causal efficacy of his mental states (e.g., one patient with MDD worries the DBS device may replace him as the "source of his thought, mood and behaviour" [Lipsman & Glannon 2013, 468]).

Each of these accounts postulates a relatively narrow conception of the self. They focus on only one or two processes in the self-pattern, and often do so without giving good reasons why other processes are excluded. As a result, they fail to capture the full range of potentially relevant DBS-induced changes. The diversity of symptoms inventoried by Schüpbach et al. (2006), Christen et al. (2012), and others listed above suggest that we need a more comprehensive conception of self to understand such changes.

Several theorists do start to move in this direction. Lipsman and Glannon (2013; Glannon 2009), for example, acknowledge that things are more complex; they suggest that in addition to changes in agency, DBS affects the patients' memories, character traits, and narrative identity. De Haan et al. (2013) propose a model that would integrate the various changes across four dimensions: (a) person; (b) world, understood as a set of affordances; (c) characteristics of person–world interactions; and (d) existential (or self-relating) stance. Francoise Baylis (2013) agrees with Schechtman about the impact of DBS on the narrative aspect of self, and she importantly takes this to be part of a relational and socially constituted concept of personal identity, to which she adds social, bodily, and agentive aspects. She excludes personality, however, which she associates with behavior, mood/affect, and cognition. Although these views move in the right direction, they still lack a more comprehensive conception adequate enough to account for DBS-induced changes.

To address such concerns Roy Dings and Leon De Bruin (2016) suggested that the pluralist and dynamical notion of self-pattern, as I have been developing it here, can provide a more adequate theoretical framework to capture all the different possible changes post-DBS. In this respect the question is whether in specific disorders, for example, in PD or OCD or MDD and/or in cases of post-DBS treatment, some of the processes that are typically part of the self-pattern are diminished, or in some cases enhanced.

The dynamics of the self-pattern are important to consider in this regard. As we've seen, in regard to human actions, for example, it is typically the case that one experiences a degree of agency—a sense of agency that involves control over one's own body when acting—typically accompanied by a sense of ownership or "mineness" for one's body and actions. Reflective of the integrated gestalt nature of the self-pattern, as we've seen, the experience of agency may be interwoven with a number of other processes, and can be modulated by more complex, relational aspects, such as social, normative factors that involve culture, gender, race, and so forth, and by specific intersubjective factors that can either diminish or enhance one's autonomy. Accordingly, the experience of agency can also be an intrinsic part of reflective (prospective and retrospective) deliberation or can be enhanced or limited by narrative or normative practices. In this regard, a qualitative study of PD that shows a reduction of the experience of agency in *reflective* deliberation or life narrative (e.g., Bramley & Eatough 2005), is not necessarily incommensurable with studies that show an enhancement of the *prereflective* sense of agency connected with motor processes using intentional binding as an indirect measure in PD patients on dopaminergic medication (Moore et al. 2010). Furthermore, if the experience of agency is diminished in MDD, this may be more closely related to problems in both the affective and the intersubjective domains (Slaby, Paskaleva & Stephan 2013), and not just reflective of motor experience as one might find in patients with OCD (Gentsch et al. 2012; Oren et al. 2016).

As I have been suggesting, it is not clear that we can determine the nature of the dynamical links among the various factors a priori, or simply by adopting a particular theory. Studying psychiatric and neurological disorders, as well as the various effects of therapies, including DBS, and mapping out the precise meshing of dynamical relations, can help us understand how selves can be integrated or disintegrated in particular cases. A phenomenological approach can contribute to that project (de Haan et al. 2015). For example, de Haan et al.'s study of OCD patients' post-DBS experiences show changes (1) in ecological affordance structure (in terms of a patient's pragmatic relations with world and others), (2) in affect (moods and feelings), and (3) in reflective, second-order evaluations about their interactions and themselves. As they suggest, "the effects of DBS on the experiences of OCD patients are global and thorough" (de Haan et al. 2013, 6). Accordingly, one can start to map out how various factors in the self-pattern relate to one another, and how they change with the DBS intervention, by tracking them in the experiences of a particular subject. De Haan et al. (2013) rightly indicate that there is "a pattern among these experiences... [where] all of these elements seem to play a role," and the task is to define this pattern more precisely. As they indicate, it is "tricky business" to try to explicate the holistic character of these kinds of experiences. "The focus on *dynamics* implies the relevance of taking into account the development and (mutually) reinforcing loops of coupled processes" (2013, 6). It is precisely changes in such loops that play a role in the development of OCD, and, as well, how OCD patients readjust following DBS treatment. The threefold method introduced in Chapter 3 is meant to address this tricky business.

7.3 Relational Autonomy

We can approach the question of autonomy from two sides. First, in this section, we can ask how the concept of autonomy maps across the numerous processes of the self-pattern. Second, in the next section, in order to see how the notion of autonomy applies to situations involving DBS treatment, we can ask what factors are involved in post-DBS changes in self-experience, personal identity, and the self-pattern.

To answer the first question, how autonomy maps across the numerous processes of the self-pattern, Miriam Kyselo (2014) provides some guidance. She asks how bodily aspects of self relate to social aspects of self, and she shows that the bodily aspects mediate the social aspects. We can think of bodily processes as including not just (1) those factors of bodily existence that involve the core biological functions of homeostasis, or those processes that allow the system to distinguish between self and non-self, but also (2) the prereflective experiential aspects that are closely related to bodily action—the first-person, prereflective experience manifest in proprioception and kinaesthetia including a *sense of body ownership* and a *sense of agency* for one's actions—and (3) affective aspects, ranging from bodily affects to what may be a typical pattern of affectivity or emotion. As we've seen in previous chapters, all of these processes are interconnected in a meshed architecture, and characterized by a set of dynamical relations. The basic self/non-self distinction is not just a non-conscious function of the biological organism, it is also something that is experienced prereflectively in terms of pro-prioception, which contributes to the senses of ownership and agency. Likewise one can think of affective experiences, widely conceived as depending on various bodily systems, including autonomic and endocrine systems, as affecting one's sense of agency and one's affordance-related perception. For example, if I am fatigued or hungry, or perhaps sad or depressed, I may not have as much motiv-ation or energy to engage in action; my sense of agency may wane, and the set of available affordances may decline. Bodily processes, affect, agency, and ecological and social affordances are all closely connected.

Kyselo (2014) considers the importance of social dimensions, and "the growing acknowledgment of the idea that cognition involves the social and is, broadly construed, also concerned with inter-subjectivity and with understanding others." This includes developmental and neurobiological processes that shape social interaction, as well as the role of narrative practices. Kyselo's worry is that by emphasizing such social aspects of selfhood, one downplays the role of the body,[2] or, by emphasizing the embodied aspects, one downplays the role of the social, leading to the conclusion (which she wants to avoid) that "[t]he self as a whole can either be embodied or social, but it cannot be both." If it could be only one of these, we would return to a deflationary conception of self. This worry disappears, however, when we examine the dynamical connections between bodily and social processes that ultimately contribute to the constitution of the self-pattern. Indeed, I've argued that intersubjective factors are endogenous to embodied practices, and that one must consider the tight relations between bodily and social pro-cesses to gain a more comprehensive account of self (Gallagher 2009b). One need only consider, for example, the effects of social (normative) constraints (imposed by either dyadic intersubjective interactions or more statically organized institu-tional structures) on one's possibilities for action and thus on one's sense of agency.[3] Such social factors constrain what agents can do, and how agents may feel about their actions.

How does autonomy figure into these tightly interwoven bodily-social factors? Kyselo problematizes this issue by reinforcing the contrast between bodily, indi-vidual autonomy, and the autonomy of the social process that emerges in social

---

[2] Although Kyselo cites de Haan (2010) in this respect, de Haan, even in arguing that the self is relational, does not deny its bodily nature or posit a tension between the bodily and the social charac-ter of the self.

[3] It is simply *not* the case that, "there is nothing social about the organismic or the moving body *per se*" (Kyselo 2014, 4). Rather, as Marcel Mauss (1979) suggested, "there is simply no such thing as a 'natural' way of walking that may be prescribed independently of the diverse circumstances in which human beings grow up and live their lives" (quoted in Ingold 2004, 335).

interaction, that is, the autonomy of the interactional process that emerges as something over and above (although not independent) of the actions of the involved individuals. It's not clear, however, that this is a problem for the enactivist view of social interaction. On the enactivist model, there is always a balanced and partial trade-off between the autonomy of the individual embodied participant and the autonomy of the process that emerges in social interaction. For the dynamical coupling of bodily individuals in social interactions to persist, both forms of autonomy are required. An arrangement that maintains an absolute individualism, lacking social recognition, undermines the individual and leads to a self-destruction of a meaningful form of individual or interactional autonomy (as philosophers from Hegel to Honneth have shown [see Gallagher 2020a]). Likewise, an interaction that overwhelms individual autonomy undermines the very possibility of interaction (De Jaegher et al. 2010). What Kyselo needs in order to resolve the seeming tension between the self as embodied individual and as social agent is the notion of relational autonomy—the idea of an autonomy that is by degree, and that exists for the individual agent only because she is socially situated (see Mackenzie & Stoljar 2000; Baylis 2011; and especially Baylis 2013 for a nuanced account of post-DBS changes in personal identity with respect to narrative, agency, and relational autonomy).

The traditional notion of autonomy is closely connected with traditional conceptions of the individual self. The most influential conception of autonomy takes Kant as the *locus classicus*, and takes autonomy to involve self-sufficiency, self-legislation, or self-determination. On this view, autonomy is an individualistic concept, framed in terms of rational-cognitive decision-making processes. Harry Frankfurt (1971), for example, conceives of autonomy as something grounded in reflective practices of deliberation that allow for the formation of second-order intentions or desires. This view is consistent with traditional models of an autonomous individual, and it unduly emphasizes an assumed ideal of rational self-awareness, for the most part ignoring the effects of embodied, situated, affective, and socially embedded aspects of action.

Within this traditional framework, narrative competency can be thought to be an important part of the precise kind of self-reflection that informs decision-making processes. Narrative can facilitate retrospective evaluation and prospective intention formation. On this view, autonomy depends on forming intentions that are consistent with one's narrative understanding of oneself. David Velleman (2007), for example, emphasizing the prospective function of narrative, argues that narrative provides a framework for testing one's formation of prior intentions and for guiding actions. Narrative competency is also thought to be important for the formation of self-identity and a more comprehensive self-understanding in individuals. We understand ourselves best in terms of our own self-narratives, and narrative "authorship" is considered a means of autonomous self-governance (Velleman 2007).

Thinking of autonomous decision-making in terms of narrative moves us in the direction of a wider account of autonomy despite the fact that, as Velleman and others portray it, narrative authorship is still a seemingly private and individual matter. One simply has to consider the developmental story of how we gain narrative competency to see that this emphasis on individual cognitive processes is off the mark. We learn to form linguistic narratives through interactions with others around the age of two to three years—specifically when caregivers elicit accounts of just-past actions or events. Young children around two to three years appropriate the narratives of others as their own. Not only does narrative competency develop and derive from our interactions with others, our narrative practices are most frequently social practices. Specifically, deliberation is not always or for the most part a lonely exercise taking place in the confines of an individual's head. It is frequently an intersubjective accomplishment where we consult with others (friends, partners, family, group members, and so forth), or engage in joint decision-making. Intentions often get co-constituted in communicative actions and interactions with others, and in such cases are not reducible to processes that are contained exclusively within one individual. Even private deliberation is informed by considerations of what others might think or how others might respond to our actions. Indeed, the kinds of things that find their way into our self-narratives, or that count as important are to some degree normatively determined. Even as adults, shared narratives, the stories of others, and the stories others tell about us, become part of our self-narrative.

Deliberations and narratives are about actions, and the actions that matter for such processes are never socially isolated events. Autonomous actions are embodied and happen in a world that is physical and social; intentions often reflect immediate perceptual and affective valences, and the effects of physical and social forces and affordances. Notions of agency, intention, and autonomy are thus best conceived in these embodied and socially situated terms. Accordingly, autonomy should be thought of as *relational*, rather than narrowly individualistic (Christman 2004; 2009). As Mackenzie and Stoljar (2000, 4) put it, we need to think of autonomy "as a characteristic of agents who are emotional, embodied, desiring, creative, and feeling, as well as rational, creatures" (also see Baylis 2011).

Individuals are embedded in social contexts, interacting with others in ways that can enhance or impoverish the control they have over their lives. Intersubjective relations, and the normative constraints that come along with those relations, as well as the various extended physical arrangements of the surrounding world, may limit or enhance our ability to act, or even what we recognize as our possibilities. Autonomy, conceived in this relational way, is thus a matter of degree—it can be won or lost, it can be enhanced or reduced by physical, social, economic, cultural factors, including our own narrative practices, and especially our relations with others. To think of autonomy in this way, however, is not to rule out the importance of embodied motor control processes. Thus, the loss or reinstatement of motor control (in PD or post-DBS, respectively), with accompanying changes in the sense of agency, can limit or increase our action possibilities.

In the context of the self-pattern, the notion of relational autonomy most neatly maps onto the way that the complex experience of agency involves not only prereflective experiential aspects (motor control and the intentional sense of achieving a goal), but also reflective (and narrative) processes involved in intention formation, and the constraints introduced by ecological and normative factors connected with physical environments, others, and social institutions. Limitations introduced in terms of any of these factors also impose limitations on autonomy. Likewise, new possibilities introduced by any of these factors can lead to an expanded degree of autonomy.

7.4 The Self-pattern in the Post-DBS Ecology of Affordances

To answer the second question, about how autonomy figures into situations involving DBS treatment, and what factors of the self-pattern are changed post-DBS, we can take some guidance from de Haan et al. (2013; 2015; 2017), who, although they don't mention the concept of autonomy, reframe the problem in terms of affordances and their variations. In some sense this may seem like a move away from questions about self and personal identity originally motivated by those who undergo specific side effects of DBS treatment. But affordances concern precisely what *I* as an individual, or *we* as a social unit can do in current circumstances; such ecological factors relate directly to affect, agency, and autonomy. In this respect, we can consider affordances to be the flip side of autonomy.

As Kiverstein, Rietveld, and Denys (2021) put it:

> There are two sides to the increased self-confidence we see in our DBS patients, corresponding to the self and the world. On the side of the world is the expanded range of possibilities that the patient is now open to engaging with—activities previously deemed impossible. On the side of the self, new ways of being are now available.... Our patients literally relate to their own existence in a new, more open way, with greater understanding of who they fundamentally are.

Specifically, given the relational nature of affordances—the fact that an affordance is defined not just in terms of (physical and social) environmental arrangements *simpliciter*, but in terms of what an agent is capable of in that environment (e.g., the agent's skill level)—affordances always imply the self-as-agent with some degree of autonomy. A specific pattern of affordances (see Figure 7.1), at the same time and in important respects, reflects a specific self-pattern.

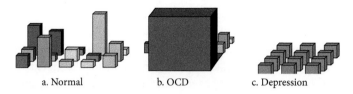

a. Normal   b. OCD   c. Depression

Figure 7.1 A schematic depiction of different fields of relevant affordances, normal vs OCD vs Depression

Note: "[T]he 'width' refers to the broadness of the scope of affordances that one perceives. This dimension relates to having a choice or action options. The 'depth' of the field refers to the temporal aspect: one not only perceives the affordances that are immediately present here and now, but one is also pre-reflectively aware of future plans and possibilities for action. . . . Lastly, the 'height' of each of the affordances refers to the relevance or importance of the affordances that one is responsive to, i.e., to the experienced solicitation or affective allure. This dimension of relevance and salience relates to motivation" (de Haan et al. 2013, 7). The different shades refer to variations in affective allure. "It is a dynamic field: to the extent that [if] either our concerns or the environment changes, the field of relevant affordances changes too" (de Haan et al. 2015, 18; also see de Haan 2020, 218–20; Dings 2018).

Source: From de Haan et al. (2013).

Consider the four dimensions of the affordance field that de Haan et al. (2017) define, that is, range, temporal proximity, salience, and affective allure.[4] I'm suggesting that, at least in some respects, the number and quality of an agent's affordances track the agent's autonomy, even if they do not entirely define it.[5] *Within certain limits*, or perhaps *ceteris paribus*, the greater number of affordances (i.e., range and temporal proximity) and the higher the quality of the affordances (i.e., salience and affective allure), the more autonomy, which relates directly to one's sense of agency. How this field of affordances might relate to the self-pattern more generally depends in some regard on the kinds of affordances available. In part the question depends on how one categorizes affordances. The four dimensions don't specify whether the affordances are physical, social, or cultural affordances, or intellectual or cognitive affordances. Clearly, for example, social affordances will relate directly to the intersubjective aspect of the self-pattern. If, as the result of depression, my intersubjective relations shrink or become impoverished, both the number and the quality (especially affective allure) of my social affordances will decrease. Likewise, physical affordances will depend on my bodily condition. Any particular condition, for example, being in a wheelchair, may rule out some

---

[4] The "field of affordances" is defined as "the affordances that stand out as relevant for a particular individual in a particular situation; i.e., the multiplicity of affordances that solicit the individual" (de Haan et al. 2013).

[5] An increased range of possible actions doesn't always mean increased autonomy. Patients undergoing a manic episode or under the influence of drugs could report an increased sense in their field of affordances, and a feeling of being overwhelmed but this would not mean an increased autonomy. Moreover, to conceive of autonomy in this way is not necessarily consistent with more traditional conceptions of agency (e.g., Frankfurt's idea that agency has to do with endorsing important desires). On that view, changing affordances does not necessarily amount to changing autonomy. Thanks to a reviewer for making this clear.

and create others. Cultural affordances may depend on my prior history, as well as my learned values, which further reflect ecological and normative factors in the self-pattern. Cognitive affordances will relate directly to my skills and capacities for memory, imagination, problem solving, and so forth, which make up the cognitive aspects of the self-pattern. Moreover, we can make the story more nuanced by considering that salience and affective allure cut across any affordance field in the same way that the affective aspect dynamically relates to all other aspects of the self-pattern.[6]

Patients interviewed by de Haan et al. (2013) provide some important insights. For example, Patient 3 expresses not only an enhanced affordance space, but also a set of positive changes in affect and evaluative reflection that appear to be dynamically linked to his expanded set of affordances, reflected in an increased sense of agency and autonomy:

> When the DBS was turned on, that was very strange! I had this pleasant feeling all of a sudden (...) Right before, I had been quite negative and then, two minutes later, I was thriving (...) Before [DBS] I saw all the restrictions, you know, from having this disorder. All the things I cannot do. (...) But after the DBS was turned on, I thought: 'oh but I *can* do this.' (5)

> With the right settings, I am in a better mood. I can immediately notice that. It's...my breathing is calmer and more relaxed (...) I feel less tense and so, well, I have less the need to do these compulsive actions. (6)

> I make plans, positive plans (...) [Before the DBS] I would not have dreamed about setting up an online store, or maybe I would have dreamed about it, but then like 'that will never work out anyway'. But now I think: 'oh, I can give it try.' (6)

These narratives reflect the dynamical nature of the self-pattern, and at the same time, the dynamical nature of the affordance space. On either register it seems possible to map out the individual differences from one patient to another in ways that can specify either an increase (as in Patient 3) or a decrease in autonomy. Generally, OCD patients who undergo DBS treatment report an increase in autonomy. De Haan et al. (2015, 8–9) indicate that a large majority of the patients interviewed

> mentioned that they dared to plan and to do things again. They used to avoid making plans, because it usually did not work out anyway because of the

---

[6] For the connection between affect and affordance see Sass and Ratcliffe (2017). They describe the EAWE category of atmospheric changes (diminished sense of reality, altered sense of meaning, disrupted feeling of familiarity, and diminished vitality and relevance) as involving changes in "existential feeling."

compulsions. Now, related to the hope and optimism, participants started to make plans, either for the next days, or even for the next years. And they also in fact dared to do more things, were less avoidant...were more interested in the world around them, and more engaged.

The world "opens up and becomes bigger"; patients are able to see "a larger range of possible actions, both immediately and in the future" (de Haan et al. 2015, 18). Patient 8, for example, reports that "the DBS certainly has done something, because I am much stronger and powerful now. And much more like, you know, this is what I want, and this is what I will pursue; making my own choices" (de Haan et al. 2015, 8).

In these cases, of course, the contrast is being made with the OCD experience, which involves a significantly different affordance space structure (see Figure 7.1). The point here, however, is that the changes that can be mapped across these various reports are simultaneously changes in the self-pattern and the affordance pattern, and they reflect varying degrees of autonomy. In each case there is a change in the sense of what the person can do, both in terms of physical and social possibilities, and how patients experience (or don't experience) this change—including changes in their sense of agency and autonomy. These changes may be significantly different for each individual (some experiencing more cognitive flexibility, and some experiencing less), reflecting difficulties in planning and organizing; some experiencing better concentration, others becoming easily distracted, and for different conditions being treated.

At the same time patients report changes in their social and intersubjective relations: they may be more expressive, assertive, and aggressive: "Many participants report that in social interactions they speak out more what they think of things, and generally express themselves more. They also stand up for themselves more, are more assertive. Some also report being more easily annoyed by other people, and being more irritable. Three participants were more aggressive, mainly in traffic" (de Haan et al. 2015, 8). This assertiveness, in turn, has implications for their social relations:

> Several participants report that they had difficulties in their relationship after DBS treatment. Their partners had to get used to their sudden changes in behaviour; in being confronted with 'a different person' as one participant described it. Moreover, many participants experience ups and downs in treatment, which makes them less predictable to their partners. Whereas participants themselves were generally happy with the changes, several noted that their partners were considerably less enthusiastic.   (de Haan et al. 2015, 11)

The idea that autonomy is relational means that the measure of autonomy is not just the individual, but how that individual's actions and interactions are configured in social contexts. If the patient turns out to be more aggressive, rather than more friendly, his social affordances and his degree of autonomy may decline even if he reports a sense that he feels more in control of his life. Likewise, if the patient finds himself involved in closer interactions with others and more reliant on them, this may signal an expansion of affordances rather than a decline in his overall autonomy. Even in the face of serious disabilities, an individual's autonomy may be sufficiently intact with the support of others, and with the right arrangement of social and institutional factors.

Some patients, following DBS, experience increased impulsivity, and this is not always a good change. For example, Parkinson's patients may become more daring, take more risks, and make more impulsive decisions (Frank et al. 2007). Different patients may reflectively evaluate these changes differently. The variations may depend on "whether or not the patient himself perceives the changes in his personality, mood, behavior, or cognition brought about by DBS as disruptive of his personal...identity" (Schermer 2011, 2). Indeed, as Schermer indicates, such changes in personality and behavior that negatively affect others, may raise problems concerning personal responsibility. How we think of autonomy will have some importance for the DBS patient, as well as for physician and family members. Indeed, patients who are not autonomous on the traditional concept might still qualify as autonomous on a relational concept given certain degrees of support from others.

To summarize, we can draw a complex map of processes and relations in the self-pattern related to what we might call the "4As": agency, affect, autonomy, and affordances. The experience of agency involves a number of variables; likewise, affective processes modulate some of these same variables. Moreover, we can conceive of changes in agency and affect in terms of both the number and quality of affordances. Autonomy, in turn, is closely tied to agency but also (as relational) to social and intersubjective factors.

The 4As are part of what we called a meshed architecture (Chapter 3), in which disruptions or interventions that effect a change in any of these factors will lead to more holistic changes. Accordingly, affective changes can modulate both my experience of agency and my field of affordances. The experience of agency and my affordance-based perception of possibilities may co-vary. For example, the higher quantity and quality of affordances available, within certain limits, the stronger my sense of agency, whereas a constriction of affordances and a decline in agency may lead to a decline in autonomy.

7.5 The Therapeutic Reconstruction of Affordances

A variety of neurological and psychiatric disorders can be understood in terms of changes to the subject's field of affordances. Understanding disorders in this way also has some implications for therapy, including the use of DBS. Clearly, however, this approach opens up considerations that go beyond neurocentric therapies like DBS or pharmaceuticals. In this respect, an affordance-based approach to therapy allows us to think about therapeutically intervening on physical, social, and cultural environments.[7]

Physical damage to the body will result in the loss, disappearance, or change of physical affordances. Consider, for example, the variations in the affordance field following limb amputation, heart attack, or stroke. Such changes may lead to new or different physical (but not only physical) affordances. For example, the affordance field of a person confined to a wheelchair can be different compared to someone who is not so confined, and these differences may be due not only to the person's wheelchair skills, but also to the design of the built environmental, as well as to differences in social and cultural attitudes on the part of others (Cole 2007). In a wheelchair, social affordances change in part because others' attitudes and expectations change.

We can also see changes in the field of affordances, for example, in the case of depression:

> [In major depressive disorder] the conative dimension of the body, that is, its affective and appetitive directedness, is lacking or missing. Normally, it is this dimension that opens up peripersonal space as a realm of possibilities, 'affordances' and goals for action. In depressive patients, however, drive and impulse, appetite and libido are reduced or lost, no [longer] disclosing potential sources of pleasure and satisfaction.   (Fuchs & Schlimme 2009, 572)

Likewise, in schizophrenic delusions, affordances change. For example, Marguerite Séchehaye (1968) in *Autobiography of a Schizophrenic Girl*, describes affordance changes for Renee, a schizophrenic patient:

> [A jug appeared to her] not as something to hold water and milk, a chair not as something to sit in—but as having lost their names, their functions and meanings; they became 'things' and began to take on life, to exist.
> (Cited in Sass 1992, 118)

In the case of OCD there is a serious constriction of the affordance field as the subject finds herself limited to one repetitive action, or one set of specific actions, and unable to move beyond that. In the case of utilization behavior (following

---

[7] An affordance-based approach to therapy is not intended as a complete account that captures everything of importance in therapeutic settings. Clearly there are other aspects, such as personal understanding and empathy, that are important but not emphasized here.

frontal damage), everything becomes a solicitation. Presented with any object (e.g., a hammer), the subject is unable to refrain from picking it up and using it.

In some cases, one might think of the task of therapy as restoring function. As Hans-Georg Gadamer puts it, "Convalescence, becoming well again, is a process of returning once more to one's accustomed form of life" (2018, 97). In some cases, however, if one is in the middle of a prolonged, chronic, or clinical condition, it seems possible that the illness itself can shape one's life so pervasively that it permanently (re)defines one's form of life. Thinking in these terms, Merleau-Ponty remarks, that "Illness, like childhood…is a complete form of existence" such that it can lead to permanent adjustments in optimal grip—that is, in the way that we pragmatically attune to the world (2012, 110). In other words, illness can redefine our field of affordances and our being-in-the-world in such a way that there is no going back. Tracking these different ways of considering illness, there are debates about whether the goal of therapy is restoration or reconstruction (Øberg et al. 2015). Given changes in one's physical-mental-affective health, Ramstead, Veissière, and Kirmayer (2016) suggest that adjustments across the affordance space can start to reshape "a field of solicitations out of the total landscape of available affordances," dynamically moving the organism toward transformations in what counts as optimal grips on various situations:

> The field of affordances thus changes dynamically along with perception-action and changes to states of the organism and environment. Responsiveness to the field, informed by states of the organism and environment, prescribe modes of optimal coupling.   (Ramstead et al. 2016, 13)

It is not just that the patient can no longer lift up a cup, sit in a chair, complete a task, or appreciate another person's emotional expression—it's rather that the world has taken on a different meaning—or that the affordance space has been reconfigured. Accordingly, therapy involves not just understanding what patients can or cannot do, and facilitating adjustments—it involves understanding their form of existence, their changed experience, their refigured self-pattern, how they are differently in-the-world, and how they are differently enabled. In this respect, I note the importance of taking a phenomenological approach—that is, an approach that attempts to understand the patient's first-person experience and their changed being-in-the-world, factors that can be worked into a "rich diagnosis" (Parnas & Gallagher 2015), with implications for therapeutic practices. Following this line of thought, in the remainder of this section I outline six (relatively unsystematic but connected) ideas that form part of an affordance-based approach to therapy, addressing the self-pattern through its ecological window, so to speak.

First, in therapeutic contexts, optimal coupling needs to be understood holistically, in terms of a form of life that involves an agent's changed self-pattern. A therapeutic evaluation (pre- and post-DBS, or any other therapy) should consider the full inventory of factors in the self-pattern. One should ask, not only what the patient can or can't do now that she could not do, or could do before, but also how such changes affect her emotional life, her sense of agency, her social relations, her personality.

Second, when Merleau-Ponty calls illness a complete form of existence, he also notes that "[t]he procedures it employs to replace normal functions which have been destroyed are equally pathological phenomena. It is impossible to deduce the normal from the pathological" (2012, 110). In that case, one needs to distinguish in the changed self-pattern between what remains undisturbed, what genuinely changes, and what may only be a compensatory rearrangement (Marcel 2003).

Third, an affordance-based therapy should understand the relations between abstract and concrete behaviors and corresponding affordances according to a gestalt principle summarized succinctly by Goldstein and Scheerer:

> Although the normal person's behaviour is prevailingly concrete, this concrete-ness can be considered normal only as long as it is embedded in and codeter-mined by the abstract attitude. For instance, in the normal person both attitudes are always present in a definite figure-ground relation.
>
> (Goldstein & Scheerer 1964, 8)

This is roughly consistent with the idea that "concrete" behavior (involving body-schematic processes and prereflective experiential processes of the self-pattern) is dynamically coupled to or meshed with "abstract" behavior (i.e., cognitive-reflective processes) in a gestalt structure. These processes are also integrated with social, cultural, and normative factors. Neurological and behavioral evidence for this can be found in experiments on intersubjective alignment and synchronic joint action, where the formation of "joint body schemas" is modulated by cultural factors. Soliman and Glenberg (2014) show that joint actions involving synchronic movements lead to an expansion of peripersonal space to include the co-actor's peripersonal space (similar to the incorporation of tools, often described in terms of an extended body schema or expanded peripersonal space—see Cardinali, Brozzoli & Farne 2009). The interesting twist is that Soliman and Glenberg looked across cultures to find differences on these measures. It turns out that the adaptation of a joint body schema is more pronounced for those who self-identify as socially interdependent in contrast to those who self-identify as individualist (see Park & Kitayama 2014). Their conclusion [enhanced by Goldstein and Scheerer's terminology]:

> Culture is not a[n abstract] psychological structure that exists apart from more mundane [concrete actions]. Rather, the psychological underpinning of culture consists of an individual's sensorimotor tuning arising from and guiding social interactions.   (Soliman & Glenberg 2014, 209)

In effect, one should not think of the normative effects of culture as a set of higher-order cognitive practices that are distinct from lower-order bodily processes. And this is true in both theoretical and therapeutic contexts. Embodied, agentive behaviors are always embedded in cultural practices, and vice versa, so that they always operate in a dynamic gestalt figure–ground relation, a meshing of normativity in sensory-motor processes. Everyday practices that involve normative factors affectively attune perception and action in a way that does not always require a reflective deliberation about what is or is not correct or what is or isn't expected behavior in each case (see Rietveld 2008). Our bodily skills and our intersubjective interactions make us normative experts.

Fourth, it is important to distinguish between differences in the patient that are either recognized by, or unrecognized by the patient. In some cases, patients recognize that they have changed, or are undergoing change, either as the result of a disorder or as the result of a type of treatment. In other cases, the patient does not recognize this change. For example, in some cases of PD or OCD treated with DBS, the patient's personality and behavior undergo significant changes of which they are not aware, even though it is evident to their loved ones or care givers (de Haan et al. 2013).

Fifth, it is beneficial to recognize and address modulations in the field of affordances that may come about not just as a result of the generative disorder, but as a result of social and intersubjective factors. This can go in two directions for purposes of therapy. (1) Social context may enhance therapeutic effects in a positive way. In cases of apraxia following stroke, for example, motor rehabilitation is improved when patients engage in actions in meaningful social contexts, in contrast to when they engage in less meaningful, non-social exercises (Marcel 1992; Gallagher & Marcel 1999). (2) Negative social contexts can complicate disorders. For example, studies of individuals with various disorders suggest that the non-social or socially limited behavior of such individuals may in part be due to the way that others treat them (McGeer 2001; Cole 2007; Krueger & Michael 2012; see, e.g., Section 3.4.4). In such cases, the reconstruction of affordances might involve reconstructing social attitudes more generally.

Finally, in the self-pattern there are no strict lines between physical (embodied), psychological, and social disorders. Working in the tradition of phenomenological psychiatry, Medard Boss (1979), for example, proposed to dissolve the traditional dualism between somatic and psychiatric illness, illuminating how the experience of illness, whether mental or physical, is always already shaped and mediated by a changed form of being-in-the-world. Likewise, following the enactivist idea that the unit of explanation is the brain-body-environment, one should not expect to be able to pull apart psychological and physical changes in many disorders.

In sum, within therapeutic contexts, agents are understood to be socially-culturally-normatively embedded. Autonomy in this regard must be understood as relational. This does not rule out the importance of self-narrative and reflective capacities, emphasized in traditional accounts of autonomy. Such capacities remain relevant for understanding responsible decision-making processes, even as such practices are situated in worldly contexts. These processes are tempered by affectivity, intersubjective interactions, and affordance-based actions in ecological and normative contexts. On the relational view, autonomy is a matter of degree as it is limited by or enabled by others and by various situations that are integrated with a patient's self-pattern. Thinking of these issues in terms of a self-pattern provides a model which supports an approach in psychiatry that involves rich diagnosis and an enriched variety of therapies—a phenomenologically informed enactivist approach that considers not just cognitive abilities, but also issues of motor performance, affectivity, intersubjectivity, ecological factors, and so forth—and that takes the brain-body-environment as the explanatory unit, including the affordances defined by the social and cultural situation of the patient.

8

Artificial Transformations
of the Self-pattern

According to Lawrence Krauss in *The Physics of Star Treck*, the speed of digital information transfer in 1996 was less than about 100 megabytes per second. He notes that at this rate "it would take about 2000 times the present age of the universe (assuming an approximate age of 10 billion years) to write the data describing a human pattern to tape!" (1996, 76–7). In the last twenty-five years we've made some progress. The fastest data transmission speed is now 319 terabits or 39,875,000 *megabytes* per second. If that's a good upload speed, and if my math is right, it would take only 50,000 years, give or take a century or two, to upload a human pattern as Krause defines it. As he defines it, however, the human pattern is not equivalent to the self-pattern, but only to something like the bodily processes of the human (namely, the information defining the position and internal structure of every atom in the human body, approximately 10^{28} kilobytes of information). The full self-pattern would seemingly include a significantly higher amount of information (assuming it can be reduced to information).

In previous chapters I have been careful to avoid a neurocentric focus, conceiving of the self-pattern as distributed across brain-body-environment. I will continue to do so in this chapter, although in scientific (and science fiction) discussions of artificial enhancements the focus is quite often just on the brain. If we add a chip here (in the brain), or a neural network there (in the brain), what happens to the self-pattern? Specifically, in considering advances in artificial intelligence (AI), and how such advances might change human practices, and thereby human nature, people usually think of placing chips in the brain. But, of course, chips are now almost everywhere (in many tools, in some bodies, and in some brains), and examples of AI applications are starting to be pervasive. In some cases they are directly relevant to psychiatry.

In this context, the most general approach is computational psychiatry. "Most general" since a computational approach, rather than a particular theory of psychopathology, can be viewed as a modeling tool that can support or test a variety of theories (Constant et al. 2022). Moreover, computational psychiatry can be applied in numerous ways. For example, in the research area of cognitive developmental robotics (Asada et al. 2001), one can use embodied artificial agents "to examine phenomenological concepts such as the self…and relate those to action and behavior" in order to model psychopathological variations "in silico" (Möller

The Self and its Disorders. Shaun Gallagher, Oxford University Press. © Shaun Gallagher 2024.
DOI: 10.1093/oso/9780198873068.003.0009

et al. 2021, 2). Alternatively, one can use machine learning techniques to identify variables with predictive values for clinical disorders and to test the efficacy of antipsychotic medications (Koutsouleris et al. 2016).

Research in such areas is moving at lightening-speed. In 2019 Fellous et al. wrote:

> The use of Artificial Intelligence and machine learning in basic research and clinical neuroscience is increasing. AI methods enable the interpretation of large multimodal datasets that can provide unbiased insights into the fundamental principles of brain function, potentially paving the way for earlier and more accurate detection of brain disorders and better informed intervention protocols. (Fellous et al. 2019, 1)

They explain that one limitation of current deep brain stimulation (DBS) systems, discussed in the previous chapter, is that they are open loop, which means that the standard DBS chip is unable to monitor and modulate neural activity in real time. In a closed-loop design neurostimulation could be determined by the implanted chip. Less than a year later Alik Widge, a psychiatrist at the University of Minnesota Medical School, described, in the popular media, the development of a closed-loop technology that will monitor and "sense brain activity moment to moment, millisecond to millisecond." It will be able to "read the brain signals and interpret and say, now is the moment when you need to deliver that single little nudge of stimulation to get that network back into its healthy state."[1]

In the terminology from the various philosophical critiques of the 1970s and 1980s, such applications would be considered forms of specialized "weak" AI. Many theorists today, however, think that we are ultimately threatened by a "strong" AI—that is, systems designed to match or exceed human intelligence. Moreover, AI has advanced so much that the older philosophical critiques (by people like Dreyfus and Searle) may be outdated (see, e.g., Schneider & Mandik 2018). Artificial *general* intelligence (AGI) is still a project rather than an existing product, but we seem to be moving forward at a fast clip.[2] In contrast to "good old-fashioned AI," which involved a bottlenecking process of symbol crunching, the more recent combination of deep, neural-network machine learning with big data, allows for the virtualization of models that deliver fast, reliable, and relatively accurate processing. The use of new mathematical tools means that the

---

[1] Local news (October 14, 2020). https://kstp.com/health-medical/first-of-its-kind-brain-chip-to-treat-mental-disorders-being-developed-at-the-u-of-m/ —accessed July 29, 2023. Also see Provenza et al. 2019; Vu et al. (2018).

[2] Shortly after I wrote the noted sentence, ChatGPT appeared on the scene in November 2022. ChatGPT is not an AGI. I confirmed this with ChatGPT. Even as a large language model, with an imperfect performance record (see van Dis et al. 2023), however, it challenges the older philosophical critiques.

weighting of data by backpropagation has improved. Perhaps surprisingly, precisely how this works, and "why neural networks work as well as they do" is, as Marcus and Davis (2019, 57) suggest, "an unsolved mystery." Deep learning, they explain, "is opaque." But so are the workings of neural networks in the brain and most psychiatric medications and therapies.

Many critics, including some leading scientists, like the late Stephen Hawking (Cellan-Jones 2014), worry about a struggle that will develop between machines and humans when AGI reaches a point of superintelligence (Bostrom 2014; Chalmers 2010). The focus of this chapter, however, is on a more cooperative relationship; that is, how AI might enhance human existence, with special reference to therapeutic practices. Specifically, whether we call it enhancement or something else, I want to ask how AI could change the self-pattern (this is the topic of the first two sections). This may range from implanting chips in the brain for therapeutic purposes (as in DBS), to using AI in creating environments designed to facilitate mental health. I'll start to explore the therapeutic context in Sections 8.3 and 8.4.

As we might expect in reference to AI, much of the discussion focuses, not just on applications involving neural enhancement, but on cognitive intelligence, pure and simple, although changes ("advances") in intelligence may have implications for social skills, empathy, and moral capacity. To be clear, I am not asking about whether an AGI system might itself have a self-pattern, and I am not concerned here about how to engineer an artificial self-pattern (for instructions, see Ryan, Agrawal & Franklin 2020, and Hölken et al. 2023). Rather, the focus is on philosophical issues involving existing human self-patterns and how they might be changed by artificial means. As David Chalmers (2010, 7) puts it:

> The potential consequences of an intelligence explosion force us to think hard about values and morality and about consciousness and personal identity. In effect, the singularity [the point at which humans can no longer predict or understand superintelligent systems] brings up some of the hardest traditional questions in philosophy and raises some new philosophical questions as well.... To determine whether we can play a significant role in a post-singularity world, we need to know whether human identity can survive the enhancing of our cognitive systems, perhaps through uploading onto new technology.

8.1 Living the Enhanced Life

The following is a thought experiment proposed by Susan Schneider (2009; repeated in Schneider & Mandik 2018). (1) A few years from now various technologies for brain enhancement are available and you purchase an internet microchip for your visual system and a working memory enhancement. (2) Sometime later nanotechnology-based therapies are able to extend your lifespan, and as time goes on you continue installing enhancements so that your basic capacities exceed present-day humans and you are considered posthuman. "At this point, your intelligence is enhanced not just in terms of speed of mental processing; you are now able to make rich connections that you were not able to make before" (Schneider & Mandik 2018, 307). You live a long life, and your enhancements continue.

> [3] It is now 2250 AD. Over time, the slow addition of better and better neural circuitry has left no real intellectual difference in kind between you and AI. Your mental operations have been gradually transferring to the cloud, and by this point, you are silicon-based. The only real difference between you and an AI creature of standard design is one of origin—you were once a natural. But you are now almost entirely engineered by technology—you are perhaps more aptly characterized as a member of a rather heterogeneous class of AI life forms.
>
> (Schneider & Mandik 2018, 307)

This seems to have been a gradual transformation, but clearly you have lost some things along the way—specifically, some factors that originally made up your self-pattern. Being-in-the-cloud is different from being-in-the-world. It's not clear what has happened to your body, but you have apparently uploaded your memories and cognitive capabilities into a machine. "You are silicon-based." You? In what sense is that you?

It may be that you begin, at (1), by incorporating some new capabilities into your brain or body, perhaps extending your cognitive powers. To the extent that this would affect memory, it would likely allow you to enhance the details of your self-narrative. That may also give you more to reflect about. If visual perception is upgraded, then perhaps you could improve your skills and refine your habitual practices. Perhaps you could walk away from your unique set of psychiatric symptoms. All of this will change your relations to others, either as a direct result of all these changes, or as a side effect (similar to a side effect in some cases of DBS). At the start of this enhancement process, all of this seems fine and manageable. We can certainly say that some things in the self-pattern have changed; other things have adjusted, and everything may be working well.

As you continue, through (2), perhaps the enhancement simply intensifies. This is described simply in terms of enriched and speedier intelligence, and it is not clear what else might be changing. Yet it is likely that there would be some changes in your affective life given that your lifespan has extended. At the very least, there may be a reduction in existential angst if this means ruling out some life-threatening diseases. This may also affect your relations to others, depending on whether your significant others did or didn't buy into the same enhancements. There may be multiple "mid-life" crises to cope with. Nonetheless, it is still possible to say that there is a kind of continuance of the self-pattern, even if some of the dynamics have changed.

At (3), however, there seems to be some major changes. Perhaps you trade in your body for the silicon cloud. This is where a lot of questions—both practical and philosophical—arise. If bodily existence is eliminated or transformed into a machine by using artificial replacement parts, and if we think of affective and emotional processes as not confined to the brain, but as involving bodily processes, can we still talk about an affective process contributing to your self-pattern? Is your locomotion in any way similar to your previous movement? Would you have a sense of agency for it, or a sense of ownership for whatever your locomotive system is? It also seems likely that your self-narrative would radically change, not just with updated content, but especially in regard to what you considered valuable enough to include, since as a machine, or as an information-based operation, rather than a biological entity, you would likely have very different interests. That would also seem to motivate some normative adjustments. And intersubjectivity or social interaction would be quite up in the air.

Schneider and Mandik admit that "enhancing by moving from carbon to silicon may not be something that preserves your conscious experience or personal identity" (309). Hence, they advise caution, since it is likely your intention had been for the enhancement to increase the quality of your life and enable your survival, but at this point it's not clear that *you* survived, or that *you* are enjoying a better life. For Schneider and Mandik, following a Lockean conception of personal identity, the question is simply whether your consciousness survived unscathed. Whatever that means, if your consciousness were to be the only thing that survived, it would still be questionable whether *you* survived if your self-pattern has changed so radically, or had failed even to upload.

8.2 Uploading the Whole Pattern

> Mind can be offloaded. It can be copied from person to robot, robot to robot, robot to robot, and so on.
>
> (Takashi Ikegami 2022)

The point is that when it comes to personal identity and survival, it may be more than an issue of consciousness or intelligence if the self or person just is the self-pattern, nothing more and nothing less. Still, in this regard, it may be possible for the pattern to be less than what one has been or what other people are, as we find in some cases of psychopathology. I may lose my memory because of Alzheimer's disease, or my sense of agency because of schizophrenia, or my self-narrative because of some form of dysnarrativa, but the self-pattern adjusts, and perhaps compensates to maintain ipse-identity. If what survives is just consciousness or just an intellect, however, it's not clear that the self-pattern does.

The notion of mind uploading (MU) is based on a Cartesian and narrow-minded conception of the mind, using "narrow" in the technical sense—specifically the idea that the mind is entirely in the head, or reducible to brain processes. Thus, the "idea behind uploading is that the person's brain is scanned, and a software [AI] model of it is constructed that is so precise that, when run on ultra-efficient hardware, it thinks and behaves in exactly the same way as the original brain" (Schneider & Mandik 2018, 310). Although the late Stephen Hawking was not a fan of superintelligent AI, he was more optimistic about MU. "I think the brain is like a programme ... so it's theoretically possible to copy the brain into a computer and so provide a form of life after death" (Hawking 2013). So maybe *not* the *late* Stephen Hawking.

MU is an AI shortcut to the cloud. On this version of the thought experiment, however, Schneider and Mandik provide the uploaded mind with an android body that one can inhabit temporarily, basically renting a body when convenient. In this case, if having (or renting) a body clarifies something about the sense of agency, it complicates the sense of ownership, even if it may make one's self-narrative more interesting. "Bodily harm matters little to you, for you just pay a fee to the rental company when your android surrogate is injured or destroyed. Formerly averse to risk, you find yourself skydiving and climbing Everest" (2018, 310). This fleshes out a certain type of multiple realizability associated with functionalism. Still, it's not clear how pain, or hunger, or fatigue, or great pleasure, or affective life more generally, figures into this scenario. It may be possible to map out with precision the neural correlates of some particular set of emotions (using advanced AI and machine learning—see, e.g., Chen, Chang & Guo 2021). But again, neural correlates, or their uploaded variants, do not constitute the full emotion pattern, so it's not clear that one would have anything like one's full affective life in the cloud. Even with an android body, affective processes, including emotional patterns, would likely be quite different, if indeed they could be instantiated in android bodies. For MU, the important thing remains cognition or consciousness; the physical entity that is capable of realizing it remains unimportant. Indeed, the android body is more an accessory than a realizer, and it would have a very different status from bodily existence in the self-pattern.

Max Cappuccio (2017, 426) has argued that, "[w]hether or not MU can deliver what it promises does not only depend on what technology is able to do, but also on the correctness of MU's metaphysical assumptions: that is, that minds are actually the kinds of 'substrate independent' things that could be extracted from a brain map, emulated by a computer, and moved from one material vessel to another." In other words, the real question is not about how advanced AI technology might become, but about the nature of the mind, or, if survival is at stake, the nature of the self, and specifically about what constitutes the identity of the mind or self. If the self is just the mind, and the mind is just a program that manipulates information, then something like MU may be possible;[3] but if the mind is constitutively embodied, and the self is a self-pattern that includes more than the mind, then it seems a much more difficult engineering problem.

The engineering models described by Chalmers (2010) (again in the form of thought experiments) are limited to methods that transfer brain operations to a computer. As Cappuccio points out, there is no material transfer; there is simply the replication of formal (syntactical) information structures (synapse A connects or communicates with synapse B, etc.) that were originally instantiated in the brain, and now instantiated in the computer. During the upload there are careful specifications about maintaining proper connections (possibly via radio signals) between your brain, which is being gradually decommissioned, and the computer which is taking over its function. Your brain gradually stops functioning altogether. At the end of the process those brain–computer connections are eliminated and there is just a completely integrated brain program in the computer. Your uploaded mind, now instantiated in the computer, seemingly exists independently from your body. Your body would continue to function only if some complex connections were maintained with the brain program in the computer. Assuming good connections, you could go about your life as normal. The mind upload engineers, however, realize that at some point these connections are eliminated (perhaps during the next power outage) and your body dies. But your mind continues once the computer is turned back on.

One very large assumption that accompanies this experiment, besides the Cartesian dualism, is the standard cognitivist supposition that the brain is representational. If we think that as human biological entities we move around a real world, perceive real objects, and respond by taking various actions, and that in this process our brains generate mental or neural representations which in some way simulate the world in a virtual format inside our heads, then the uploaded program should be able to generate the same kind of simulations due to its complete parity of informational structure. Even if we think that this is the way the brain works (something that is currently under debate in what has been called the "representation wars" [Clark 2015]), representations or simulations are not generated ex nihilo. Rather, the representation is supposedly what it is because your brain is coupled to your body, and your body is coupled to a complex environment, and there is a complex information flow that the brain manipulates. Decoupled from the body, would the brain, or could the uploaded program, continue to generate representations without input? If so, then not only is your mind replicated in silicon, but your world (or some kind of world, albeit, a simulated world) is also.

---

[3] For a functionalist account of the possibility of a virtual person, framed in terms of Searle's critique of AI, and with reference to psychopathologies like Dissociative Identity Disorder, see Cole (1991).

Cappuccio worries about whether your identities—both ipse- and idem- (or numerical) identity—are maintained, and rightly suggests that this depends on how we conceive of the components of your cognitive system. Clearly this may already beg the question if we limit considerations to just cognitive systems rather than self-patterns. Cappuccio includes cognitive function, consciousness, and mental content as candidate components of the system. I've been arguing that both ipse- and idem-identity depend on more than this, with the implication that if one wants to upload and re-constitute one's identity in a computer program one has to think about the complexities involved in bodily, affective, intersubjective, ecological, and normative details of the self-pattern. Cappuccio gets at some of these details by expanding the initial list of components to include what enactive and extended versions of embodied cognition would require. He specifically focuses on the idea that bodily existence counts as a requirement. He argues that what he calls the "ultra-Functionalism" involved in the MU hypothesis, that is, the idea that "the set of formal structures and processes that exhaustively map one's brain activity can be relocated from one substrate to another remaining just one and the same set," is inconsistent with such embodied approaches (2017, 432ff.):

> [Ultra-functionalism] posits criteria of continuity and identity of a mind that are extrinsic to its physical and functional constituents, and unrelated to the specific contextual integration of the mind-body-world system; on the contrary, [embodied mind approaches imply] that individual identity, real status (existence), and…causal powers of a mind exist only in relation to its bodily implementation: not only the existence, but also the very essence of one's mind depends on the contingent circumstances of its material realization; and the essence of mental functions itself is codetermined with the contingencies of its existential constitution.   (438)

We can complete this idea by acknowledging that all processes in the self-pattern are materially realized, and that the material processes involved are not simply in the brain, but include extra-neural, bodily, and environmental and social processes. A self-pattern does not exist in the abstract. It exists in the dynamical set of relations that make it a pattern and are materially realized in a way that cannot be uploaded autonomously or *in abstracto*.

8.3 Real AI and AI-guided Psychotherapy

Although thought experiments can help to clarify some philosophical issues, and although there are reports that researchers are working on MU technology in Silicon Valley and at Oxford University (see Laakasuo et al. 2018; and Schneider

& Mandik 2018, respectively) there are real-life applications of AI that can bring us down from the clouds, or back to earth, where they have real effects on self-patterns.

We engage everyday with technology in which sophisticated AI is already at work. I recently traded in my twenty-year-old fossil-fuel vehicle for a new EV which came with an already fully developed "frontal cortex" in the form of numerous AI enhancements. It does some things that I used to do. For example, it steers around curves and keeps me in the same lane; it slows down if I get too close to the car in front of me; it automatically brakes to avoid collision. With the fob in my pocket it turns on lights when I walk near it. It also anticipates my actions. For example, it unlocks the door when my hand moves near the door handle. Its built-in GPS makes suggestions about where to stop for coffee. There are a number of other things it can do, but I don't yet fully understand how to activate all of its features. My sense of agency during the act of driving has declined a little. This is not a self-driving car, but I imagine that my sense of agency could decline further in such a vehicle. Agency would at least get distributed. There has also been some adjustment to my affective system since I've had to learn to quash my fear and to trust the technology while on the highway.

These are minor adjustments. But AI is becoming pervasive, and a lot of minor adjustments could add up to some major changes. Some advances in AI can clearly change societal structures that shape our own normative sensibilities. To stay with the self-driving car example, a German ethics commission on AI and self-driving cars expressed some consternation about the idea that such cars will be programed to abide by traffic laws, robbing its human passengers of the kind of autonomy that would enable them to break such laws:

> One manifestation of the autonomy of human beings is that they can also take decisions that are objectively unreasonable, such as a more aggressive driving style or exceeding the advisory speed limit. In this context, it would be incompatible with the concept of the politically mature citizen if the state wanted to create inescapable precepts governing large spheres of life, supposedly in the best interests of the citizen, and nip deviant behaviour in the bud by means of social engineering. Despite their indisputable well-meaning purposes, such states of safety, framed in absolute terms, can undermine the foundation of a society based on humanistic and liberal principles.
>
> (Ethics Commission 2017, 20; cited in Simanowski,
> Brodmer & Chase 2019, 425–6)

Commenting on this concern, Simanowski, Brodmer, and Chase (2019, 426) remark, "[Such things as pre-programmed speed limits] may not greatly bother behaviorists or technocrats, but it does require a fundamental change in our view of human beings, as practical constraints render criteria like subjectivity and free will absurd." This is also clearly an issue in regard to the kind of algorithms that we find invading our web browsers and search engines, or the ones that we are welcoming on our smart phone apps, starting with face recognition.

Consider also how AI technologies may change our intersubjective inter-actions. Not only is there CCTV everywhere, but I may have it installed in the high-tech eyeglasses I'm wearing. How do you feel about being videoed? Moreover, why should I go through all of the mating rituals of dating when I can benefit from the algorithms that run dating apps that will tell me who is a good match. Indeed, it's not clear why I need to be involved in this at all. Yuval Noah Harari (2017) wonders why these apps shouldn't communicate and decide: "my Cortana [Microsoft's virtual assistant] may be approached by the Cortana of a potential lover, and the two will compare notes to decide whether it's a good match—completely unbeknown to their human owners" (2017, 347; cited in Simanowski, Brodmer & Chase 2019, 426).

How precisely will decisions be made about joint actions when your team includes an artificial agent that may have more information than other members of the team? Will AI caregivers reduce the loneliness of seniors, or comfort infants in the right way? Will we be better off if our workplace manager is an AI system? Or if we are wearing very smart exoskeletons that do a lot of the heavy lifting for us? Or, if our workplace is nothing other than a computer interface? How do we relate to an expert system rather than a physician doing our medical diagnosis (see Jiang et al. 2017; Yu, Beam & Kohane 2018); or how comfortable are we with AI-guided robotic surgery, or with AI-guided psychotherapy?

One of the early first attempts at creating a natural language program that could run a simple psychotherapeutic encounter was ELIZA (running DOCTOR). ELIZA was a rule-based chat system that would basically turn anything you said into a question that was repeated back to you, with the idea of getting you to elu-cidate. If you say "cheeseburger," it says, "Tell me about cheeseburger." If all goes well, you seemingly talk your way to a cure. ELIZA doesn't diagnose anything—not even an eating disorder. Rather it simply emulates a Carl Rogers style of talk therapy that mirrors whatever the analysand says (Bassett 2019). It runs a rule that basically asks you to elucidate, with the goal of "self-actualization." Although ELIZA seems somewhat primitive compared to current AI deep-learning chat-bots, there are anecdotal reports that subjects appreciated the encounter.[4] As Caroline Bassett puts it, "if humans found ELIZA useful perhaps it was as a mir-ror, a listening surface which enabled forms of self-examination, self expression, or self re-narrativization. If users found something revealing in their interactions

---

[4] Using a different computer-assisted interview program, the Primary Care Evaluation of Mental Disorders (PRIME-MD), Kobak et al. (1997, 910) found that "patients were more willing to admit symptoms of certain psychiatric disorders to the computer than to the primary care physicians.... The sensitivity, specificity, and positive predictive value of the computer for these disorders were high, indicating a high level of accuracy."

with ELIZA then that something was their own: ELIZA never did, and does not now, deliver injunctions, suggestions—or nudges; and has no program to promulgate" (2019, 809). ELIZA itself (or herself) doesn't have a goal, and there is no trajectory involved; it's not committed to anything. But if interacting with ELIZA could change the analysand's self-pattern, what should we think of the more sophisticated AI projects of today and tomorrow?

Consider one further example of the use of AI in therapeutic contexts. We noted (in Section 4.4) that borderline personality disorder (BPD) is characterized by four "structurally intertwined" instabilities involving self-reflective/narrative processes, affectivity (emotion dysregulation), intersubjective relations, and alienation from bodily self-experience—all of these reflecting dynamical and holistic relations among these various aspects of the self-pattern (Schmidt 2021, 225). Moreover, these instabilities may also have add-on effects for an individual's sense of agency, and reflect developmental disruptions due to environmental, economic, and early social factors. In self-narratives, BPD patients tend to reflect an incoherent or fragmented identity, to interpret situations in a rigid way, and to interpret others in a negative way. Problems with intersubjective relations tend to spill over into the therapeutic context where some patients mistrust the therapist and resist therapy, leading to high dropout rates (Martino et al. 2012).

Judit Szalai has proposed that AI-supported interventions, combined with behavioral or narrative therapy, could address these issues. Specifically, AI programs in natural language processing "could help patients re-author their self-narratives into more coherent and meaningful sequences, in which they view themselves more like agents and less subject to external control, as well as assign more consistent roles to others" (Szalai 2021, 491). The intervention focuses on finding inconsistencies in narratives, failures to properly self-attribute agency, or misattributions of negative intentions to others. As part of a therapeutic process, this would entail the use of AI, computer-based communication technology (a chatbot)—"a natural language processing-based AI device that asks targeted questions, offers conversational prompts, and processes the affective tone and content coherence," and mimics human interaction—to supplement sessions with the therapist. This type of system could even include the capacity for pattern recognition of postural and gestural cues indicative of emotional states.

The system is meant to facilitate the patient's reflective processes and the reframing of self-narrative. The benefit of such a system would not only be economical, but could reduce motivation for the patient's antagonistic responses to the therapist, assuming the patient does not perceive the AI system as a person. Szalai also notes that patients are more willing to reveal information to "virtual humans" than to the human therapist. The use of AI in this context is not meant to solve all problems; nor is it meant to replace the therapist, and it cannot be the complete therapeutic process.

Depending on how one defines having a goal or an intention, current chatbots may be designed to have a goal, and to recognize its interlocutor's goal. Is this an improvement over ELIZA? In contrast to ELIZA, a conversational agent of this sort is on a trajectory, and not simply responding to the momentary phrase. Peter Wallis and Bruce Edmonds discuss a "Belief, Desire and Intention" (BDI) architecture that tends to rigidly stay on course, or "overcommit" to a predetermined goal. "For computer systems that do things...from autonomous cars to conversational agents, a critical issue is to balance reactive decision making against deliberative behaviour. Rather than naively re-planning atomic actions at every instant, a...BDI commits to time-extended actions" (Wallis & Edmonds 2021, 3). This, however, leads to an inflexibility so that if one inputs "cheeseburger" one doesn't get the empathetic response "Tell me about your cheeseburger"; one rather gets an error message with instructions to start over. To build more flexibility into the system Wallis and Edmonds suggest that the system recheck to confirm that it is on the right trajectory—that it is working on the correct goal. If the system is on track to book a flight reservation and you say "cheeseburger," it may be able to switch to a menu that provides information about reserving a special meal on the flight, or about in-airport dining—perhaps even asking "Do you want to order a special meal?" The machine "guesses" or predicts how the trajectory is changing. This may or may not work. Wallis and Edmonds suggest that this is comparable to a ToM approach to reading minds. The machine recognizes a behavior (a phrase), and then infers an intention.

One should note, however, there is an important tradeoff between trust (or distrust) relevant to social interaction, or specifically to human therapist–patient relations, and expectations of reliability in regard to artificial systems or mechanisms. The distinction between trusting others and relying on a tool or instrument has been made by Katherine Hawley (2014). In contrast to another person, an instrument cannot be dishonest or try to hide something, or try to mislead me in some circumstances; it is incapable of betraying me. In the human–human therapeutic situation it is imperative that the therapist gains the trust of the patient. It's not clear that by substituting impersonal reliability (in the case of an AI chatbot, for example) we gain an improved therapy. The rigidity noted by Wallis and Edmonds is not easily fixed and may be persistent in such systems, introducing issues of sustainability. Artificial systems may fail or may work differently than expected in changing circumstances (so-called counterperformativity in the field of economics [Bamford & MacKenzie 2018]). "Reliability tends to be short term, not only because mechanisms sometimes break down, but oftentimes because circumstances (including human inclinations) change" (Gallagher & Petracca 2022, 16–17).

An alternative approach, proposed by Wallis and Edmunds, and drawn from the enactivist idea of direct social perception, is to design a system to directly recognize a trajectory (a goal or intention) in the interlocutor's action by recognizing when its own behavior could be complementary, thus forming a "multi-agent trajectory." As I understand it, the trick is to get the artificial agent to recognize what the other's action or expression affords, that is, to register it in terms of its own possible response with a high probability weighting for appropriateness. Seemingly, that would mean understanding how one can transform, via machine learning, embodied communicative actions, including facial expressions, gestures, vocal intonations, within a rich worldly context, into an AI architecture capable of responding with similar features. "Implementing this on a computer is beyond us at the moment and we expect more work needs to be done understanding what the philosophers mean by 'primary and secondary intersubjectivity'" (Wallis & Edmonds 2021, 9).

The challenge may be glimpsed in the differences that show up when we use a much simpler technology that mediates communication in the psychotherapeutic setting—that is, the use of computer-based communication software for online therapy where real humans are on either end of the communication. The lack of embodied presence requires a variety of adjustments in verbal and nonverbal behavior, and a displacement of what are usually non-intentional, prereflective aspects onto reflective ones (García, Di Paolo & De Jaegher 2021). That is, changes in communicative and intersubjective interaction dynamics can lead to changes in other aspects of the self-pattern that will likely not be neutral with respect to the success of the therapy.

If computer-based technologies are not yet perfectly enactive, they are nonetheless re-ordering the world, and as a result, re-ordering self-patterns. There are at least two ways to explain this—two interpretations. The first is consistent with the assumptions involved in the previous discussion of AI enhancement and MU; the second is more aligned with an approach based on embodied-enactive cognition.

As an example of the first interpretation, consider Luciano Floridi's (2011, 550) suggestion that these everyday AI technologies involve "self construction, significantly affecting who we are, who we think we are, who we might become, and who we think we might become." He argues that by approaching this re-ordering of self via a concept of information, we can view it as an engineering project of self construction, where advances in AI are solving the various challenges facing this project—such as those that involve "communication, coherence, rationality, successful interaction with the environment, coordination and collaboration with other agents, to mention the most obvious—[these] are just AI translations of classic issues in the philosophy of the self" (551). By introducing an information theoretic model, Floridi conceives of self-generating boundaries (or "membranes") moving "from the corporeal, to the cognitive to the consciousness membrane," gaining an increased degree of virtualization. Selves, on this view, are the result of such encapsulations, "although of informational rather than biochemical structures." Data start out as streams of physical patterns, which can be processed/encoded by an emerging cognitive system, which, in turn, becomes a self-aware system "once data become repurposable information, including conventional meanings" (559), which includes narrative meaning. This issues in a "mental homeostasis," a unity of self, that if it breaks down does not result in a further boundary, but in schizophrenia.

For Floridi, then, whether we conceive of self-identity in terms of consciousness or narrative, it "is achieved through forms of information processing" (2011, 555). We could think of this in the information-theoretic terms of predictive processing, where self-boundaries can be defined as a series of Markov blankets that delineate self and non-self, and where self is whatever is inside the blanket or boundary. Floridi describes it as a detachment or encapsulation, but on some versions of the predictive processing account Markov blankets describe coupling dynamics between organism and environment, an idea more consistent with enactive-embodied accounts (Gallagher & Allen 2018)—which leads to the second interpretation.

The second interpretation holds that our encounters with AI technologies are embodied encounters; we materially engage with such technologies in our social-cultural-normative practices. Such engagements have consequences for our experiential senses of agency and ownership, our pragmatic behaviors and habits, our affective lives, our intersubjective relations, as well as for our cognitive, reflective, and narrative practices. To say that such technologies change information structures may be an abstract way of saying that they change the real dynamics of the self-pattern.

Although there is a plethora of ethical questions generated by these technologies, not all of them lead to ethical problems; some may greatly improve our lives. One way or the other, however, that is, for better or for worse, they are all capable of colonizing self-patterns.

8.4 Therapeutic Uses of Virtual Reality

Pursuing both the "for better" option, and the second, embodied-enactive interpretation outlined in the previous section, we should consider the use of AI applications in clinical settings intended to enhance therapeutic treatment of psychiatric disorders. The use of advanced technology has had numerous applications in therapy, allowing for a more holistic treatment involving not just the brain (using medications, or DBS), and not just cognitive processes (using talk or cognitive therapy), but also body-based, action-oriented therapies, such as robotic-assisted rehabilitation following stroke or brain injury (Bergamasco et al. 1994; Frisoli et al. 2007; 2009), or the use of specialized virtual environments in the treatment of psychopathologies. Uses of virtual reality (VR) in general, and

VR-based therapies not only have the potential to change the way we move and interact, they can lead to adjustments in the self-pattern, and change the patient's affordance space (Kljajevic 2021; Luxton 2014; Nagaraj et al. 2022; Torous et al. 2021; these studies explore a broad range of possibilities and limitations of the use of AI and VR in therapeutic situations, including discussions of self, social interaction, emotion recognition, and gesture recognition).

In line with John Dewey's advice to physicians in his 1937 lecture in St. Louis, to treat not just the body, but also the environment, numerous applications using VR, and the creation of artificial and mixed environments, have been used to treat a variety of disorders, such as phobias, anorexia nervosa, and schizophrenia. In this regard, Röhricht et al. (2014) suggested the relevance of VR and mixed reality (MR) simulated environments to address environmental and social factors in the context of therapy. In a "mixed reality clinic" environments can be created where participants interact with both physical (real) and digital (virtual) objects in an integrated way (Milgram & Kishino 1994). The construction of VR and MR environments in a clinical setting, enhanced by AI applications, can introduce novel (more thoroughly embodied/enactive and environmentally situated) aspects into the therapeutic process (in this context, referred to as digital psychiatry; Burr et al. 2020; Torous 2017).

VR has been used in a variety of medical contexts. For example, Cole et al. (2009) employed a virtual arm to reduce phantom limb pain for amputation patients. There are also psychotherapeutic applications of VR and MR that address a variety of anxiety disorders: acrophobia (Emmelkamp et al. 2002; Rothbaum et al. 1995), arachnophobia (Carlin et al. 1997), and a variety of eating disorders such as anorexia (Riva et al. 1999), as well as post-traumatic stress disorder (Difede et al. 2007).

As Röhricht et al. (2014) note, the efficacy of such treatments is most often explained in terms of brain plasticity; on enactivist principles it may be better explained in terms of overall system plasticity (what Malafouris [2013] calls "meta-plasticity"), where system includes the various factors and processes of the self-pattern. Again, understanding the system as a dynamical gestalt, means that changes to any one of these integrated factors (changing behaviors, changing intersubjective interactions, changing cognitive practices, changing narratives, changing ecological factors, etc.) will generate changes in the system as a whole, leading, in the therapeutic context, to meta-plastic readjustments that address the disorder.

Consider the idea of a psychotherapeutic practice that incorporates MR design to replicate a particular environment (based perhaps on a patient's drawing or photographs), or to expose a patient to an object or set of objects (Röhricht et al. 2014). For example, employing advanced avatar technology, one could introduce an avatar that resembles a particular person typically encountered by the patient. The patient (or the patient and therapist together) could walk into an MR environment where an avatar, run on an advanced AI system, enters into interaction with the patient. The use of avatars in virtual environments have been shown to elicit significant changes in bodily and affective experiences, including the experience of peripersonal and extrapersonal space (Pasqualini et al. 2018), indicating a change in ecological and social affordances.

Or consider the possibility that a therapist and patient could co-construct a mixed reality environment that replicates the patient's delusional reality. Could the virtual construction and then deconstruction of that delusion have positive therapeutic effects? To be clear, this is no longer science fiction (see Freeman et al. 2017 for a comprehensive review). For example, avatar-based therapy is being used at University College London to allow patients with schizophrenia to control a hallucinated voice (Rus-Calafell et al. 2018). The patient contributes to the creation of a computer-based avatar, by choosing the face and voice of the entity they believe is talking to them. The system allows the therapist to speak to the patient through the avatar in real time, synchronizing the avatar's lips with its speech. The therapist encourages the patient to oppose the voices and gradually teaches the patient to take control of them.

VR has also been used to diagnose paranoid schizophrenia (Freeman 2008). A neutral social situation is presented using a virtual scenario, for example, a five-minute ride on the London underground metro. Individuals who experience auditory hallucinations in social situations report voices in the virtual metro. Likewise, those at high risk for psychosis, or who experience persecutory delusions, report persecutory thoughts about the neutral avatars in these settings:

> The interactions of patients in the social world are key to understanding and treating psychosis.... [T]he virtual world can be altered to determine the environmental elements that increase the likelihood of delusional ideas, hallucinations, or social difficulties. For example, paranoid ideation may partly depend on the size of a room, whether the person feels 'trapped' in the situation, the distribution and distance of other people, the amount of eye contact, the facial expressions of other people, and the level of background noise.
>
> (Freeman 2008, 607–8)

All of these factors are easily adjusted in a smart digital environment. Embodied immediacy, intersubjective relations, and cultural contextualization, all complicate, but also form crucial parts of therapeutic processes as interventions on the self-pattern (see Adery et al. 2018).

From the perspective of the self-pattern, all of these interconnected factors, and not just a person's brain or mental interior, or not just the person's social environment, or not just the person's affective existence, must be taken into account when attempting to alleviate stress and/or change patterns of self-regulatory responses to a range of challenging, or distressing or problematic or traumatic/adverse events.

Technology-based intervention models can incorporate features of a variety of therapies, including movement therapies, and more complex psycho-dramatic scenic enactments of past or present real-life scenarios (Röhricht & Priebe 2006), where patients explore spatial relationships in a safe, contained space, or engage with others in joint actions. Common symptoms of boundary loss and somatic depersonalization can be addressed by creating safe spaces within the virtual environment, the borders of which can be adjusted by the subject, shaping a place as open or closed as required.

Most of the examples I've mentioned are currently experimental, and my intention is not to endorse any of them. Rather, the point is that the concept of self-pattern as outlined in previous chapters can offer more precision in explaining just what such technologies may be changing in regard to our self-identities. Just as pervasive everyday AI may already be leading to unintended consequences for self-identities, more specialized AI systems could be put to work in a targeted therapeutic fashion to address various disorders in the factors and processes that make us who we are.

9

Mindfulness in the Self-pattern

As many philosophers have pointed out, there is a tension between the everyday belief in a coherent and persisting self—who I am—and specific philosophical and scientific insights that suggest that there is no substantive self. Resolving this tension in favor of holding tightly to the idea of a self, as an existential investment, is, from a Buddhist perspective, not a good thing. It leads to restless struggle, dissatisfaction, anxiety, or what is generally called suffering (*Dukkha*). This has personal, existential significance and not just philosophical significance. It also has relevance for psychiatry. Mindfulness meditation practices have been shown to have general health benefits, including stress reduction, the reduction of depression relapse, improved wellbeing (Cahn & Polich 2006; Godfrin & van Heeringen 2010; Carmody & Baer, 2008), and even enhanced immune response (Grossman et al. 2004). This evidence has been balanced by data showing that mindfulness practices are not always good for everyone (American Psychiatric Association 2013), and may lead to a form of depersonalization that approaches a form of psychopathology. In this chapter we'll discuss some of these claims. We start, however, with a philosophical focus on questions about the nature of self and the relevance of the concept of self-pattern for such issues.

At least in some Buddhist practices the self is treated as an illusion which is to be avoided. A non-Buddhist view, however, might argue that eliminating the self, eliminating suffering, engaging in a disinterested non-judgmental attitude that leads to a self-less existence, is to move closer to a non- or less-than-human existence. Human existence is complicated and such things as struggle and grief are valuable, or reflect what we take to be valuable; they are part of what makes life interesting and indeed, what makes us human.

What many Buddhists consider to be an illusion, however, is the self, conceived of as an independent entity, over and above the various factors that characterize human existence. Rupert Gethin (1998, 145), for example, suggests that the Buddhist view of the no-self "is not an absolute denial of self as such, but a quite specific denial of self as an enduring substance." Likewise, George Dreyfus (2011, 124) characterizes the Abhidharma tradition as holding that the self is not substantial, but rather, a "construct that comes to be only in dependence on complex configurations of multiple mental and material events (the aggregates)." In this respect, according to Evan Thompson (2020), who makes clear how complicated Buddhist views of the no- or non-self (*anattā* in Pāli, *anātman* in Sanskrit) are, this doesn't mean that what we call the self is not real in some sense (also see

The Self and Its Disorders. Shaun Gallagher, Oxford University Press. © Shaun Gallagher 2024.
DOI: 10.1093/oso/9780198873068.003.0010

Mackenzie 2011 for a Madhyamaka perspective on this issue). Thompson references the concept of the self-pattern as we have been developing it, and he suggests that Buddhist thinking about the self is consistent with thinking of self as a real processual pattern. "The way I like to put this idea is that a self is an ongoing process that enacts an 'I' and in which the 'I' is no different from the process itself, rather like the way dancing is a process that enacts a dance and in which the dance is no different from the dancing" (Thompson 2020, 39).

In this chapter I'll consider how the notion of a self-pattern and Buddhist practices of meditation, and concepts such as the no-self and the five aggregates (*khandha*) can be mutually enlightening, and also enlightening for our understanding of psychopathology and therapy. What effects do mindful meditative practices have on the self-pattern? Can the notion of a self-pattern give us a way to conceive of a no-self view?

9.1 Buddhist Psychology and the Self-pattern

It has been suggested that the Buddhist conception of the five aggregates (*khandha, skandhas*) correlates in some respects with the notion of self-pattern.[1] The aggregates are considered to be impersonal psychophysical processes that in some way give rise to a sense of self and agentive control. The general consensus, from a Buddhist perspective (but also in Western philosophy arguably from the time of John Locke's writing on personal identity, as well as in recent neuroscience), is that the self is not a substantial soul (as in Plato), or a thinking thing (as in Descartes). The latter views are considered mistaken (*miccha-ditthi; sakkaya-ditthi*), views that mistakenly identify one of the aggregates as self—which is, more generally, the wrong attitude to take in one's personal existence. Consider, then, that within a self-pattern, understood as a dynamical gestalt, and much like an autopoietic entity, there is no element that operates as a self or agent per se. Following Scott Kelso on this point, "patterns in general emerge in a self-organized fashion, without any agent-like entity ordering the elements, telling them when and where to go" (1995, 1). If there is no self within a self-pattern, and if what you are or what I am, just is a pattern, is this a way to understand the Buddhist concept of no-self?

[1] The idea was first suggested to me by Sean Smith, after a talk I gave on the dynamics of the self-pattern at the Philosophy Graduate Conference at the University of Toronto in 2018. The idea was further developed by what I will call the Lorentz group. Since 2019 I've been working with this interdisciplinary research group that originated at the Lorentz Center in Leiden, at a meeting entitled "Mechanisms of meditation and consequences for clinical practice." We have focused on Buddhist concepts of meditation and self. This group includes Henk Barendregt, Prisca Bauer, Aviva Berkovich-Ohana, Kirk Warren Brown, Fabio Giommi, Ivan Nyklíček, Brian Ostafin, Antonino Raffone, Heleen Slagter, Fynn-Mathis Trautwein, and David Vago. Much of what I have to say concerning Buddhist perspectives is informed by working with this group, although any misunderstandings are definitely my own. (See Gallagher et al. 2023; Giommi et al. 2023.)

The five *aggregates*, as explicated in Buddhist psychology (*Abhidharma*), tend to provide identity, and are those aspects we tend to preserve (e.g., Anuruddha 2000; Dalai Lama 1966; Davis & Thompson 2013; Harvey 1995; 2013). They are interpreted as corresponding to the following categories of experiences:

(1) bodily or material forms experienced in different sense modalities (*rūpa*)
(2) feelings/sensations (with specific valence—positive/negative, pleasurable/ painful; *vedanā*)
(3) cognitive discernments (*saññā, saṃjñā*; e.g., perceptual differentiation, categories, with practical [action-related] implications)
(4) dispositional formations and habitual volitional states (*saṅkhāra, saṃskāra,* e.g., emotions, motives, intentions)
(5) consciousness (*vijñāna, viññāṇa*), that is, awareness of an object and discrimination of its components and aspects.

The important point emphasized by such accounts is that one cannot find the self in any one of these aggregates; nor is there a self in the totality of the aggregates. As Varela, Thompson, and Rosch (1991, 69) pose it: "Each aggregate taken singly is transitory and impermanent; how, then, are we to combine them into something lasting and coherent?" We're left with a pattern of processes, but no agent or self behind the pattern.

Accordingly, on some views, the dynamic, temporal, and enactive characteristics of the self-pattern align well with the core Buddhist notion of non-self, as found in early Buddhist teachings (Analayo 2010) and the Theravada, especially Visudhimagga, traditions (Anuruddha 2000). According to such teachings the non-self is one of the *three characteristics* or marks of experience or existence together with *impermanence* (*anicca, anitya*) and *suffering* (Analayo 2012; Dunne 2011; Harvey 1990). Non-self does not mean the negation of the self, as if there is first a self that then gets negated. There is rather a dynamically changing process, a pattern of phenomena and processes which are simultaneously or sequentially occurring and that are ordinarily linked to a self-awareness understood as a witnessing (Albahari 2006). This is a dynamic pattern, following causal laws and conditions of nature, in which there is no reification of a self as a separate and permanent entity (Christoff et al. 2011).

Clearly there is no one-to-one correlation between the five aggregates and processes or elements of the self-pattern, and it would be artificial to try to map one set of aggregates onto the other.[2] Still there is some obvious meshing that reflects more complex dynamical integrations where, on the one hand,

---

[2] Likewise, it would be difficult to find any one-to-one mapping between changes in the self-pattern under various forms of mindfulness training, and changes in neuronal processing. There is, however, evidence of such alteration in the function of neural regions and networks supporting self-awareness (Dahl et al. 2015; Hölzel et al. 2011; Millière et al. 2018; Vago & Silbersweig 2012).

behavioral, intersubjective, narrative, and ecologial factors in the self-pattern involve a range of conditions that relate to all five aggregates. On the other hand, there are selective connections where aggregate (1), bodily form, relates directly to processes involving embodied, experiential, and ecological factors; (2), feelings/sensations, relates to affective factors; (3), cognitive, to cognitive, reflective, and narrative processes; (4), habitual states, to affective, reflective, behavioral and ecologial factors; and (5), consciousness, to experiential, reflective, cognitive, and ecological processes. Moreover, just as we have described dynamical relations among the processes of the self-pattern, so the aggregates are said to interrelate.

There are different ways to think of these interrelations. For example, one might think of them as arranged in a nested or cascading order, or in a more organic relation, or as a reciprocal network. Varela, Thompson, and Rosch suggest the nested view: "Consciousness is the last of the aggregates, and it contains all of the others. (Indeed, each of the aggregates contains those that precede it in the list)" (Varela et al. 1991, 67). Evan Thompson attributes this view to Varela's teacher, Trunga Rinpoche. Thompson prefers the analogy of the hand and its fingers: "the five aggregates, as traditionally presented as distinct elements, are organically related. This may also include reciprocal relations since, the aggregates can't function independently (feeling requires a basis in [bodily] form, perception requires feeling, consciousness requires them all, and they require consciousness)" (Thompson, personal correspondence).

The notion of self-pattern, even if it eschews the idea of a hierarchical or cascading order, can help us understand how aggregate self-organizing processes can be integrated in a dynamical gestalt, but can also become rigid or inflexible. As we'll see, the notion of rigidity or inflexibility in the self-pattern will be important for understanding transdiagnostic processes that contribute to the generation and maintenance of psychopathological symptoms and disorders (Giommi et al. 2023). According to Buddhist psychology, affective aspects of craving or attachment with respect to any one aspect of the self-pattern is what continually reinforces the development of rigid habits. The experience of a self as something permanent or unchanging is regarded as an illusion. As Miri Albahari (2006, 51) puts it: "On the Buddhist position, we are to understand that the witnessing subject makes the (deeply mistaken) assumption of being a self through its very act of assuming various *khandās*." It is this illusory assumption that leads to an unhealthy attitude (*sakkaya-ditthi*) (Analayo 2010; Harvey 1990).

The Buddhist remedy to this attitude comes from a systematic training and practice of meditation. Continuous cultivation of mindfulness facilitates the insight or realization of non-self. Specifically, mindfulness practices promote changes in self-related processing that reduce the effects of self-narrative while enhancing an awareness of the present moment (Farb et al. 2007; Dunne 2015;

Wielgosz et al. 2019).[3] If, as suggested in previous chapters, narrative processes reflect all of the other factors of the self-pattern, they reflect at best, according to Buddhist teachings, an uncertain (and perhaps a false) coherency. The reduction of narrative in meditation practices leads to what one might consider a content-free reflective process.

Emptiness (*suññatā*, *śūnyatā*), which is closely related to the notion of non-self (Analayo 2012; Conze 1953; Dunne 2011), would, according to Buddhist psychology, characterize the metastable, transient processes of the self-pattern as a whole (Kelso et al. 19954; Varela 1997). If this in some way supports the emptiness or non-self view, it may also motivate some Western philosophical worries. Even if there is no agent or self that drives the self-pattern, Western philosophers may be inclined to think that there must be an agentive person, as the ongoing whole that emerges from or enacts itself in the processes and dynamical connections of the self-pattern—an emergent agent capable of bodily actions, intersubjective interactions, social engagement and cultural practices, a person who has affective/emotional experiences, and is capable of cognition, reflection, and narrative. Indeed, Buddhist psychology acknowledges that in ordinary human experience the self-pattern and its constituent processes are subject to being identified with a self to which we are attached, based on the mistaken attitude that posits a permanent self. According to this view, in meditative practice, insight into the dynamical nature of the self-pattern enables an understanding of the "true nature" of the pattern itself, namely, that neither the self-pattern nor the various elements of the self-pattern, constitutes a self in any substantive sense.

On the one hand, narrative or reflective capacities do not have agency in themselves; on the other hand, narrative may loop into and influence our actions. In that case, illusory views and attitudes concerning self-identity influence perceptual and action processes with a tendency to sculpt or crystallize preferences, habits, views, emotional reactivity patterns, fears, desires, aversions, delusions, or judgments, which then form and sustain an overly rigid self-pattern. Stable meanings, perspectives, and habits, which may serve useful functions in human life, come at the cost of stress, dissatisfaction, anxiety, lack of clarity about oneself and others, emotional confusion, and other afflictions and emotional vulnerabilities. In part, to avoid this type of rigidity, mindfulness practices aim to reduce the role of self-narrative and enhance the minimal aspects of prereflective experience. Some Buddhist styles of meditation actually target such shifts as a primary goal of practice (Dunne 2015; Wielgosz et al. 2019).

---

[3] On Buddhist views, meditative insight on non-self can lead to a liberating "breakthrough," giving way to an "unshakeable wellbeing" (Amaro 2019), that is, a change in the affective factors of the self-pattern, with a dramatic reduction of negative or unwholesome experiences (such as existential anxiety, stress, greed, hatred, and unhappiness), and the enhancement of salutary or virtuous experiences (such as equanimity, wisdom, love, compassion, and happiness) (Barendregt 1988; Mahasi Sayadaw 2016).

9.2   Flexibility in the Self-pattern: Meditation-based Interventions and Therapy

William James, who described consciousness as having a flow structure that seemingly contained substantive perchings and transitive flights, quoted G. E. Moore in regard to the attempt to provide a phenomenology of this structure. "The moment we try to fix our attention upon consciousness and to see what, distinctly, it is, it seems to vanish. It seems as if we had before us a mere emptiness. When we try to introspect the sensation of blue, all we can see is the blue; the other element is as if it were diaphanous. Yet it can be distinguished, if we look attentively enough and know that there is something to look for" (Moore 1903, 450 cited in James 1904, 479). James then immediately adds a quotation from Paul Natorp: "Consciousness is inexplicable and hardly describable, yet all conscious experiences have this in common that what we call their content has this peculiar reference to a center for which 'self' is the name" (Natorp 1888, 14; cited and translated in James 1904, 479). James goes on to take issue with this view suggesting that reflection introduces a freeze-framed dualism and comes to alight on and attach itself to the substantive perchings that are always gathered to form a self. The flow becomes too fixed.

Buddhist teachings reject both the fixity and the flow. The idea that consciousness is a flow is a phenomenological claim made by both James and Husserl, for example. In the meditation tradition, however, the phenomenological claim is that experience is discontinuous—"a moment of consciousness arises, appears to dwell for an instant, and then vanishes, to be replaced by the next moment" (Varela et al. 1991, 73).[4] In Buddhist teachings, of course, the issue is not just a phenomenological one; it has implications for living a healthy life. Mistaken attitudes are said to lead to an experienced inflexibility in the self-pattern, correlated to unhealthy attachment or overinvestment (Gombrich 2005). Arrangements in the self-pattern take on a condition of "rigidity," as one might find in destructive emotional states (in Buddhist teaching, the "three poisons," i.e., greed, hatred, and delusion), or in disorders such as depression, or OCD. Self-narrative, as just indicated, reflects and reinforces this rigidity. Buddhist psychology calls this a mental (or conceptual) *proliferation* (*papañca, prapañca*), a reiteration or elaboration of thoughts that run through many cycles of conceptualization and narration (Giommi et al. 2023; Ñāṇananda 1997).

A significant body of research has identified "transdiagnostic" cognitive and behavioral processes, that is, features of psychopathology that manifest across a

---

[4] Varela et al. also provide a footnote to indicate that this is a view that has been under debate in Buddhist schools as much as in Western philosophy (1991, 265n17). Truly, the vanishing and replacement might itself be viewed as a flow process by some. Others might view it less as a stream (as described by James Joyce) and more like a shower of atoms or raindrops (as described by Virginia Woolf) (see Gallagher 1998, 182–3).

diversity of psychiatric disorders (Harvey et al. 2004). These processes include self-focused attention (Baer 2007), a type of hyperreflexivity, repetitive negative thinking (Ehring & Watkins 2008), inflexibility, and automaticity, which tend to generate distress or disability in the various modalities of attention, memory, thinking (rumination), affectivity (worry); avoidance behaviors; perfectionism; intolerance to uncertainty; neuroticism; impulsivity; compulsivity, and so forth (Morris & Mansell 2018; Schultz & Searleman 2002). Rigidity is "the tendency to develop and perseverate in particular cognitive or behavioral patterns, [where] such patterns [are] continuously employed in situations where the pattern is no longer effective" (Morris & Mansell 2018, 3). In some cases, such rigidity in thought, emotion, and behavior indicates a lack of contextual sensitivity (Kashdan & Rottenberg 2010), and involves difficulty in switching from one way of responding to a different way of responding.

Various conditions express this rigidity in different ways. Depression, for example, is marked by a rigidity or lack of flexibility evidenced in rumination, wherein self-narratives, commonly negative, become automated and perseverative, accompanied by depressed mood which becomes chronic. In the case of substance addiction, as we saw earlier (Section 5.5), there are disturbances in the self-pattern involving sense of agency and control. In this regard, dual-process perspectives on addiction (Noel, Brevers & Bechara 2013) propose that appetitive processes involving constant thinking about use, craving, and overt behaviors to obtain and consume become automatized and rigidly linked to substance-related cues (Berridge & Robinson 2016; Wiers et al. 2017). Another example is the phenomenon of dissociation found in the case of psychological trauma (van der Hart, Nijenhuis & Steel 2006). Dissociation involves a lack of integration among different processes in the self-pattern; a "division of personality [that] involves two or more insufficiently integrated dynamic *but excessively stable* systems" (Nijenhuis & van der Hart 2011, 422). Rigidity and a lack of systemic complexity are the primary features of this dissociation:

> Adaptation requires systemic complexity, that is, the ability of a (sub)system to develop new actions that fit changed inner and outer conditions, as well as the ability to continue previously developed effective actions when conditions are unchanged. Living systems that are too stable do not adjust their actions to altered circumstances. As overly stable (sub)systems, dissociative parts often engage in fixed actions that may have worked previously but that do not fit transformed conditions.   (Nijenhuis & van der Hart 2011, 422)

This kind of rigidity or inflexibility appears to be a modification of the dynamical and changing processes of the self-pattern. Thinking of this in terms of the self-pattern suggests a process-oriented perspective on psychopathology and in psychotherapy where the focus is on increasing flexibility (Giommi et al. 2023).

Meditation-based interventions (MBIs) can address such learned and habitual inflexibility. We can think of meditation as a form of training that involves attending to, monitoring, and self-regulating oneself in ways that affect a rearrangement of the self-pattern. MBIs include a diversity of practices based on their core aims and techniques (e.g., Dahl, Lutz & Davidson 2015; Travis & Shear 2010). The most well-known practices involve focused attention, that is, sustaining one's attention on a particular object or sensation such as one's breath, and open monitoring, that is a form of meta-awareness engaged in non-judgmental, non-selective awareness of the present moment. In addition, a more intersubjective-focused practice aims at cultivating compassion toward oneself and others. Mindfulness meditation often combines these three types of practices, either in a single session or over the course of a practitioner's training.

In psychotherapeutic contexts, these practices have been put to use in programs of mindfulness-based stress reduction (MBSR) (Kabat-Zinn 2013; Lutz et al. 2015) and in mindfulness-based cognitive therapy (MBCT), which combines cognitive therapy with mindfulness practices (Segal, Williams & Teasdale 2013). Despite some differences in these approaches, the therapeutic aim of mindfulness meditation is to reestablish flexibility in the self-pattern—to open up its dynamics. Indeed, several studies have provided some initial evidence that mindfulness may increase flexibility in the self-pattern by showing correlations between mindfulness practice and the weakening of connections between self-related processes, creating opportunities for more flexible interactions between those processes (Giommi et al. 2023). For example, mindfulness has been associated with a weakening of the association between behavior-related self-perceived disability and feelings of affective distress (Nyklíček et al. 2015). Furthermore, those with higher self-reported mindful states on a day-to-day basis showed weaker associations between cognitive rumination and both negative and positive affect; likewise, a higher level of mindful self-acceptance weakens the link between reflection and affect (Blanke et al. 2020).

Besides research showing the beneficial effects of MBIs on affective processing, particularly in regard to anxiety and depression (e.g., Goldberg et al. 2022; 2018), on addiction-related behaviors (Li et al. 2017) and eating disorder behaviors (Turgon et al., 2019), there is also some evidence that mindfulness can alter cognitive processing through what has been described as cognitive decentering. In decentering, meditators switch "to a perspective within which negative thoughts and feelings [are] seen as passing events in the mind that [are] neither necessarily valid reflections of reality nor central aspects of the self" (Segal et al. 2013, 36). It's a form of "disidentifying from [not just negative thoughts, but] the entire play of inner experience" (Kabat-Zinn 2013, 297). Meditators "disidentify with narrative and conceptual senses of self" but may continue to identify with minimal aspects of the experiential process (Britton et al. 2021, 7). Attending to the present moment and decentering accomplish a shift in one's experiential perspective from a rigid mental absorption in self-referential thought, or a running mental commentary about one's experience, to a monitoring of or a prereflective living in that experience. This practice results in less perseverative cognition, such as worrying and rumination, and a reduction of the emotional salience of ruminative thought, processes which are important contributors to anxiety and depression (Bernstein et al. 2019; Wielgosz et al. 2019; see Britton et al. 2021 for a review of empirical evidence).

Initial practices of focused attention and open monitoring (*Samatha/Shamata* practices) aim to achieve a settling and calming of the mind, less controlled by one's narrative and conflicting emotions. This opens up new experiential processes that run counter to mind-wandering (Mrazek et al. 2012), and leads to a stronger sense of bodily existence, being more aware of sensory and bodily experience in the present moment. This enhancement of embodied awareness can lead, at the same time, to a reduction of emotional reactivity (Killingsworth & Gilbert, 2010), to a more flexible attunement to others and the surrounding environment, to shifts in what counts as important in one's self-narrative, and a reduction of rigidity in the narrative process (Farb et al. 2007; Hölzel et al. 2011; Vago & Silbersweig 2012). Such practices involve a transformation—a type of "deconstruction" and reconstruction that builds on the sense of interconnection with others and the world (Dahl et al. 2015).

In these initial effects of meditation, the flexibility introduced into the self-pattern clearly does not entail a complete dissolution of self-related structure. Indeed, one requires a reformation or a consolidation of habit within the self-pattern to support meditative practice. It cannot be a deconstruction of all habit. Specifically, meditation is said to foster improvements to reflective processes, enabling sharper and subtler forms of reflection, allowing a non-reactive discernment of experience which can become habitual and faster (Raffone & Barendregt 2020; Schoenberg & Vago 2019). With reflective meditation practice, subjects can free themselves from entanglement with affective processes that typically bias judgments. They can short-circuit the slow narrative process of self-integration, attuning reflection closer to an ongoing temporal presence, enhancing and transforming experience (Lutz et al. 2015; Dahl et al. 2015; Vago & Silbersweig 2012). One thus loosens the inclination to identify with all the other aspects of the self-pattern. There is specifically a dampening down of psychological, cognitive, and narrative processes, and a re-arrangement in which the reflective capacity which initiates mindful-awareness becomes a more habitual reflexive practice, an ongoing mindfulness, that operates as a minimal form of witnessing-consciousness, replacing the ingrained habits of psychological identity, and enhancing the flexibility of the self-pattern. This is said to be a type of freedom from self (Anālayo 2010). It leads to a more minimal integration, which, instead of constantly building and adjusting narratives, allows the subject to live more in the ongoing experiential flow, or simply the presence of consciousness.

The promotion of flexibility is characterized not simply by the effect on individual aspects of the self-pattern, but by the way it affects the system dynamics reflecting changes in the functional coupling of the different processes of the self-pattern. If these transitions effect a more flexible reorganization of the self-pattern, others purportedly cause more radical changes. For example, transitioning to a state of deep absorption (*samadhi*), meditators may experience the absence of continuity in the stream of consciousness (Sayadaw 2016). These are states that can lead to disintegration of the self-pattern. In such experiences, bodily processes tied to the differentiation between self and non-self, may be disturbed. For example, prolonged sitting in a still position reduces proprioception and multi-sensory integration, responsible for a sense of self location (Park & Blanke 2019), and this can entail a diminishment of the sense of ownership, an experience of expanded body boundaries, a corresponding feeling of unity and connectedness with everything, and, correlatively, an annihilation, a feeling of self-loss and emptiness (Yaden et al. 2017). *Samadhi* or full absorption may involve more subtle experiences of silence, stillness, spaciousness, or emptiness.

On the one hand, such experiences may then lead to a transformative form of mindfulness, involving feelings of energy, joy, tranquility, and so forth (Goleman 1977). On the other hand, when not accompanied by the proper flexibility, this deeply altered experience can sometimes lead to intensified aversive emotional states (e.g., fear, panic, and disgust), giving rise to the so-called "dark night of the soul" (Hunt 2007). In some cases, it could also result in dissociative states or delusions (van der Kolk, Brown & van der Hart 1989).

9.3 Adverse Effects of Mindfulness

The use of MBSR and MBCT in therapeutic practices involves an attempt to undo the habitually ingrained inner process of self-identification to a point where one's experiences become non-personal, thereby "disidentifying with the entire play of inner experience, whether it be the breath, sensations, perceptions, thoughts or feelings" (Kabat-Zinn 2013, 297). Rather than saying "I-Me-Mine" in regard to mental and bodily states, the proposal is to use the present-participle so as to avoid an expression of ownership: "we say 'I *have* a headache' or 'I *have* a cold' or 'I *have* a fever', when it would be more accurate to say something like 'the body is headaching' or 'colding' or 'fevering'" (Kabat-Zinn 2013, 282; see Segal et al. 2013, 194). The suggestion is that the therapeutic effect of this reorientation is a feeling of liberation "to see that your thoughts are just thoughts and that they are not 'you' or 'reality'" (Kabat-Zinn 2013, 69).

Such therapeutic practices, and more generally, meditation practices, are not without their critics (for recent evaluations, see Canby et al. 2021; Cullen et al. 2021;

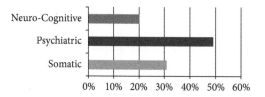

Figure 9.1 Proportion of broad types of meditation adverse events
Source: Farias et al. (2020, CC-BY license).

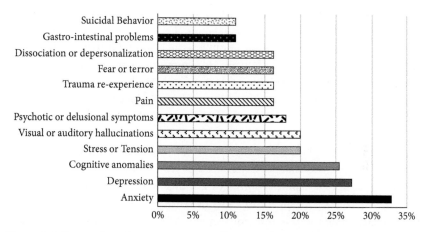

Figure 9.2 Proportion of most common meditation adverse events
Source: Farias et al. (2020, CC-BY license).

and Van Dam et al. 2018). Farias et al. (2020) reviewed eighty-three studies of meditation practices (primarily mindfulness and transcendental meditation) and found that 8.3 percent of practitioners experience adverse effects, such as anxiety, depression, cognitive anomalies, and less frequently, gastrointestinal problems and suicidal behavior. Cognitive anomalies, for example, reported in fourteen studies, included thought disorganization, amnesia and memory problems, and perceptual hypersensitivity. Moreover, adverse effects "may occur in individuals with no previous history of mental health problems" (Farias et al. 2020, 374; see Figures 9.1 and 9.2).

Indeed, in the DSM-4 section on depersonalization disorder one finds the following statement:

Voluntarily induced experiences of depersonalization/derealization can be a part of meditative practices that are prevalent in many religions and cultures and should not be diagnosed as a disorder. However, there are individuals who initially induce these states intentionally but over time lose control over them and may develop a fear and aversion for related practices.

(American Psychiatric Association [APA] 2013, §300.6, p. 304)

As indicated, adverse effects do not occur in all meditators, and the results are mixed about whether there is an association between length of meditation practice and frequency of adverse effects. For example, some studies suggest that in some cases, attempting to reach a state of no-self may cause disorientation and anxiety, similar to that experienced in dissociative disorders in post-traumatic stress disorder (e.g., Fingelkurts & Fingelkurts 2018), a clinical condition in which a non-self experience following a traumatic event may trigger a deep lasting fear (Bryant 2019). Otis (1984) found a positive association with psychiatric or psychopathological conditions, with increased symptoms of anxiety, confusion, and depression in the most experienced transcendental meditators (also see Shapiro 1992). In contrast, Schlosser et al. (2019) found no significant correlation.

Lindahl and Britton (2019), in their Varieties of Contemplative Experience (VCE) study, collected reports, based on semi-structured interviews with meditation practioners, exploring somatic, perceptual, cognitive, affective, conative, social experiences, and changes in the sense of self. They report that "six discrete changes in sense of self were reported by Buddhist meditators: change in narrative self, loss of sense of ownership, loss of sense of agency, change in sense of embodiment, change in self–other or self–world boundaries, and loss of sense of basic self" (2019, 157). In some cases, subjects who were predisposed to depersonalization disorder and who started meditation practice went into such nonpersonal states as a "dark night of the soul," but then failed to come out. The results of the VCE survey included:

- 72 percent of surveyed meditators (n = 68)—long-term practitioners (Theraváda, Zen, and Tibetan practices) and some mindfulness teachers—reported changes in sense of self;
- 55 percent of those reported associated distress;
- 45 percent reported impairment in functioning.

Lindahl and Britton explore each kind of change in the self-pattern. For example, changes to the narrative aspect involved becoming more aware of one's self-narrative leading to a questioning, revision, or even abandoning of that narrative, sometimes accompanied by a "disintegration or dissolution" of personal identity. One Zen meditator reported:

[A]ll day long I saw how all my actions were reinforcing this story that I had told myself, and it was really deflating and unsettling and just made me kind of sad. [...] And this story that I was telling myself was the very thing that was preventing me from being with my experience. [...] I would build these stories up about what I thought practice was or who I would be when I practised, but my real life didn't match that narrative that I had told myself.

(Lindahl & Britton 2019, 163)

Another Theravāda meditator reports: "I was deeply wounded in the sense of my identity. I felt that my identity was threatened. I would walk, and I would feel that I forgot my past" (164). This person goes on to report how his practice interfered with memory and sense of agency. Others report interference with their social interactions. It's notable, however, that these reports are themselves self-narratives that in some sense can count as revisions to their former identities.

Changes (both positive and negative) in experiences of the body, self-location, personal space, and body boundaries were frequent, including feelings of disembodiment, "out-of-body" experiences, and changes in the body schema or body image. This kind of "profoundly diminished sense of embodied, vital self-presence" overlaps with some psychiatrically defined disordered experiences (Parnas & Henriksen 2016, 78). In such experiences the bodily self either might extend to incorporate the world, or lapse into indifferentiation. One Theravāda meditator reported:

I read a paper on schizophrenia he [Louis Sass] wrote, and I just saw this paper and thought, "Fuck, I have schizophrenia." It sounded so like schizophrenia. Like: hyper-reflectivity, hyper-awareness, diminished feeling from inside because all this stuff...It was like I was observing my body from outside, everything felt strange, the whole atmosphere looked different. And then there was also the loss of self that came with it.   (Lindahl & Britton 2019, 169)

Lindahl and Britton discuss such changes to ipseity (what they call the "basic self," or what I have been calling the prereflective experiential aspect of the self-pattern), and the related sense of ownership and sense of agency: "Practitioners experiencing a loss of sense of ownership described feeling that their body, body parts, thoughts, or emotions no longer belong to them, sometimes to the extent that they are experienced as impersonal, as belonging to no one" (164–5). One example from a Theravada meditator described a negative rather than an insightful experience:

I didn't have a sense of my body belonging to a "me." There wasn't a sense of "me" there. I could feel my hand—there was a feeling of a hand, but it didn't feel like my hand. Yeah, [it] didn't feel like my hand, my chest, my head. [...] There are so many ways to have insight into selflessness where there's a kind of clarity. This was not that at all.   (165)

Another described it as a kind of depersonalization where feelings and thoughts seemed unreal "or not to belong to oneself" (165). Reflecting the idea that self-narrative provides a sense of unity, feelings were experienced as unconnected because "I didn't have a story behind it" (166)—it was experienced as something without reasons.

Meditation practitioners also reported a loss of the sense of agency; "actions that were typically voluntary now felt involuntary and beyond their control," or felt as if they were on automatic pilot; and this was sometimes experienced as adopting unusual body postures, or in some cases a sense that someone else was "performing actions through the practitioner's body" (166). Some reported these experiences as positive Buddhist insights; others reported them as negative experiences, or as disturbing.

I'll discuss some philosophical issues related to changes in ipseity or the no-self experience in the next section. Here, however, the VCE study suggests that we should think of psychopathology as operating at the extremes of self-pattern arrangements, where rigidity or inflexibility is on one problematic side, and depersonalization, or complete disorganization is on the other. Indeed, a diminished sense of self is considered a risk factor for psychopathology (Raballo et al. 2018). Lindahl and Britton note that in some percentage of cases, meditators experience distress and impairment of everyday life, and these were "most likely to accompany changes in basic self and least likely to accompany changes in sense of self–other or self–world boundaries" (2019, 175). Practitioners had more problems with changes in self-experience that overlapped with known changes in psychopathologies, for example, loss of the sense of agency or changes in ipseity, where changes are more akin to depersonalization (Albahari 2011, 102). Crucially, as Lindahl and Britton suggest, "the greater number of dimensions of selfhood attenuated by meditation—that is, the more 'global' the change in sense of self—the more likely the experience was to be associated with impairments in functioning or, in Albahari's words, to be 'debilitating'" (2019, 177; see Britton 2019; Lindahl et al. 2020).

9.4 Deconstructing the Self and No-self

A final area of concern involves the idea of the no-self, non-dual states, or states of full absorption and what happens to prereflective self-awareness, or ipseity. In extreme cases of absorption, if even this minimal type of witnessing can be lost, one implication is that it would not be possible to report on what the experience is like (Gallagher 2020c; Josipovic & Miskovic 2020; Metzinger 2020). This is a concern that is also raised by some Buddhist philosophers (e.g., Dignāga and Dharmakīrti in the sixth century CE—see, e.g., Thompson 2010). If one can report such states, arguably, what is still left in the no-self state is a first-person perspective. On some interpretations, a prereflective self-awareness is still operative and functions as a minimal witnessing consciousness (Albahari 2011; Gupta 1998), which enables some post-state reporting. Some theorists suggest that this witness consciousness is continuous with the meditational process itself, but as a non-conceptual, non-dual reflexive awareness (Dunne 2015; Rabjam 2007).

Is a minimal self-awareness still possible in a no-self experience? To develop an answer, I'll first focus on prereflective experiential self-awareness (*Svasaṃvedana*), as it is contrasted with reflective or narrative processes within the self-pattern. Phenomenologists explain minimal prereflective self-awareness as a structural feature of the flow of consciousness reflecting its intrinsic temporality (Gallagher & Zahavi 2021; 2020). Husserl (2001), not unlike William James (1890), argues that in any moment of consciousness we are aware not only of a knife-edge present moment, but we retain a little bit of our just-past experience, and we anticipate (or "protend") a little bit of what is just about to happen. If this were not the case we would never be able to perceive a melody or understand a sentence (we would literally hear only one note or word at a time, unconnected with any other note or word). On Husserl's phenomenological account, the flow of experience is unified across short time trajectories by the retentional-protentional structure intrinsic to it. Similar to accounts of working memory, Husserl suggests that in the current moment we retain the previous few seconds of perception of a temporal object, such as a melody.

Importantly, retention (as well as protention) involves a double intentionality. Retentional consciousness of a melody, for example, retains (1) the just-past phase of consciousness (Husserl calls this the "longitudinal intentionality" of retention) which includes (2) the just-past awareness (the just-past "primal impression") of the previous note ("transverse intentionality"). The previous notes of the melody are retained by way of retaining the previous moments of correlated experience. This means that we are aware, not just of the melody as it develops, but of our experience (of the melody) as it unfolds, and indeed, the former depends on the latter, that is, transverse intentionality depends on longitudinal intentionality. Retention thus constitutes a form of minimal (very short-term) self-awareness, understood not as an awareness of *a self*, but as an intrinsic aware-ness of one's ongoing experience. This is a first-person prereflective self-awareness which does not take one's experience as an object; rather it is an intrinsic struc-tural feature of one's experience of any object, including objects that endure or that, like a melody, involve succession. On the one hand, if one agrees that we actually hear melodies as they unfold, the implication that goes along with this is that there is a perceiver who is at least minimally or prereflectively self-aware. On the other hand, if one denies that there is a retentionally constituted minimal self-awareness (e.g., Georges Dreyfus [2011] who, in defending a no-self perspective, allows for a synchronic (momentary) prereflective self-awareness, but not for a diachronic self-awareness), it would imply that we do not actually hear melodies.

Joel Krueger (2011, 37) quotes the Buddhist scholar Dharmakírti to this effect: "If cognition were not itself perceived, perception of an object is never possible." This would seem to apply to a temporal object, such as a melody, and not just a momentary object in a momentary perception.

For the phenomenologist this intrinsic, diachronic (longitudinal) prereflective awareness of experience constitutes a basic sense that this ongoing experience is *my* experience (providing a sense of mineness, or ownership for that experience), and that this experience is distinct from the object experienced (e.g., the melody)—reflecting a self/non-self distinction. This structure of consciousness is similar to what Neisser (1988) calls the embodied ecological aspect of self. For example, when I move, I am aware of changes in my perceptual field and at the same time, re*flexively* (but not re*flectively*) aware that I am moving. When I am engaged in action, this structure also provides a sense that I am the one acting, which also involves anticipating (protending) where the action is heading—a sense of agency. All of this is what we have called the prereflective experiential aspect of the self-pattern.

To be clear, retention does not involve an explicit act of recollection; it is distinct from episodic memory which is required to recall a melody that has faded from retentional consciousness. On this view, however, my reflective report or memory of an experience depends on my having been retentionally self-aware at the time of the original experience. If, when listening to a melody, I was not prereflectively aware of listening to the melody, I would not be able to recall listening to the melody.

Is it possible to reach a state of no-self through meditative practice that escapes this minimal prereflective self-awareness? And does the emphasis in meditation to focus on the bare present in some way discount the intrinsic temporality of consciousness (see Stone & Zahavi 2022 on this point)? Do we arrive at something even less than minimal prereflective self-awareness? Do we find some experience without the sense of mineness involved? And even if there is a sense of mineness in the now moment, is that momentary sense necessarily connected with other moments such that it forms something like a unified identity across successive experiences? More generally, however, since minimal self-awareness is not some free-floating process unrelated to other aspects of the self-pattern, we also need to ask how meditative practice affects the dynamical connections between prereflective self-awareness and that pattern.

What, then, is the experience of no-self? If the notion of a self-pattern gives us a coherent way to talk about a self—one that may even be consistent with the Buddhist notion of aggregates, which are themselves not thing-like real selves, but processes that make up a self-pattern—then, we have to flip Hume's question around; that is, instead of explaining how, despite not being a self, we have an idea that we are a coherent self, we instead have to explain how, despite being a self-pattern, we can talk about being no-self. Recent attempts to address this issue have focused on the distinction between the minimal self and the narrative self. As we've seen, there is general agreement that in the experience of no-self, the narrative aspect is not operative. We can expand this now to say that through various forms of meditation practice, not only the narrative, but the rest of the elements of the self-pattern—the behavioral, affective, intersubjective, psychological/cognitive, reflective, ecological, and normative factors—are diminished or changed in some respect. Meditation practice, however, is still in some sense embodied, although experienced body boundaries are relaxed with a diminished distinction between self and non-self, and practices are designed to disidentify with one's body. As Kabat-Zinn puts it, "Whatever you are, 'you' are definitely not your body" (2013, 297).

To the extent that meditation may move the meditator into a non-dual or no-self experience, can't we still ask about the minimal experiential aspect of prereflective self-awareness, and the sense that this is *my* experience (sense of ownership or mineness)? It is difficult to get an answer to this question. One reason is, as Hölzel et al. (2011, 547–8) note, because the concept of no-self "is rather difficult to operationalize" and has "yet to be rigorously tested in empirical research" (also see Britton et al. 2021). Indeed, George Dreyfus suggests that the description of a non-dual awareness is beyond conceptualization, and a challenge for philosophical analysis. "It may be experienced directly or evoked indirectly by helpful metaphors and instructions on how to reach such a state, but it cannot be described. Hence, we may find it difficult to articulate a view of subjectivity based solely on this level of analysis" (2011, 128).

On the one hand, notwithstanding this difficulty, some Buddhist practitioners claim that in the no-self state, there is no prereflective self-awareness or sense of mineness.[5] On the other hand, as we mentioned, phenomenologists claim that if prereflective self-awareness is missing, then we are not conscious at all. In that case, it's not clear that one could report on the no-self experience. More precisely, there would be *no experience* of no-self.

Consider an empirical study by Dor-Ziderman et al. (2016) which focuses on the sense-of-(body)-boundaries (SB)—the fundamental division of the field of experience into bodily self versus world. They collaborated with a long-term meditation practitioner, practicing in the Satipatthana and Theravada Vipassana traditions, who was able to repeatedly produce graded SB experiences, from:

- SB1, the experience of a normal sense of body boundary, to
- SB2 a state that still involved a minimal self-awareness, where the SB began to dissolve, and finally to
- SB3 which the researchers defined as "a selfless mode of awareness where the sense of ownership [mineness] disappeared."

---

[5] Millière and Newen (2022) provide an analysis that is consistent with this idea. They argue that the original non-self experience does not contain a self-awareness (or *de se* content); the first-personal aspect found in the report is added by the constructive memory process. They do not deny, however, that there is an experiencing subject of the original experience.

They recorded brain activity using magneto-encephalogram (MEG). In the SB2 (minimal self) condition—beta-band power decreased across ventral medial prefrontal, medial posterior, and lateral parietal regions; and in the S3 (selfless) condition—there was attenuation of beta-band activity in the right inferior parietal lobule. The experimenters also used a method of phenomenological interviews to explore the specifics of these experiences (Dor-Ziderman et al. 2016—referencing Petitmengin 2006; 2014).

Here are the meditator's reports on the SB3 condition (self-less, non-dual, or no-self mode of experience)—(from Ataria et al 2015; Dor-Ziderman et al. 2013). First, we have a proviso: "it is quite hard to put it into language, because I don't know that we have a language for [it]." Second, however, a set of negative descriptions:

[T]here is no center...there's really no address. I have no idea where I am in stage three, it's all background, I'm not there basically, just world, so there's no real location at all in stage three...the body is so spread that it's very difficult to know where it is and what it is.

It was emptiness, as if the self fell out of the picture. There was an experience but it had no address, it was not attached to a center or subject...

I become absorbed into the background, meaning the whole world without any separate entity...dropping distinctions, dropping interest in any boundaries or limits, dropping habit, and automatic sensori-reality.

[T]here's no personal point of view, it's the world point of view, it's like the world looking, not ME looking, the world is looking.

[T]here is no sense of mine there is no sense of me....There is no sense of controlling.

Third, we get a set of positive descriptions:

Like in a dream. Like I'm not awake now but dreaming. Sensations of all kinds of things flickering....A sort of meditative phenomena and flickering of light and darkness—difficult to describe in words.

Floating above the entrance door, between the room and the lab...

There was a feeling of a shift in alertness, a cessation of reflectivity. A different kind of quiet.

Nave et al. (2021) conducted a larger study of forty-six advanced meditators who reported SB3, or something approaching SB3 (characterized as SB-, for a dissolution of self-boundary) in a variety of ways: "A sense of floating in some sky consciousness"; "There's something very delicate, very innocent there, vulnerable. I can't explain"; "An experience without an observer interfering, discerning;

'Like leaning back inside the head'; 'It's a puddle and there's no…it's not solid anymore. There's no longer me. It…[seven seconds of silence] it stops being separate. It's not me melting on the bed. There's no me and there's no bed. It all melts together"; "Some sort of intergalactic blackness […] completely still and deeply serene" (13, 16). "There's a field of sensuality, and it's not bounded. […] I'm not located anywhere. I am not. It contributes to the dissolution. There's no sense of observer. No witness. […] It didn't lose the sense of being-part-of, not entirely. […] There's a sense of flow and it is going through something" (19).

We can find similar descriptions in the reports of deep states of no-self from meditators in Lindahl and Britton's (2019) VCE study:

> Then I became very small in my own being. […] I was gone, I was lost—there was nothing there. I didn't believe I even had a shadow. I didn't believe anyone could even really see me.   (171)

> […] I'm kind of wondering which sensation is it that tells me that I don't really feel like I'm here? I can't really identify that, right? Maybe, it's somewhere.…When you feel angry, right, there's a sensation of anger. But there's no real sensation of not-being-here. […]   (172)

> […] Those experiences that I related about what I would call *kenshō* experiences, there was no viewer in those.   (170)

As the researchers also acknowledge, "changes at this basic level of selfhood can be very difficult to describe, and can include references to 'not being there', 'disappearing', or 'not existing'" (2019, 171).

The problem is this: If we can get these descriptions of the experience that is a purportedly non-dual, self-less experience, then, according to the phenomenologists, there still must be some minimal prereflective self-awareness present. If one says, "there is no I in this experience," and then goes on to describe what one experiences, it's like saying "I wasn't there, but here's what it was like." Or, "this is the experience I had, but it wasn't my experience."

A neurophenomenological study by Fingelkurts, Fingelkurts, and Kallio-Tamminen (2021) documents eight different meditation-induced changes in what they define as a triadic self-pattern that includes (1) the prereflective experiential self (which they also call the "witnessing observer"); (2) the embodied (sensory-motor and affective) agent; and (3) the cognitive-reflective-narrative aspect. Throughout all eight changes, most of them involving bodily changes (e.g., changes in body boundary or body image, and in some cases involving the sense of being disembodied), the prereflective experiential self retains a relatively constant functional integrity—in some cases undergoing a slight down-regulated modulation, and in other cases a slight up-regulated modulation (as measured by EEG recordings, phenomenological reports, and a battery of questionnaires). The researchers rightly note that even when the aspect of witnessing decreased slightly, it is this prereflective experience that "may explain why the participant was still able to report" the various experience states (2021, 26).

Some versions of Buddhist doctrine allow for this minimal experiential self-awareness in the no-self experience. In contrast to one report that there is no observer, or no witness, another meditating subject reports: "There's still a witnessing happening and that witnessing is what's left of me... it's like knowing it is happening without an object, or without a specific object" (Ataria, Dor-Ziderman & Berkovich-Ohana 2015, 142). In some regard, however, if the only process of the self-pattern that is left is prereflective self-awareness, then, strictly speaking, there is no self-pattern (understood as a pattern of different elements) left. Indeed, one might call that no-self, but no-self with a prereflective self-awareness. This is one possible interpretation.

Here's an explanation by the Buddhist scholar John Dunne (2011, 74) who uses the term "reflexive awareness" to refer to what phenomenologists call prereflective self-awareness characterized precisely as an awareness that does not take the self as an object (Gallagher & Zahavi 2020):

> For practitioners to experience a non-dual state, however, there must be some form of knowing or experiencing that is not structured by subject–object duality. This form of knowing is 'reflexive awareness' (Skt. *Svasa mvitti*, Tib., *rang rig*), and it does not receive a robust theoretical treatment until the works of Dharmakírti and his major commentators (seventh to ninth centuries). Once a clear account of reflexive awareness is in place, Buddhist authors now have the tools to speak of truly non-dual meditative states, namely, those in which the meditator experiences consciousness in its true form as utterly devoid of subject–object structuring. And this is precisely the type of practice that emerges historically as Mahámudrá in India by the end of the first millennium (C.E.).
>
> (Dunne 2011, 74)

On this description, a minimal prereflective (reflexive) self-awareness is still intact, although a reflective awareness that involves the subject-object structure is absent.

We can think of this in terms of Hume's famous introspective search for the self:

> For my part, when I enter most intimately into what I call *myself*, I always stumble on some particular perception or other, of heat or cold, light or shade, love or hatred, pain or pleasure. I never can *catch myself* at any time without a perception, and never can observe any thing but the perception.   (emphasis added)

There's a certain type of mistake that Hume never makes in his introspective practice. He never wanders into someone else's set of experiences; he doesn't stumble by mistake into his neighbor's stream of consciousness. Structurally, this would be impossible. That is, part of the very structure of experience, as the phenomenologists suggest, includes a first-person, prereflective self-awareness that allows me to say that "I catch myself." Neither the catcher nor the one who is caught is equivalent to a substantial self, or even to a fully complex self-pattern. Yet, the possibility of reporting on non-self states suggests there is always some degree of prereflective self-awareness with some degree of implicit mineness and affectivity in such "non-dual," or "self-less" processes. Mindfulness, even no-self mindfulness, is never mindless.

This is not to say that minimal prereflective self-awareness is not changed. The studies cited above suggest that the phenomenology of SB dissolution in meditation practice entails changes in sense of agency, sense of ownership, body sensations, first-person perspective, sense of time, and self–other distinction (Ataria et al. 2015; Nave et al. 2021). These are all aspects of prereflective self-awareness.

Here is a second interpretation. It is noted that affectivity does not disappear. The meditators were able to report heightened or positive emotion in the SB3 (or SB-) condition (Nave et al. 2021, 22, 26). Someone is experiencing this emotion, even if in SB3 there is a dissolution of various aspects of the self-pattern (narrative, cognitive, reflective, intersubjective, ecological, normative). Moreover, it is just a fact that the meditator is still functioning as a bodily existence even if there are modulations in the sense of body boundaries. This is also reflected in reports of "floating" in an egocentrically defined space, for example. Accordingly, even in SB3, not only is some form of prereflective self-awareness still operative, but some modified instantiation of the self-pattern that includes affectivity and bodily existence is still in place. Given that bodily existence, affect, and prereflective self-awareness are still in place, on this second interpretation, a self-pattern is still operative.

10

The Cruel and Unusual Phenomenologies of Torture and Solitary Confinement

Organized practices of violence in genocide, terrorism, slavery, rape, torture, and violent criminality continue to exist on a significant scale. There has always been and continues to be an overabundance of examples to point to, from atrocities committed in ancient battles, to the contemporary decimation of populations in modern warfare, from medieval crusades and pogroms to the Nazi holocaust and more recent instances of genocide, from continuing instances of enforced labor and slavery to the continuing violence of systemic racism, from everyday reports of rape and violence against women and children, to the increasing pandemic of school shootings and mass murders in some societies. Counting victims doesn't help, since the abstractions involved in statistics tend to have neutralizing effects on our understanding of what this violence means. Thinking too much about the experiences of the victims (and of their families), however, could easily lead to depression. Yet it seems important to consider the effects of such violence on those who survive the trauma.

Discussions of violence and psychiatry often focus on questions about whether psychiatric patients can be violent (e.g., Rueve & Welton 2008; Swanson 2021). In this final chapter I want to turn this issue around and explore how violent practices (by individuals and by institutions) can lead to trauma and psychiatric illness. I'll explore extreme cases in which the trauma is so severe that there is a complete breakdown of the self-pattern, especially where breakdowns involve failures and distortions of intersubjective processes. I'll start by looking at some phenomenological accounts of trauma associated with torture. Such accounts start with a focus on bodily processes involved in such experience. Within this phenomenological framework I want to broaden the analysis by considering the effects of violent trauma on the self-pattern as a whole. In this respect the importance of intersubjective processes will come into view. If intersubjective interaction clearly plays a significant role in therapeutic success, it is also clear that when intersubjective interaction is eliminated or perverted, the dynamics of the self-pattern can be totally undermined and can lead to psychopathologies. The penal practice of solitary confinement, which excludes the individual from intersubjective interaction, is one that completely disrupts the self-pattern, the effects of which can manifest as extreme psychiatric disorders. Although there is a growing professional and popular awareness about the effects of solitary confinement,

The Self and its Disorders. Shaun Gallagher, Oxford University Press. © Shaun Gallagher 2024.
DOI: 10.1093/oso/9780198873068.003.0011

there is still disagreement about whether solitary confinement should be considered a "cruel and unusual punishment." Indeed, there is no consensus on the
definition of the term "cruel" in the use of that legal phrase. I'll argue that a close
examination of the phenomenology, psychology, and psychopathologies of torture and solitary confinement, and their effects on the self-pattern, can provide
the basis for a clear moral consensus on the meaning of "cruelty."

10.1 Violence and Bodily Existence

Phenomenology provides a good starting point for considering the effects of traumatic violence by focusing on the body. Thiemo Breyer, for example, offers a phenomenological analysis of violence as a "violation of experiential structures" (2017,
737), which begins by focusing on bodily existence. Phenomenologists distinguish
between the body understood as the lived body (*Leib*), or the body-as-subject,
experienced from a first-person perspective, and the body-as-object (*Körper*),
which is the body understood from a third-person perspective. One's body can be
experienced from both perspectives. As Breyer explains, citing Husserl:

> Insofar as it is the same bodily unity that is sensing and being sensed, the human
> organism 'is reflexively related to itself' it is the subject and the object of the
> same overarching process of experience—of perceiving and being perceived,
> acting and being acted upon.   (Breyer 2017, 738)

In this particular experiential structure, the perceiving body-as-subject, typically
functions without taking itself as an object. The experience of pain, however, can
motivate a reflexivity in which we start to experience our bodies as both subject
and object, and in some cases, "the body [can become] both hostile and our own"
(Améry 1980, 64). Accordingly, the body may turn from being the medium of our
enactive engagement with the world "to being an 'enemy', having its own dynamics that go against our intentions" (Breyer 2017, 738). If in normal circumstances
this ambiguity of subject-object stays in the background, in cases that involve
pain, our coping may involve a kind of negotiation or flexible reconciliation
between these two poles. In extreme cases, however, and certainly in cases of the
extreme violent imposition of pain, "such flexibility of perspectives and therefore
the possibility for reconciliation are destroyed" (2017, 739).

The United Nations' *Convention Against Torture and Other Cruel, Inhumane, or
Degrading Treatment or Punishment* (1987) defines torture as the "severe pain or
suffering, whether physical or mental" deliberately inflicted on a person. Breyer
focuses on the infliction of physical rather than psychological torture. He follows
Buytendijk (1948) in differentiating pain and suffering, where "suffering refers to
the [psychical] reflectivity as surplus over and above sheer pain" (Breyer 2017,

742). The imposition of pain in torture, reorients attention to the body in an immediate presence (Leder 1984, 255), but reduces the experiential/relational distinction between body-as-subject and body-as-object (Plessner 1970, 132). It also undermines one's enactive engagement with the world, so that, as Breyer suggests, being locked into one's body the "I can" of affordances collapses, so that, "the freedom of kinaesthetic movement and perceptual exploration, is transformed into an 'I cannot"' (Breyer 2017, 743). We can start to see here that, any attempt to bracket off psychical suffering from bodily pain does not work. The effects of torture are not limited to body understood in a purely physical or objective way; they point to impacts on affective processes and intersubjective relations as well as habitual behavior and the sense of agency:

> This 'I cannot' becomes a quasi-transcendental background for all the experiences to come during captivity. The certainty of not being able to change the situation and to be utterly dependent on the will and action of those in power goes hand in hand with the uncertainty of the outcome. Being exposed in this way, the awareness of one's vulnerability is drastically heightened.
>
> (Breyer 2017, 743–4)

There is, Breyer suggests, a "pathic character" to torture, which destroys the practical "horizons of previously acquired experience and habitualities" (744).

A similar interpretation can be found in Yochai Ataria's phenomenological studies of torture (Ataria 2016; 2018; 2019a,b; Ataria & Gallagher 2015). Drawing on numerous phenomenological sources, Ataria argues that what changes under traumatic conditions of torture involves the normal inconspicuous fluidity and immersion of the body in the world, where typically there is no confusion between proprioception and the perception of other things (see, e.g., Fuchs & Schlimme 2009; Ratcliffe 2008). In the case of torture, however, everything changes as a direct consequence of what is done to the body. Ataria cites Solzhenitsyn's description of torture in the Gulag where the simplest and least expensive method of torture involved forcing prisoners to stand for long periods of time, and preventing them from sleeping to the point when their body would betray them:

> The system created a situation in which the prisoner's body was the enemy. It is important to stress that there was no defined enemy: the system was almost passive, simply creating an unbearable situation in which the prisoner's body became the source of suffering.   (Ataria 2019b, 32)

An extreme form of such torture can be found in the phenomenon of the *Muselmann* during the holocaust.[1] These prisoners, who were near death due to

---

[1] *Muselmann*, the German word for Muslim, came to be used among concentration camp inmates to describe prisoners dying of starvation or exhaustion who no longer possessed the will to live. Some

exhaustion and starvation, experienced helplessness and a profound alienation and disownership toward their bodies. In the case of the *Muselmann* the body-as-object is experienced as alien, comes to be felt as belonging to the captors, and is perceived as a tool to inflict suffering and pain on the *Muselmann* himself. His body becomes an enemy, which may, in turn, lead to suicidal inclinations, even after liberation from the camp.

Typically, disownership is defined, in the context of pathologies such as somatoparaphrenia (following a stroke), as the feeling that a body part—an arm or a leg—is alien: "It does not feel like a part of their body, although the patients *can acknowledge* that it is contiguous with the rest of their body. They experience that the *body part* does not belong to them" (de Vignemont 2011, 90, emphasis added). According to de Vignemont (2010; 2007), there are three different kinds of body disownership:

(1) experiencing a limb as alien, yet still believing that the limb belongs to you, as in the case of anarchic hand syndrome (Della Sala, Marchetti & Spinnler 1994);

(2) experiencing a limb as alien and also believing that the limb does not belong to you; the limb may seem to belong to someone else, as in somatoparaphrenia (Vallar & Ronchi 2009); and

(3) experiencing a limb as part of your body, but nevertheless believing that the limb does not belong to you, as in body integrity identity disorder (First 2005).

In all of these cases, however, disownership is defined narrowly, with reference to limbs and not the entire body. Yet, it seems that at least in some cases of depersonalization it is possible to refer to a sense of disownership toward the entire body (Sierra et al. 2005; Simeon & Abugel 2006). Similarly, it has been suggested that during extreme trauma subjects can feel this kind of complete somatic dissociation (Scaer 2014).

Under conditions endured by the *Muselmänner* in the Nazi concentration camps, the prisoner may develop just this kind of disownership toward his entire body. He becomes a pure object, or a kind of device, and loses any subjective dimension of embodiment:

scholars suggest that the term arose as a result of the similarity between the near-death prone state of a concentration camp *Muselmann* and the image of the Muslim at prayer, prostrate on the ground (Agamben 1999; Levi 1993). The *Muselmänner* could not stand up for more than a short period of time and therefore could not work. Since only the healthy and those capable of work could pass the frequent selections conducted by the Nazis, the *Muselmänner* were among the first to be sentenced to death (Sofsky 1996). Descriptions of individuals in this situation can be found in accounts given by survivors like Primo Levi (1959), Robert Antelme (1992; first published in 1947), Jean Améry (1980), and Imre Kertész (2004).

The *Muselmann* makes mechanical movements without any reason, no longer controlling his own body; he is beaten without offering any kind of resistance: at most they would beat me, and even then they could not truly do much harm, since for me it just won some time: at the first blow I would promptly stretch out on the ground and would feel nothing after that, since I would meanwhile drop off to sleep.   (Kertész 2004)

This body-disownership is characterized by (1) total numbness: blunted senses and emotions, and as a result the loss of the ability to be touched, and the loss of what Merleau-Ponty (2012) calls the "reversibility" implicit in self-touch, which is a prerequisite for feeling alive (Slatman 2005). (2) Lack of awareness: The *Muselmann's* level of awareness drops, in some cases to zero, with the effect that he can drop into a state of unconsciousness even while being beaten. (3) Loss of identity: When looking at the mirror, Antelme describes the following experience: "I saw a face appear. I'd forgotten about that" (Antelme, 1992, 51–2). Accordingly, the *Muselmann* becomes faceless, a nobody. Memories disappear: "I forget, every day I forget a little more, one gets farther away, one drifts" (Antelme 1992, 108). (4) Loss of future perspective: "But who can seriously think about tomorrow?" asks Levi (1959, 156). Antelme adds that in the concentration camps one simply could not "use the future tense" (1992, 95).

In cases of torture and severe trauma, then, it is possible that an experiential dissociation from one's whole body can be realized. This dissociation is sometimes thought to be a defense mechanism (e.g., Keleman 1989; Morgan et al., 2001; Nijenhuis, Vanderlinden & Spinhoven 1998; van der Hart et al. 2004). On one interpretation, such processes of defense work via a trade-off. That is, by giving up some degree of the sense of ownership over one's body, one gains a sense of agency in other areas (e.g., an ability to engage in mental exercises or distractions). Essentially, this trade-off enables a traumatized subject to maintain a limited sense of control over some aspects of existence during acute stress, even if he has less control over his own body (Ataria 2015).[2] Activating this kind of defense mechanism, however, takes a significant amount of (cognitive and emotional) energy. As the person weakens, physically and psychologically, the defense mechanism may start to fail. Ataria suggests that in cases of severe and prolonged trauma (as in the torture experienced by the *Muselmann*) we should, at least theoretically, consider the possibility that this dissociative defense mechanism can itself collapse. In this case, there is a change in the quality of the disownership experienced toward the entire body, which also has an effect on the sense of agency. The *Muselmann* is unable or unwilling to resist or engage in any form of self-defense, and the subject's senses of agency and body ownership move into a

---

[2] Ataria and Neria (2013) provide descriptions of this process from interviews with former prisoners of war.

more negative range (Ataria & Gallagher 2015). Specifically, everything (all objects, and all others, including fellow prisoners [Levi 1959]), and even one's own body, which is experienced as not one's own, are organized to produce suffering and pain. One's own body is not only *not* one's own, but becomes identified as an object designed, like any other in the camp, to inflict pain. Kertész (2004) calls it "being at war with myself." In some cases, the subject accepts and internalizes the idea that he must be annihilated (see Améry 1980). It's notable that Primo Levi, Améry, and many others (including Paul Celan and Bruno Bettelheim, to mention only a few well-known names) committed suicide after liberation. Indeed, Améry felt that he had to finish the Nazis' work (Ataria 2019a).

10.2 The Phenomenology of Intersubjectivity

Both Ataria and Breyer recognize that the effects of torture go beyond the body, and both point to a disruption in intersubjective relations. Breyer points to the practice of solitary confinement as an example of torture that is obviously a disruption or deprivation of intersubjectivity. I'll return to a discussion of this practice. Clearly, however, that is only one type of violent disruption of intersubjectivity. The experience of pain imposed by others in torture involves a different type, namely a "border violation of my self by the other, which can be neither neutralized by the expectation of help nor rectified through resistance" (Améry 1980, 33). Such situations of one-on-one torture, according to Breyer (2017), destroy, not just the body, but the relational structure of subjectivity. Ataria points to a third type of intersubjective disruption, which is something like the opposite of solitary confinement. He cites Aleksandr Solzhenitsyn's description of the horrendous conditions involved when, in the gulag, as a means of torture, too many prisoners are pushed into a cell (eighteen people in a cell designed for one; or 140 prisoners in a cell designed for twenty-five): "In this impossible situation, the people who are imprisoned together and in exactly the same situation torture one another by their very presence. Furthermore, one's sense of boundaries collapses" (Ataria 2019b, 31). Here Ataria cites de Haan and Fuchs (2010, 329) who emphasize the importance of the sense of boundary: "the loss of self is often accompanied by a feeling of being somehow too open to the world, of having a too 'thin skin,' [leading] to experiences of transitivism, of the permeability of boundaries between the self and others, or the self and the world, [so that] other people and the world may be experienced as intrusive, invading the personal sphere."

These considerations point to some classic phenomenological concepts related directly to understanding intersubjectivity in the self-pattern. I review these concepts in the remainder of this section. In the next section I'll show how these concepts are reinforced by developmental studies. Finally, I'll consider the effects of solitary confinement, when subjects are deprived of intersubjective contact.

Phenomenological approaches to philosophy, psychology, and psychiatry have been keen to incorporate the principles of embodied and enactive conceptions of intersubjective interaction (e.g., Fuchs & Schlimme 2009; Fuchs & De Jaegher 2009; de Haan 2020; Gallagher 2001; 2020a; Ratcliffe 2006). Even in its classic form, phenomenology emphasizes the idea that intersubjective relations are intrinsically constitutive for human experience. I'll briefly discuss three concepts from phenomenology directly relevant to this idea: being-with, transcendental intersubjectivity, and intercorporeity.

Heidegger (1962) provides an analysis of human existence in which being-with (*Mitsein*) is part of the very structure of human existence, shaping the way that we are in the world. According to this notion, the social dimension is not an external add-on or supplement to our existence. Being-with does not signify that we are in-the-world first, and then because of that we come to be with others. Indeed, Heidegger argues that our social nature does not depend on empirically encountering others; it is rather an a priori structure—the fact that others are in the world only has significance because our existence is pre-structured as being-with. If one happens to be alone, or has always been alone, one still has the structure of being-with—and "only as being-with can [one] be alone" (1988, 238). Heidegger goes on to further emphasize that this particular way of being-with co-determines other aspects of our existence, including our relations with the world around us: "By reasons of this *with-like* [*mithaften*] being-in-the-world, the world is always the one that I share with Others. The world of [human existence] is a *with-world* [*Mitwelt*]" (1962, 155/118). According to Heidegger, one encounters others primarily through one's various projects, and even in terms of what one pragmatically perceives. One's projects equally implicate other people—as co-workers, intended recipients, and so on. Accordingly, the world in which we find ourselves cannot be extricated from our relations with other people—it is permeated with social relations. Heidegger also makes the point that being-with shapes our own self-experience. One's *own* existence is something that one experiences in the kinds of pragmatic projects that one shares with others.

In effect, one doesn't come to have a social constitution by way of interacting with others; one is "hard-wired" to be other-oriented, and this is an existential characteristic that makes human existence what it is. The term "hard-wired" is not a term that Heidegger would have used. I introduce it, however, to indicate the possibility of something going wrong in regard to being-with (see below). To the extent that the *Mitsein* structure is damaged, it damages the very core of the individual's human existence.

The notion of an existential sociality is not only relevant to questions about social cognition and our relations to others. According to Husserl, the very *objectivity* of the world *as experienced* depends on others. This is what he refers to as transcendental intersubjectivity (e.g., Husserl 1959, 449; 1968, 295). Intersubjectivity is transcendental, in the sense that it is a condition of possibility for us to experience anything like a coherent and meaningful world, and specifically to experience it as real and objective. This latter point is what Husserl's concept of transcendental intersubjectivity adds to Heidegger's notion of *Mitsein*. The analysis Husserl gives is based on the perception of our immediate environment. We see things, not as mere surfaces, but as multi-sided objects based on an implicit reference to the (real or potential) perceptual perspectives that others can take on the same objects. Our basic experience of the world as having reality or objectivity depends on a kind of tacit confirmation by others:

> Thus everything objective that stands before me in experience and primarily in perception has an apperceptive horizon of possible experience, including my own and that of others. Ontologically speaking, my perception of the world is, from the very beginning, part of an open but not explicit totality of possible perceptions [that others may also have]. The subjectivity belonging to this experience of the world is open [or transcendental] intersubjectivity.
>
> (Husserl 1973a, 289; translated in Gallagher & Zahavi 2021, 139)

The idea that something may go wrong with the basic structures of being-with or transcendental intersubjectivity was followed up in the tradition of phenomenological psychiatry, as found in the classic works of Jaspers (1997), Minkowski (1970), Blankenburg (1971), and others. A certain form of derealization, for example, can be analyzed as a disruption of transcendental intersubjectivity, to the point that real things may no longer feel real or familiar, or as fully objective as they should. A significant privation of intersubjectivity, accordingly, may lead to an erosion of the sense of reality (although, to be sure, not all forms of derealization are due to such privation). Such experiences, found in instances of schizophrenia, may also be closely tied to the phenomenon of depersonalization. As previously noted, phenomenologists have analyzed some of the symptoms of schizophrenia (including autistic aspects of schizophrenia) as involving very basic disruptions in self-experience or ipseity (e.g., Sass & Parnas 2003). "Such experiences may also involve dissociative features, in which one experiences a pathological, subjective detachment from the external world, an estrangement from one's body and even from mental processes" (Varga 2012, 103). On this view, the loss of a basic intersubjective dimension of existence can lead to the loss of the sense of worldly realness, as well as disturbances in prereflective self-awareness, the sense of ownership, and/or the sense of agency.[3]

---

[3] As Ciaunica et al. (2021) point out, in the case of depersonalization, the self-alienation occurs across a number of different processes: "(a) detachment from one's body or body parts ([involving] sensory and bodily aspects of the self); (b) detachment from one's subjective feelings and emotions (experiential aspects); and (c) disconnection from one's personal stories, memories, thoughts and future plans, often described by sufferers as a lack of a narrative or a 'plot' in one's life." See Adrien et al. (2023) for a review of the effects of PTSD on the sense of agency across a number of symptoms.

In terms of our actual engagement with others, being-with and transcendental intersubjectivity are cashed out in very basic sensory-motor processes involved in our bodily interactions with others. Merleau-Ponty calls this "intercorporeity": "There is...between this phenomenal body and the other person's phenomenal body such as I see it from the outside, an internal relation that makes the other person appear as the completion of the system" (2012, 368). For Merleau-Ponty, our perception of others is interactional rather than observational, and the actions of others elicit the activation of our own motor systems. These processes involve the kind of motor resonance often described in the mirror neuron literature; but for Merleau-Ponty this is more than a brain event; he emphasizes the dynamic embodied interchange that one finds in the affective attunement that occurs between interacting agents. A good example of intercorporeity can be found in the experiment conducted by Soliman and Glenberg (2014) (see Section 7.5), showing the emergence of a joint body schema in processes of joint action. In this regard, Merleau-Ponty suggests that the borders of the transcendental and the empirical become indistinct—we should not think of the facticity of embodied being with others as external to subjective experience or cognition, but the place where the mind happens, or as he dramatically puts it, where "the transcendental descends into history" (1963, 107). The best way to see the details of this kind of embodied intersubjectivity is by looking at developmental studies.

10.3 Taking a Developmental Perspective

The *interaction theory* of social cognition draws on the work of phenomenologists, but also the developmental studies of primary and secondary intersubjectivity (Trevarthen 1979; also see Hobson 2004; Reddy 2008; Rochat 2001). As previously indicated (in Chapter 3), primary intersubjectivity involves the sensory-motor capacities that shape our interactions with others from the very beginning. From early infancy, for example, infants are capable of actively interacting with others. Throughout the first year of life, infants develop an enactive perceptual access to the emotional and intentional states of others. At two months, for example, second-person *interaction* with others is evidenced by the timing of their movements and emotional responses. Infants "vocalize and gesture in a way that seems [affectively and temporally] 'tuned' to the vocalizations and gestures of the other person" (Gopnik & Meltzoff 1997, 131). Further evidence for this is provided by still face experiments (Tronick et al. 1978) and contingency studies (Murray & Trevarthen 1985) where infants become significantly upset when faced with unresponsive behavior or mis-timed responses from the mother—processes that disrupt basic intercorporeity.

The concept of secondary intersubjectivity (Trevarthen & Hubley 1978) is associated with the advent of joint attention during the first year. Infants start to notice how others pragmatically engage with the world and they begin to co-constitute the meaning of the world through interactions with others in joint actions. Pragmatic and social contexts start to matter, and they enter into situations of participatory sense-making (De Jaegher & Di Paolo 2007). Secondary intersubjective processes are ways of cashing out the phenomenological concepts of *Mitsein* and transcendental intersubjectivity.

The important point made by interaction theory is that both primary and secondary intersubjectivity are not only early developing, characterizing our existence from infancy, but they remain essential aspects of our continued adult existence with others. Moreover, in processes of primary intersubjectivity we develop and continue to sustain a relational sense of self. That is, a sense of self that is intricately coupled to others, which we have called the intersubjective aspect of the self-pattern. If one's primary, most basic, prereflective experiences of self-ownership and agency are tied to one's embodied, sensory-motor, proprioceptive processes, these processes are also fully involved in intersubjective interactions from the start. We are, as Lisa Guenther (2013) puts it, *relationally constituted*. Again, all of these intersubjective dimensions are reflected later (at two–four years of age) in the way we start to form our self-narratives.

Since the capacities of primary and secondary intersubjectivity are not left behind, but continue to characterize and contribute to our mature adult behavior, in some ways they come to be transformed through our rich communicative and narrative practices. Behavioral analyses of social interactions in joint actions and shared activities, in working together, in communicative practices, and so on, show that adult agents continue to unconsciously coordinate their movements, gestures, and speech acts (Issartel et al. 2007; Kendon 1990; Lindblom & Ziemke 2008). In communicative practices we coordinate our perception-action sequences; our movements and gestures are coupled with changes in velocity, direction, and intonation in the movements, gestures, and utterances of the other speaker. Such processes can vary across different circumstances, as demonstrated in numerous empirical studies (e.g., Goodwin 2017).

Furthermore, the social interaction which characterizes primary and secondary intersubjectivity goes beyond each participant; it results in something (the creation of meaning) that goes beyond what each individual qua individual can bring to the process (De Jaegher et al. 2010). As we have been arguing, these interactive practices shape who we are, our identities, our meaningful experiences of the world, and what we take to be valuable or not so valuable.

Consider a case in which intersubjective interaction is disrupted in early life. During the Ceauşescu regime in Romania young children were left in orphanages, often because of the extreme poverty of their parents. Peter Hobson (2004) summarizes the conditions in these orphanages:

- Infants were confined to their cots, without toys or other playthings, fed by bottles that were sometimes left propped up for use.

- Little sustained, interpersonal exchange; no opportunities to establish relationships with caregivers.
- The physical environment was also extremely harsh, and it was not uncommon for children to be washed by being hosed down with cold water.

Children who were adopted from these orphanages lacked the reciprocal to-and-fro of social exchange, they showed limited social awareness and empathy, they found it difficult to maintain social interaction, and they would rarely turn to their adoptive parents for security and comfort (Hobson 2004).

Studies by Michael Rutter et al. (1999; 2007) showed that a small but much higher than expected proportion of these children developed an atypical (or quasi) form of early childhood autism. A variety of studies found severe problems with social relationships and communication involving:

- Poverty of eye-to-eye gaze and gestures in social exchanges
- Limited language and to-and-fro conversation
- Preoccupations with sensations and other cognitive characteristics of autism—including strong interest in abnormal patterns and objects (but at the same time including problems in perception of gestalt).

Additional studies show:

- Emotional difficulties sustained through childhood (Colvert et al. 2008)
- Negative effects on motor development in children who were psychosocially deprived in these orphanages (Levin et al. 2014)
- Disruptions in the development of the neural circuitry involved in the recognition of facial expressions, due to psychosocial deprivation (Parker & Nelson 2005).

Rutter et al. drew the tentative conclusion that prolonged experience of such terrible social and non-social privation was responsible for these quasi-autistic symptoms. Hobson is less tentative: the circumstances of these institutions led to a form of induced autism. Autism (naturally occurring or induced) involves "a disorder of the system of child-in-relation-to-other" (Hobson 2004, 203).

By looking at studies of naturally occurring autism we can be more specific about some of the embodied aspects that underpin intersubjectivity. As noted above (Section 3.4.3) there is extensive evidence to suggest that ASD involves problems with basic sensory-motor processes that support primary intersubjectivity. Long-standing research based on the analysis of videos of infants younger than one year and later diagnosed with autism shows asymmetries or unusual sequencing in crawling and walking, as well as problems and delayed development in lying, righting, sitting (Teitelbaum et al. 1998). Experimental studies by Elizabeth Torres et al. (2013) show disrupted patterns in re-entrant (afferent, proprioceptive) sensory feedback that usually contributes to the autonomous regulation and coordination of motor output. From an early age, this feedback supports volitional control and fluid, flexible transitions between intentional and spontaneous behaviors.

Torres shows that across the entire autistic spectrum there is a disruption in the maturation of this form of proprioception, accompanied by behavioral variability in motor control. In clear contrast to typically developing individuals, the normalized peak (micro-movement) velocity and noise-to-signal ratios of all participants with ASD, including adolescents (fourteen–sixteen years old) and young adults (eighteen–twenty-five years old), across different ages and across verbal or non-verbal status, remain in the region corresponding to younger typically developing children. For a person with ASD, noise overpowers signal in the motor system. Proprioceptive input is random (unpredictable), noisy (unreliable), and non-diversified; autistic subjects accordingly have difficulty distinguishing goal-directed from goal-less motions in most experimental tasks, and difficulty anticipating the consequences of their own impending movements in a fine-tuned timely fashion (Torres et al. 2013, 16). It's also unlikely they could apply fine-tuned discriminations to the actions and emotional facial micro-expressions of others during real time social interactions.

To be clear, appealing to the data on motor problems in ASD is not meant to suggest an equivalency between individuals with ASD and those who have a form of induced or quasi-autism. Rather, the point is simply that some of the same motor difficulties that correlate with problems in social or intersubjective experience can be found in both groups. Furthermore, both of these groups are, or come to be, embedded in socially rich environments, which may provide them with important support for compensating against such differences in motor attunement. This clearly differentiates them from prisoners in solitary confinement who may develop similar motor problems (see below). Children who show signs of quasi-autism often improve once they are introduced into social and caring environments; likewise, some individuals with ASD who engage in sensory-motor therapies improve their social performance and achieve a relatively high level of intersubjective activity. The important point, here, is that motor problems that can undermine social interaction can be induced by social and physical privation.

10.4 Solitary Confinement

Borsboom and Cramer (2013, 104) suggest that "in almost any mental disorder, significant social effects...exist; in general, prolonged severe problems lead to a greater degree of social isolation." This also operates in reverse: prolonged social isolation can lead directly to severe mental disorders. The institutional practice of solitary confinement demonstrates this reversal. Solitary confinement may differ from one prison to the next in the precise details of how it is carried out. The common element is some high degree of isolation—the reduction or complete elimination of intersubjective contact between the prisoner and others for a significant amount of time. One example of the practice is found in the Security Housing Unit of Pelican Bay State Prison in California:

> [Some prisoners were] isolated for ten or more years in an eight by ten foot windowless cell for twenty-two and a half to twenty-four hours a day. Time spent outside of the cell was limited to an empty outdoor exercise yard with twenty foot high concrete walls and no windows. Plaintiffs were not permitted contact visits with family, friends, or attorneys, and the only phone calls permitted were 'bereavement calls' when a family member passed away.   (Guenther 2018, 74)[4]

Prisoners who are subjected to solitary confinement show symptoms, and they describe a phenomenology that is not equivalent to either ASD or induced autism but reflects similar motor problems and often times more extensive and serious disruptions of experience. Lisa Guenther (2013), looking at the phenomenology associated with solitary confinement, describes it as becoming "unhinged": "[Prisoners subjected to solitary confinement] see things that do not exist, and they fail to see things that do. Their sense of their own bodies—even the fundamental capacity to feel pain and to distinguish their own pain from that of others—erodes to the point where they are no longer sure if they are being harmed or are harming themselves" (2013, xi). There is a long list of experiences associated with solitary confinement: anxiety, fatigue, confusion, paranoia, depression, hallucinations, headaches, insomnia, trembling, anger, apathy, stomach and muscle pains, oversensitivity to stimuli, feelings of inadequacy, inferiority, withdrawal, isolation, rage, anger, and aggression, difficulty in concentrating, dizziness, distortion of the sense of time, severe boredom, and impaired memory (Smith 2006; see Cloud et al. 2015; Hastings et al. 2015).

Peter Smith notes: "whether and how isolation damages people depends on duration and circumstances and is mediated by prisoners' individual characteristics; but for many prisoners, the adverse effects are substantial" (2006, 441). He documents high rates of mental illness resulting from solitary confinement, starting in the nineteenth century. Hearing about new practices of solitary confinement in

---

[4] The United Nations Standard Minimum Rules for the Treatment of Prisoners, known as the Nelson Mandela Rules, define extended solitary confinement as torture. New York State banned solitary confinement in its state prisons for lengths in excess of fifteen days (starting in 2022). Solitary has been banned for juvenile offenders in federal prisons (but not in all state prisons). The popular press reports that over sixty thousand inmates were housed in solitary confinement at the start of 2020. Many prisoners are kept in solitary for years. One prisoner in New York State had been in solitary for over thirty years.

American prisons, delegates from Europe came to learn about it. One visitor, the author Charles Dickens, refered to solitary confinement as "slow and daily tampering with the mysteries of the brain…immeasurably worse than any torture of the body" (1957, 99; cited in Guenther 2013, 18).

Studies of 100 inmates in California's Pelican Bay Supermax prison found 91 percent of the prisoners suffering from anxiety and nervousness; 70 percent "felt themselves on the verge of an emotional breakdown"; 77 percent experience chronic depression (Haney 2003, 133). One prisoner reported the following experience:

I went to a standstill psychologically once—lapse of memory. I didn't talk for 15 days. I couldn't hear clearly. You can't see—you're blind—block out everything—disoriented, awareness is very bad.   (Cited in Grassian 1983, 1453)

Another confirmed sensory disturbances:

Melting. Everything in the cell starts moving; everything gets darker, you feel you are losing your vision.   (Cited in Grassian 1983, 1452)

And another confirmed memory problems:

Memory is going. You feel you are losing something you might not get back.
(Cited in Grassian 1983, 1453)

A systematic review of the phenomenology of solitary confinement reveals symptoms that involve serious bodily and motor problems, derealization, and self-dissolution (or depersonalization).

Bodily and motor problems. Dickens, when visiting an American prison, was curious about the trembling of the prisoners in solitary confinement—"their nervous ticks, their difficulty in meeting his eye or sustaining conversation, their cringing posture and nervousness" (Guenther 2013, 19). To Dickens' observation a prison guard replied:

Well it's not so much a trembling, although they do quiver—as a complete derangement of the nervous system. They can't sign their names to the book; sometimes they can't even hold the pen…sometimes they get up and down again twenty times in a minute.…Sometimes they stagger as if they were drunk, and sometimes are forced to lean against the fence, they're so bad.
(Dickens 1957, 105–6)

Dickens adds that the prisoner's sensory awareness, their capacities to see and hear clearly, to make sense of their perceptions were diminished: "That it makes the senses dull, and by degrees impairs the bodily faculties, I am quite sure" (Dickens 1957, 108–9). Guenther is right that "it is precisely at the level of bodily perception, sensibility and affectivity that prisoners find their relation to the world undermined" (2013, 154).

It's a question open to future empirical investigation whether this kind of undermining of embodiment is similar to the sensory-motor problems described by Torres (2013) in terms of disrupted patterns in the peripheral nervous system—disruptions of the re-entrant (afferent, proprioceptive) sensory feedback that usually contribute to the autonomous regulation and coordination of motor output, as well as to primary intersubjectivity. The observed symptoms do seem similar: poverty of eye-to-eye gaze and gestures in social exchanges; limited language and to-and-fro conversation; a variety of sensory-motor problems.

Derealization. One also finds, correlatively, reports from prisoners in solitary confinement reflecting derealization—undermining their relation to the world. Thus, the experience of object boundaries becomes uncertain:

> It becomes difficult to tell what is real and what is only my imagination playing tricks on me...the wire mesh on [the] door begins to vibrate or the surface of the wall seems to bulge.
>
> (Guenther 2013, 35; citing Grassian 1983; Shalev 2009)

As Guenther suggests, in solitary confinement the transcendental intersubjective basis of the experience of the world as real and objective is structurally undermined (2013, 35). It completely closes down the possibility of secondary intersubjectivity and therefore of participatory sense making, undermining the capacity to sustain meaning. These problems with derealization, and with sensory-motor processes, correlate with depersonalization and the dissolution of the self-pattern.

Self-dissolution. Christensen, in a study of a woman who experienced solitary confinement in Denmark, writes: "The person subjected to solitary confinement risks losing her self and disappearing into a non-existence" (1999, 45; cited and trans. by Smith 2006, 497). It's important, however, to specify precisely what aspects of self are at stake in such a statement. Depersonalization-derealization disorder (DPD) is characterized as affecting the sense of bodily boundaries (including disembodiment, detachment from one's body or body parts, lack of a sense of body ownership), preflective experiential and affective processes (lack of subjective feelings or emotional numbing), as well as cognitive and narrative abilities (where the subjects may experience a disconnection from their self-narrative, memories, and future plans, described as a lack of a narrative flow in one's life). Derealization, involving the feeling of being cut-off from the world, or experiencing the world as not real, correlates with these various changes in the self-pattern (Ciaunica, Charlton & Farmer 2021; Sierra & Berrios 2001; Sierra & David 2011).

Lisa Guenther (2013, xiii) points to a more central role for intersubjectivity when she asks: "How could I lose myself by being confined to myself? For this to be possible, there must be more to selfhood than individuality.... Solitary confinement works by turning prisoners' constitutive relationality against themselves." That is, solitary confinement disrupts the *relational* aspects of both ecological and intersubjective processes in the self-pattern by disrupting primary and secondary intersubjectivity, and the intercorporeity essential to social interaction.

The practice of solitary confinement is not, as some of the original prison administrators thought, a way for the prisoner to return into self—"The inmate was expected to turn his thoughts inward"—a rehabilitation by means of an isolation of oneself with oneself (Smith 2006, 456; see Guenther 2013, xvi). Such a proposal reflects a traditional concept of self as an isolated individual substance or soul that gains self-knowledge through a practice of introspection. If, in contrast, the self-pattern is relational, then solitary confinement, by undermining intersubjective relationality, leads to a destruction of the self. Stripping away the possibility of primary intersubjectivity—leading to the experience of depersonalization not unlike some symptoms of schizophrenia—disrupts basic prereflective ipseity.

Dysnarrativa. It also affects one's *narrative* capacity. Self-narrative depends on having something to narrate, and having someone to whom to narrate. In addition, as I argued in Section 5.6, self-narrative practices require capacities for temporal integration, first-person self-reference, autobiographical memory, and reflective metacognition. As it turns out, all four capacities are under threat in the context of solitary confinement. Among the commonly reported symptoms that result from solitary confinement are distortions in the sense of time, which can clearly affect the capacity for temporal integration; basic disruptions in bodily integrity, so that differentiation between self and non-self is compromised (Guenther 2013, xi); impaired memory; and cognitive difficulties (concentration, confusion), with serious consequences for metacognition.

The evidence reviewed above suggests that solitary confinement negatively affects, not just bodily and intersubjective processes, but most if not all of the processes involved in the self-pattern. Reports from prisoners, medical personnel, psychologists and psychiatrists suggest serious problems with embodied existence (e.g., physical health and motor problems), prereflective experiential processes (e.g., sensory problems, ambiguity in the sense of ownership), affective processes (e.g., depression, anxiety), intersubjective or relational aspects (which comes with the situation of being isolated), psychological/cognitive and reflective aspects (e.g., lack of concentration, confusion), narrative capacities (e.g., memory problems, distortions in temporal integration), ecological aspects (e.g., lack of control over personal property, derealization, and the relatively dire conditions of the prison cell), and normative aspects (e.g., involving the dissolution of "practical identity" or any sense of worth; the absence of social roles or social status). A breakdown in some significant number of these aspects would be sufficient to alter, or even eradicate the pattern that constitutes self in any particular case.

10.5 Cruel and Unusual

Solitary confinement is a practice that constitutes a "total institution," in the sense proposed by Erving Goffman (1961, 6)—an all-encompassing practice that disrupts everyday structures and introduces control where all tasks and functions are conducted on a regulated schedule in an unchanging place. Goffman was describing mental hospitals, where, arguably, patients were made worse rather than better. Goffman's book, *Asylums: Essays on the Social Situation of Mental Patients and Other Inmates,* as noted by Zahavi and Loidolt (2022), was cited in legal briefs and judicial rulings, and helped to establish changes in mental health policy and patients' rights. Zahavi and Loidolt align Goffman's efforts to the work of phenomenological psychiatrists, like Franco Basaglia and Franz Fanon, who engaged in critical phenomenology with the aim (and sometimes success) of changing institutions. I suggest that putting the concept of self-pattern to use in its psychiatric context can support the development of a critical phenomenology of solitary confinement (as in Guenther's 2013), with the aim of changing such a total institution.

A number of legal declarations prohibit cruel punishments. The Eighth Amendment to the United States Constitution (1791), for example, declares: "cruel and unusual punishments [shall not be] inflicted." From the beginning, however, the wording was thought "too indefinite," or "to have no meaning in it."[5] It is still difficult to find a clear definition of "cruel" in the legal domain. Radin (1978, 992) recommends that the courts "search for a deeper moral consensus on the meaning of cruelty in order to determine whether a specific punishment comports with current standards of decency." Rather than searching, as Radin suggests, legal history, legislation, referenda and opinion polls, however, I suggest that an analysis, which combines philosophical and scientific methods, including phenomenology, psychology, psychiatry, developmental psychology, and neuroscience, can be used to explicate the specific experiences of those who undergo such punishments, and can thereby help us form a deeper moral consensus.[6]

In 1972, United States Supreme Court Justice William Brennan, in *Furman v. Georgia* (408 U.S. 238; 1972), a case involving the death penalty, defined four principles that determine when a punishment is cruel and unusual:

1. When the severity is *degrading* to human dignity (including torture).
2. When a severe punishment is "obviously inflicted in wholly *arbitrary* fashion."

---

[5] Granucci (1969, 842), who provides a fine-grained history of the phrase, cites representatives to the First Congress, Smith and Livermore, respectively.

[6] This is clearly a different hermeneutical procedure than found in most legal considerations where appeal is often to historical meaning or to evolving moral standards on such questions.

3. When the severe punishment "is clearly and totally *rejected throughout society.*"
4. When a severe punishment is "patently *unnecessary.*"

Unlike the first principle, principles 2, 3, and 4 are easier to measure or define. It's not clear, however, that on their own, arbitrariness, social rejection, and lack of necessity define the concept of cruelty. Justice Brennan thus suggests that these principles need to be applied in a convergent fashion. That the concept of "cruelty" (or "degrading to human dignity")[7] remains obscure can be seen in how it is glossed in the following explanation:

> [These criteria are] interrelated, and, in most cases, it will be their convergence that will justify the conclusion that a punishment is "cruel and unusual." The test, then, will ordinarily be a cumulative one: if a punishment is *unusually severe*, if there is a strong probability that it is inflicted arbitrarily, if it is substantially rejected by contemporary society, and if there is no reason to believe that it serves any penal purpose more effectively than some less severe punishment, then the continued infliction of that punishment violates the command of the Clause that the State may not inflict inhuman and uncivilized punishments upon those convicted of crimes.   (Brennan 1972, 239; emphasis added)

The severity of punishment that is degrading to human dignity is explicated simply as when the severity is "unusually severe." Without dismissing the other three principles, I want to suggest that the phenomenology of the self-pattern, in the context of solitary confinement, provides a clearer interpretation of the first principle, along with the concepts of *cruelty* and *degrading of human dignity*; an interpretation that on its own should be sufficient for disqualifying solitary confinement as an acceptable punishment.[8]

The concept of self or person that the liberal tradition sets up as having dignity and demanding respect is a standard that treats the self as a stand-alone

---

[7] The concept of dignity is not well defined in the law either (see McDougal et al. 1980). Pellegrino (2008, xi) states: "there is no universal agreement on the meaning of the term, human dignity." The term in used in a variety of ways, but it is often associated with the concept of respect for the human person.

[8] There is no universal agreement that solitary confinement need be considered cruel and unusual punishment. Thus, Bonta and Gendreau (1990), who discount phenomenological and qualitative studies in favor of more objective and experimental ones, conclude: "solitary confinement may not be cruel and unusual punishment under the humane and time-limited conditions investigated in experimental studies or in correctional jurisdictions that have well-defined and effectively administered ethical guidelines for its use" (361). Bonta and Gendreau's study, however, has been subject to widespread criticism (see, for example, the critique by Jackson [2002]). Furthermore, most psychiatric studies of solitary confinement have condemned the practice (Grassian 1983; Haney 2003). Note that scientific research of prison conditions, including solitary confinement, is very difficult to undertake, given security constraints. Most studies of solitary confinement are commissioned as part of lawsuits (e.g., Grassian and Haney, for example, have both testified as expert witnesses).

individual cognitively capable of autonomous deliberation and decision (see, e.g., Code 2011). Both phenomenology and science show this to be an abstraction that fails to recognize the intersubjective *relational* nature of the self, further complicated by embodied, experiential, and affective dimensions, as well as by narrative, ecological, and normative aspects of human existence. Solitary confinement degrades human dignity by literally degrading (if not destroying) the person's self-pattern, in all of its processes, starting with the deeply relational dimension of intersubjectivity. Ethically and practically speaking, this multi-dimensional, relational self-pattern is the only viable concept of self that the liberal tradition should use to measure its own practices pertaining to dignity, respect, and justice. To the extent that dignity is associated with the possibility of self-respect, which exists relationally, that is, as something that depends on the respect that others have for you, and that you have for others, if we destroy the coherency of the self-pattern, or a sufficient number of the processes that constitute the self-pattern, it would be difficult to argue that we are respecting the person in any moral sense, and not degrading the dignity of the human being.

In this chapter I've focused on torture and solitary confinement, two practices that lack any kind of moral justification. What's clear from these extreme practices is the intrinsic connection between personal health and social health. The analysis could easily pursue a variety of pragmatic implications. Ugelvik et al. (2022), for example, arguing for prison reform, suggest that the phenomenology of pathology parallels the phenomenology reflective of prison practices. Following Drew Leder (2018), they focus on disruptions that are common to both illness or pathology and prison life: disruptions of embodiment, worldly involvement (or spatiality), self-image/identity, and both social and temporal dimensions. These are, perhaps, alternative ways of describing some of the disorders that emerge in the self-pattern as the result of changes to processes that range from bodily to intersubjective and normative factors. The most general implication is that psychiatric cures cannot be framed exclusively in terms of the individual person. Rather, consistent with John Dewey's message to the College of Physicians in St. Louis in 1937, because the person is relational in a very deep sense, cures must address social, cultural, and institutional arrangements.

References

Abney, D. H., Paxton, A., Dale, R., & Kello, C. T. (2014). Complexity matching in dyadic conversation. *Journal of Experimental Psychology: General* 143(6): 2304–15.

Adery, L. H., Ichinose, M., Torregrossa, L. J., Wade, J., Nichols, H., Bekele, E., Bian, D., Gizdic, A., Granholm, E., Sarkar, N., et al. (2018). The acceptability and feasibility of a novel virtual reality based social skills training game for schizophrenia: Preliminary findings. *Psychiatry Research* 270: 496–502.

Adler, J. M., Chin, E. D., Kolisetty, A. P. & Oltmanns, T. F. (2012). The distinguishing characteristics of narrative identity in adults with features of borderline personality disorder: An empirical investigation. *Journal of Personality Disorders* 26: 498–512.

Adrien, V., Linson, A., Trousselard, M., and Schoeller, F. (2023). Agency in post-traumatic stress disorder: Implications for therapy. *Psyarxiv.com.* https://psyarxiv.com/j2pwk/download?format=pdf

Agamben, G. (1999). *Remnants of Auschwitz*, trans. D. Heller-Roazen. New York: Zone Books.

Agid, Y., Schüpbach, M., Gargiulo, M., et al. (2006). Neurosurgery in Parkinson's disease: The doctor is happy, the patient less so? In *Parkinson's Disease and Related Disorders* (409–14). Vienna: Springer.

Albahari, M. (2011) Nirvana and ownerless consciousness, in M. Siderits, E. Thompson, and D. Zahavi (eds), *Self, No Self? Perspectives from Analytical, Phenomenological, and Indian Traditions* (79–113). Oxford: Oxford University Press.

Albahari, M. (2006). *Analytical Buddhism.* London: Palgrave Macmillan.

Alonim, H. A., Lieberman, I., Tayar, D. & Scheingesicht, G. (2021). A retrospective study of prodromal variables associated with autism among a global group of infants during their first fifteen months of life. *International Journal of Pediatrics and Neonatal Care* 7 (2): 178–185.

Alonim, H. A., Lieberman, I., Tayar, D., Scheingesicht, G. & Braude, H. D. (2020). A comparative study of infants and toddlers treated with The Mifne Approach intervention for autism spectrum disorder, in *Autism 360°* (277–300). New York: Academic Press.

Alonso, P., Cuadras, D., Gabriels, L., et al. (2015). Deep brain stimulation for obsessive-compulsive disorder: A meta-analysis of treatment outcome and predictors of response. *PLOS One* 10(7): e0133591. PMID26208305

Amaro, A. (2019). Unshakeable well-being: Is the Buddhist concept of enlightenment a meaningful possibility in the current age. *Mindfulness* 10(9): 1952–6. https://doi.org/10.1007/s12671-019-01179-7

American Psychiatric Association [APA] (2013). *Diagnostic and Statistical Manual of Mental Disorders (DSM-5)*: 4th edn. Arlington, VA: American Psychiatric Association.

Améry, J. (1980). *At the Mind's Limits*, trans. S. Rosenfeld and S. P. Rosenfeld. Bloomington: Indiana University Press.

Anālayo, B. (2012). Right view and the scheme of the four truths in early Buddhism: The Sayukta-āgama parallel to the Sammādihi-sutta and the simile of the four skills of a physician. *Canadian Journal of Buddhist Studies* 7: 11–44.

Anālayo, B. 2010. From grasping to emptiness: Excursions into the thought-world of the Pali Discourses. *Buddhist Association of the United States.* https://www.buddhismuskunde.uni-hamburg.de/pdf/5-personen/analayo/from-grasping.pdf

Andreasen N. C. (2007). DSM and the death of phenomenology in America: An example of unintended consequences. *Schizophrenia Bulletin* 33(1): 108–12.

Andreasen, N. C., Paradiso, S. & O'Leary, D. S. (1998). "Cognitive dysmetria" as an integrative theory of schizophrenia: A dysfunction in cortical-subcortical-cerebellar circuitry? *Schizophrenia Bulletin* 24(2): 203–18.

Andringa, E. (1996). Effects of "narrative distance" on readers' emotional involvement and response. *Poetics* 23: 431–52.

Antelme, R. (1992). *The Human Race*, trans. J. Haight and A. Mahler. Marlboro: Marlboro Press.

Anuruddha, B., Bhikkhu, N., & Maha Thera, D. (2000). *A Comprehensive Manual of Abhidhamma: the Abhidhammattha Sangaha of Ācariya Anuruddha*. Pariyatti Edition. Buddhist Publication Society.

Appleby, B. S., Duggan, P. S., Regenberg, A. & Rabins, P.V. (2007). Psychiatric and neuro-psychiatric adverse events associated with deep brain stimulation: A meta-analysis of ten years' experience. *Movement Disorders* 22(12): 1722–8. doi:10.1002/mds.21551; PMID17721929

Apps, M. A. & Tsakiris, M. (2014). The free-energy self: A predictive coding account of self-recognition. *Neuroscience & Biobehavioral Reviews* 41: 85–97.

Aquinas, Thomas. (1485). *Summa Theologiæ*, trans. Fathers of the English Dominican Province. New York: Benzinger Brothers, 1911.

Araujo, H. F., Kaplan. J. & Damasio, A. (2013). Cortical midline structures and autobi-ographical-self processes: An activation-likelihood estimation meta-analysis. *Frontiers in Human Neuroscience* 7: 548. doi: 10.3389/fnhum.2013.00548

Armstrong, P. B. (2020). *Stories and the Brain: The Neuroscience of Narrative*. Baltimore: Johns Hopkins University Press.

Arnsten, A. F. & Li, B. M. (2005). Neurobiology of executive functions: Catecholamine influences on prefrontal cortical functions. *Biological Psychiatry* 57(11): 1377–84.

Asada, M., MacDorman, K. F., Ishiguro, H. & Kuniyoshi, Y. (2001). Cognitive develop-mental robotics as a new paradigm for the design of humanoid robots. *Robotics and Autonomous Systems* 37: 185–93.

Asai, T. & Tanno, Y. (2007). The relationship between the sense of self-agency and schizo-typal personality traits. *Journal of Motor Behavior* 39(3): 162–8. https://doi.org/10.3200/JMBR.39.3.162-168

Ataria, Y. (2019a). Total destruction: The case of Jean Améry, in Y. Ataria, A. Kravitz & E. Pitcovski (eds), *Jean Améry* (141–57). Cham: Palgrave Macmillan.

Ataria, Y. (2019b). Becoming nonhuman: The case study of the gulag. *Genealogy* 3(2): 27–40.

Ataria, Y. (2018). *Body Disownership in Complex Posttraumatic Stress Disorder*. New York: Palgrave Macmillan.

Ataria, Y. (2016). When the body becomes the enemy: Disownership toward the body. *Philosophy, Psychiatry, & Psychology,* 23, 1–15.

Ataria, Y. (2015). Dissociation during trauma: The ownership-agency tradeoff model. *Phenomenology and the Cognitive Sciences* 14(4): 1037–53.

Ataria, Y., Dor-Ziderman, Y. & Berkovich-Ohana, A. (2015). How does it feel to lack a sense of boundaries? A case study of a long-term mindfulness meditator. *Consciousness and Cognition* 37: 133–47.

Ataria, Y. & Gallagher, S. (2015). Somatic apathy: Body disownership in the context of torture. *Journal of Phenomenological Psychology* 46(1): 105–22.

Ataria, Y. & Neria, Y. (2013). Consciousness-body-time: How do people think lacking their body? *Human Studies 36*: 159–178.

Austin, J. L. (1961). *Philosophical Papers*. Oxford: Clarendon Press.

Baer, R. A. (2007). Mindfulness, assessment, and transdiagnostic processes. *Psychological Inquiry* 18(4): 238–42.

Baier, A. (1985). *Postures of the Mind: Essays on Mind and Morals*. Minneapolis: University of Minnesota Press.

Baillargeon, R., Scott, R. M. & He, Z. (2010). False-belief understanding in infants. *Trends in Cognitive Sciences* 14(3): 110–18.

Baillin, F., Lefebvre, A., Pedoux, A., Beauxis, Y., Engemann, D., Maruani, A., Amsellem, F., Bourgeron, T., Delorme, R. & Dumas, G., 2020. Interactive psychometrics for autism with the human dynamic clamp: Interpersonal synchrony from sensory-motor to socio-cognitive domains. *Frontiers in Psychiatry* 11: 510366.

Baird, A. (2019). A reflection on the complexity of the self in severe dementia. *Cogent Psychology* 6(1): 1574055.

Bamford, A. & Mackenzie, D. (2018). Counterperformativity. *New Left Review* 113: 97–121.

Baptista, A., Cohen, D., Jacquet, P. O. & Chambon, V. (2020). The ecological origins of self-disturbance in borderline personality disorder. Preprint doi: 10.31234/osf.io/g84ur

Baran, N. M. (2019). Reductionist thinking and animal models in neuropsychiatric research. *Behavioral and Brain Sciences* 42: 11–12.

Barandiaran, X. E. & Di Paolo, A. E. (2014). A genealogical map of the concept of habit. *Frontiers in Human Neuroscience* 9: 1–7.

Barclay, C. R. & DeCooke, P. A. (1988). Ordinary everyday memories: Some of the things of which selves are made, in U. Neisser and E. Winograd (eds), *Remembering Reconsidered: Ecological and Traditional Approaches to the Study of Memory* (91–125). Cambridge University Press. https://doi.org/10.1017/CBO9780511664014.005

Barendregt, H.P. (1988). Buddhist Phenomenology, Part I, *Proceedings of the Conference on Topics and Perspectives of Contemporary Logic and Philosophy of Science*, Cesena, Italy, January 7-10, 1987, (Ed. M. dalla Chiara), Clueb, Bologna, 1988, 37–55.

Bargh, J. (1994). The four horsemen of automaticity: Awareness, intention, efficiency, and control in social cognition. In R. S. Wyer & T. K. Srull (Eds.), *Handbook of Social Cognition* (Vol. 1, pp. 1–40). Hillsdale, NJ: Erlbaum.

Barlas, Z. & Obhi, S. S. (2014). Cultural background influences implicit but not explicit sense of agency for the production of musical tones. *Consciousness and Cognition* 28: 94–103.

Barlow, D. (2002). *Anxiety and its Disorders*. New York: Guilford Press.

Baron-Cohen, S., Leslie, A. M. & Frith, U. (1985). Does the autistic child have a "theory of mind"? *Cognition* 21(1): 37–46.

Barrett, L. F., Quigley, K. S. & Hamilton, P. (2016). An active inference theory of allostasis and interoception in depression. *Philosophical Transactions of the Royal Society B: Biological Sciences* 371(1708): 20160011.

Bartlett, F. (1932). *Remembering: A Study in Experimental and Social Psychology*. Cambridge: Cambridge University Press.

Barton, D. A., Esler, M. D., Dawood, T., Lambert, E. A., Haikerwal, D., Brenchley, C., et al. (2008). Elevated brain serotonin turnover in patients with depression: Effect of genotype and therapy. *Archives of General Psychiatry* 65(1): 38–46.

Bassett, C. (2019). The computational therapeutic: exploring Weizenbaum's ELIZA as a history of the present. *AI & Society* 34(4): 803–12.

Baum, K., Hackmann, J., Pakos, J., Kannen, K., Wiebe, A., Selaskowski, B., Pensel, M. C., Ettinger, U., Philipsen, A., & Braun, N. (2022). Body transfer illusions in the schizophrenia spectrum: A systematic review. *Schizophrenia* 8(1): 1–14.

Baylis, F. (2013). "I am who I am": On the perceived threats to personal identity from deep brain stimulation. *Neuroethics* 6: 513–26. doi:10.1007/s12152-011-9137-1; PMID24273621

Baylis, F. (2011). The self in situ: A relational account of personal identity, in J. Downie and J. J. Llewellyn (eds), *Being Relational: Reflections on Relational Theory and Health Law* (109–31). Vancouver: UBC Press.

Bayne, T. & Pacherie, E. (2004). Bottom-up or top-down: Campbell's rationalist account of monothematic delusions. *Philosophy, Psychiatry, & Psychology* 11(1): 1–11.

Bechtel, W. (2020). Rethinking psychiatric disorders in terms of heterarchical networks of control mechanisms, in K. S. Kendler, J. Parnas, and P. Zachar (eds), *Levels of Analysis in Psychopathology: Cross-Disciplinary Perspectives* (24–46). Cambridge: Cambridge University Press.

Bechtel, W. & Huang, L. T. (2022). *Philosophy of Neuroscience.* Cambridge: Cambridge University Press.

Beckner, M. (1959). *The Biological Way of Thought.* Berkeley: University of California Press.

Becquet, C., Cogez, J., Dayan, J., Lebain, P., Viader, F., Eustache, F. & Quinette, P. (2021). Episodic autobiographical memory impairment and differences in pronoun use: study of self-awareness in functional amnesia and transient global amnesia. *Frontiers in Psychology* 12. doi: 10.3389/fpsyg.2021.624010

Bedwell, J., Gallagher, S., Whitten, S. & Fiore, S. (2011). Linguistic correlates of self in deceptive oral autobiographical narratives. *Consciousness and Cognition* 20: 547–55.

Beer, R. D. (2020). Bittorio revisited: Structural coupling in the Game of Life. *Adaptive Behavior* 28(4): 197–212. doi: 10.1177/1059712319859907

Beni, M. D. (2016). Structural realist account of the self. *Synthese* 193: 3727–40.

Bergamasco, M., Allotta, B., Bosio, L., Ferretti, L., Parrini, G., Prisco, G. M.,...& Sartini, G. (1994). An arm exoskeleton system for teleoperation and virtual environments applications, in *Proceedings of the 1994 IEEE International Conference on Robotics and Automation* (1449–54). Piscataway, NJ: IEEE.

Berlin, I. (1969). *Four Essays on Liberty.* Oxford: Oxford University Press.

Bermúdez, J. L. (2017). Ownership and the space of the body, in F. de Vignemont and A. Alsmith (eds), *The Subject's Matter: Self-consciousness and the Body* (117–44). Cambridge, MA: MIT Press.

Bermúdez, J. L. (2015). Bodily ownership, bodily awareness and knowledge without observation. *Analysis* 75: 37–45. doi: 10.1093/analys/anu119

Bermúdez, J. L. (2011). Bodily awareness and self-consciousness, in S. Gallagher (ed.), *Oxford Handbook of the Self* (157–79). Oxford: Oxford University Press.

Berna, F., Göritz, A. S., Schröder, J., Martin, B., Cermolacce, M., Allé, M. C.,...& Moritz, S. (2016). Self-disorders in individuals with attenuated psychotic symptoms: Contribution of a dysfunction of autobiographical memory. *Psychiatry Research* 239: 333–41.

Bernal, A. L. (2001). Concordancias Discordantes: Caracterizacíon del Relato Autobiogr'afico de Pacientes con Diagnòstico de Esquizofrenia. Dissertation. Universidad del Valle, Escuela de Psicolog'ia, Santiago de Cali, Colombia.

Bernieri, F. J., Davis, J. M., Rosenthal, R. & Knee, C. R. (1994). Interactional synchrony and rapport: Measuring synchrony in displays devoid of sound and facial affect. *Personality and Social Psychology Bulletin* 30: 303–11.

Bernstein, E. E., Heeren, A., & McNally, R. J. (2019). Reexamining trait rumination as a system of repetitive negative thoughts: A network analysis. *Journal of Behavior Therapy and Experimental Psychiatry* 63, 21–27.

Bernstein, N. A. (1984). Some emergent problems of the regulation of motor acts, in H. T. A. Whiting (ed.), *Human Motor Actions: Bernstein Reassessed* (354–5). Amsterdam: North-Holland.

Berridge, K. C., & Robinson, T. E. (2016). Liking, wanting, and the incentive-sensitization theory of addiction. *American Psychologist 71*(8), 670.

Berthoz, A. (2000). *The Brain's Sense of Movement*, trans. G. Weiss. Cambridge, MA: Harvard University Press.

Berti, A. & Pia, L. (2006). Understanding motor awareness through normal and pathological behavior. *Current Directions in Psychological Science* 15: 245–50. doi: 10.1111/j.1467-8721.2006.00445.x

Bhat, A. N., Landa, R. J. & Galloway, J. C. (2011). Current perspectives on motor functioning in infants, children, and adults with autism spectrum disorders. *Physical Therapy* 91(7): 1116–29.

Bhat, A. N., Parr, T., Ramstead, M. & Friston, K. (2021). Immunoceptive inference: Why are psychiatric disorders and immune responses intertwined? *Biology & Philosophy* 36: 27. https://doi.org/10.1007/s10539-021-09801-6

Bilek, E., Stößel, G., Schäfer, A., Clement, L., Ruf, M., Robnik, L., et al. (2017). State-dependent cross-brain information flow in borderline personality disorder. *JAMA Psychiatry* 74: 949–57.

Billon, A. (2013). Does consciousness entail subjectivity? The puzzle of thought insertion. *Philosophical Psychology* 26(2): 291–314.

Billon, A. & Kriegel, U. (2014). Jaspers' dilemma: The psychopathological challenge to subjectivity theories of consciousness, in R. Gennaro (ed.), *Disturbed Consciousness* (29–54). Cambridge, MA: MIT Press.

Bird, G. & Cook, R. (2013). Mixed emotions: The contribution of alexithymia to the emotional symptoms of autism. *Translational Psychiatry* 3(7): e285–5.

Bitbol, M. & Gallagher, S. (2018). Autopoiesis and the free energy principle. *Physics of Life Review.* doi.org/10.1016/j.plrev.2017.12.011

Blanke, E. S., Schmidt, M. J., Riediger, M. & Brose, A. (2020). Thinking mindfully: How mindfulness relates to rumination and reflection in daily life. *Emotion* 20(8): 1369.

Blanke O. (2012). Multisensory brain mechanisms of bodily self-consciousness. *Nature Reviews Neuroscience* 13: 556–71. doi: 10.1038/nrn3292

Blanke O. & Metzinger T. (2009). Full-body illusions and minimal phenomenal selfhood. *Trends in Cognitive Sciences* 13(1): 7–13.

Blankenburg, W. (1971). *Der Verlust der Natürlichen Selbstverständlichkeit: Ein Beitrag zur Psychopathologie Symptomarmer Schizophrenien.* Stuttgart: Ferdinand Enke.

Bluhm, R., Cabrera, L. & McKenzie, R. (2020). What we (should) talk about when we talk about deep brain stimulation and personal identity. *Neuroethics* 13(3): 289–301. https://doi.org/10.1007/s12152-019-09396-6

Bolis, D., Balsters, J., Wenderoth, N., Becchio, C. & Schilbach, L. (2017). Beyond autism: Introducing the dialectical misattunement hypothesis and a Bayesian account of intersubjectivity. *Psychopathology* 50(6): 355–72.

Bolton, D. & Gillett, G. (2019). *The Biopsychosocial Model of Health and Disease.* Cham: Palgrave Macmillan.

Bonta, J. & Gendreau, P. (1990). Reexamining the cruel and unusual punishment of prison life. *Law and Human Behavior* 14(4): 347.

Boria, S., Fabbri-Destro, M., Cattaneo, L., Sparaci, L., Sinigaglia, C., Santelli, E., Cossu, G. & Rizzolatti, G. (2009). Intention understanding and autism. *PLOS One* 4(5): e5596.

Borsboom, D. (2017). A network theory of mental disorders. *World Psychiatry* 16(1): 5–13.

Borsboom, D. & Cramer, A. (2013). Network analysis: An integrative approach to the structure of psychopathology. *The Annual Review of Clinical Psychology* 9: 91–121. 10.1146/annurev-clinpsy-050212-185608

Borsboom, D., Cramer, A. O. J. & Kalis, A. (2019). Brain disorders? Not really: Why network structures block reductionism in psychopathology research. *Behavioral and Brain Sciences* 42: 1–63. doi: 10.1017/S0140525X17002266

Bortolotti, L. (2010). *Delusions and Other Irrational Beliefs*. Oxford: Oxford University Press.

Bortolotti, L. & Broome, M. (2009). A role for ownership and authorship in the analysis of thought insertion. *Phenomenology and the Cognitive Sciences* 8(2): 205–24.

Boss, M. (1979). *Existential Foundations of Medicine and Psychology*. New York: Aronson.

Bostrom, N. (2014). *Superintelligence: Paths, Dangers, Strategies*. Oxford: Oxford University Press.

Botvinick, M. & Cohen J. (1998). Rubber hands "feel" touch that eyes see. *Nature* 391: 756. doi: 10. 1038/35784

Bourdieu, Pierre (1977). *Outline of a Theory of Practice*. Cambridge: Cambridge University Press.

Bovet, P. & Parnas, J. (1993). Schizophrenic delusions: A phenomenological approach. *Schizophrenia Bulletin* 19: 579–97.

Bramley, N. & Eatough, V. (2005). The experience of living with Parkinson's disease: An interpretative phenomenological analysis case study. *Psychology & Health* 20(2): 223–35.

Bregman, A. S. & Rudnicky, A. I. (1975). Auditory segregation: Stream or streams? *Journal of Experimental Psychology: Human Perception and Performance* 1: 263–7.

Brennan, J. (1972). *Furman v. Georgia*. 408 U.S. 257–306.

Brennan, S. E. & Hanna, J. E. (2009). Partner-specific adaptation in dialog. *Topics in Cognitive Science* 1: 274–91. doi:10.1111/j.1756-8765.2009.01019.x

Breyer, T. (2017). Violence as violation of experiential structures. *Phenomenology and the Cognitive Sciences* 16(4): 737–51.

Brezis, R.-S., Noy, L., Alony, T., Gotlieb, R., Cohen, R., Golland, Y. & Levit-Binnun, N. (2017) Patterns of joint improvisation in adults with autism spectrum disorder. *Frontiers Psychology* 8:1790. doi: 10.3389/fpsyg.2017.01790

Brincker, M. & Torres, E. B. (2013). Noise from the periphery in autism. *Frontiers in Integrative Neuroscience* 7: 34.

Bringmann, L. F., Albers, C., Bockting, C., Borsboom, D., Ceulemans, E., Cramer, A.,... Wichers, M. (2022). Psychopathological networks: Theory, methods and practice. *Behaviour Research and Therapy* 149: 104011.

Britton, W. B. (2019). Can mindfulness be too much of a good thing? The value of a middle way. *Current Opinion in Psychology* 28: 159–65.

Britton, W. B., Desbordes, G., Acabchuk, R., Peters, S., Lindahl, J. R., Canby, N. K., Vago, D. R., Dumais, T., Lipsky, J., Kimmel, H., Sager, L., Rahrig, H., Cheaito, A., Acero, P., Scharf, J., Lazar, S. W., Schuman-Olivier, Z., Ferrer, R. & Moitra, E. (2021). From self-esteem to selflessness: An evidence (gap) map of self-related processes as mechanisms of mindfulness-based interventions. *Frontiers in Psychology* 12: 730972. doi: 10.3389/fpsyg.2021.730972

Bronstein, J. M., Tagliati, M., Alterman, R. L., et al. (2011). Deep brain stimulation for Parkinson's disease: An expert consensus and review of key issues. *Archives of Neurology* 68(2): 165–5. doi: 10.1001/archneurol.2010.260; PMID20937936

Broome, M. (2005). Suffering and eternal recurrence of the same: The neuroscience, psychopathology and philosophy of time. *Philosophy, Psychiatry, & Psychology* 12(3): 187–94.

Brown, H., Adams, R. A., Parees, I., Edwards, M. & Friston, K. (2013). Active inference, sensory attenuation and illusions. *Cognitive Processing* 14(4): 411–27.

Brown, T. (2020). Building intricate partnerships with neurotechnology: Deep brain stimulation and relational agency. *IJFAB: International Journal of Feminist Approaches to Bioethics* 13(1): 134–54.

Bruineberg, J., Kiverstein, J. & Rietveld, E. 2016. The anticipating brain is not a scientist: The free-energy principle from an ecological-enactive perspective. *Synthese* 195 (6): 2417–2444. https://doi.org/10.1007/s11229-016-1239-1

Bruineberg, J. & Rietveld, E. (2014). Self-organization, free energy minimization, and optimal grip on a field of affordances. *Frontiers of Human Neuroscience* 8: 599. doi: 10.3389/fnhum.2014.00599

Bruner, J. S. (2002). *Making Stories: Law, Literature, Life.* Cambridge, MA: Harvard University Press.

Bruner, J. S. (1990). *Acts of Meaning.* Cambridge, MA: Harvard University Press.

Bruner, J. S. (1986). *Actual Minds, Possible Worlds.* Cambridge, MA: Harvard University Press.

Bruner, J. S. & Kalmar, D. A. (1998). Narrative and metanarrative in the construction of self, in M. D. Ferrari and R. J. Sternberg (eds), *Self-Awareness: Its Nature and Development* (308–31). New York: Guilford Press.

Bryant, R. A. (2019). Post-traumatic stress disorder: A state-of-the-art review of evidence and challenges. *World Psychiatry* 18(3): 259–69.

Buhrmann, T. & Di Paolo, E. (2017). The sense of agency—a phenomenological consequence of enacting sensorimotor schemes. *Phenomenology and the Cognitive Sciences* 16(2): 207–36.

Bundesen, B. (2021). The affective resonance processes in creative writing-groups: Retroaffective restructuring of the self in creative writing for people suffering from schizophrenia-spectrum disorder. *InterCultural Philosophy* 1: 59–72.

Bunge, M. (1979). The mind-body problem, information theory, and Christian dogma. *Neuroscience* 4: 453.

Bunge, M. (1977). Emergence and the mind. *Neuroscience* 2: 501–10.

Bu-Omer, H. M., Gofuku, A., Sato, K. & Miyakoshi, M. (2021). Parieto-occipital alpha and low-beta EEG power reflect sense of agency. *Brain Sciences* 11(6): 743.

Burdick, A. P., Foote, K. D., Wu, S., Bowers, D., Zeilman, P., Jacobson, C. E., Ward, H. E. & Okun, M. S. (2011). Do patients get angrier following STN, GPi, and thalamic deep brain stimulation. *Neuroimage* 54: S227–32. PMCID3014411. NIHMS247959

Burr, C., Morley, J., Taddeo, M. & Floridi, L. (2020). Digital psychiatry: Risks and opportunities for public health and wellbeing. *IEEE Transactions on Technology and Society* 1(1): 21–33.

Buytendijk, F. J. J. (1948). *Über den Schmerz.* Bern: Hans Huber.

Cahn, B. R. & Polich, J. (2006). Meditation states and traits: EEG, ERP, and neuroimaging studies. *Psychological Bulletin* 132(2): 180.

Caixeta, M., Chaves, M., Caixeta, L. & Reis, O. (1999). Emotionally loaded narrative increases dyslogia in schizophrenics. *Arquivos de Neuro-Psiquiatria* 57(3A): 695–700.

Caldwell, C. (2014). Mindfulness and bodyfulness: A new paradigm. *Journal of Contemplative Inquiry* 1: 77–96.

Campbell, J. (2016). Validity and the causal structure of a disorder, in K. S. Kendler and J. Parnas (eds), *Philosophical Issues in Psychiatry IV: Psychiatric Nosology* (257–73). Oxford: Oxford University Press.

Campbell, J. (1999). Schizophrenia, the space of reasons, and thinking as a motor process. *The Monist* 82(4): 609–25.

Cameron, K., Ogrodniczuk, J.,& Hadjipavlou, G. (2014). Changes in alexithymia following psychological intervention: A review. *Harvard Review of Psychiatry* 22(3): 162–78. https://doi.org/10.1097/HRP.0000000000000036

Canby, N. K., Eichel, K., Lindahl, J., Chau, S., Cordova, J. & Britton, W. B. (2021). The contribution of common and specific therapeutic factors to mindfulness-based intervention outcomes. *Frontiers in Psychology* 11: 3920.

Capps, L., Kehres, J. & Sigman, M. (1998). Conversational abilities among children with autism and children with developmental delays. *Autism* 2: 325–44.

Capps, L. & Ochs, E. (1997). *Constructing Panic: The Discourse of Agoraphobia*. Cambridge, MA: Harvard University Press.

Cappuccio, M. L. (2017). Mind-upload: The ultimate challenge to the embodied mind theory. *Phenomenology and the Cognitive Sciences* 16(3): 425–48.

Cardinali, L., Brozzoli, C. & Farne, A. (2009). Peripersonal space and body schema: Two labels for the same concept? *Brain Topography* 21(3): 252–60.

Carel, H. (2016). *Phenomenology of Illness*. Oxford: Oxford University Press.

Carlin, A. S., Hoffman, H. G. & Weghorst, S. (1997). Virtual reality and tactile augmentation in the treatment of spider phobia: A case report. *Behaviour Research and Therapy* 35(2): 153–8.

Carmody, J. &d Baer, R. A. (2008). Relationships between mindfulness practice and levels of mindfulness, medical and psychological symptoms and well-being in a mindfulness-based stress reduction program. *Journal of Behavioral Medicine* 31(1): 23–33.

Caspar, E. A., Cleeremans, A. & Haggard, P. (2015). The relationship between human agency and embodiment. *Consciousness and Cognition* 33: 226–36.

Cattaneo, L., Fabbi-Destro, M., Boria, S., et al. (2008). Impairment of actions chains in autism and its possible role in intention understanding. *Proceedings of the National Academy of Sciences of the United States of America 2008* 104: 17825–30.

Cellan-Jones, R. (2014). Stephen Hawking warns artificial intelligence could end mankind. *BBC News Broadcast* December 2, 2014. https://www.bbc.com/news/technology-30290540)

Chalmers, D. (2010). The singularity: A philosophical analysis. *Journal of Consciousness Studies* 17: 7–65.

Chambless, D. L., Goldstein, A. J., Gallagher, R. & Bright, P. (1986). Integrating behavior therapy and psychotherapy in the treatment of agoraphobia. *Psychotherapy: Theory, Research, Practice, Training* 23(1): 150.

Charon, R. (2006). The self-telling body. *Narrative Inquiry* 16(1): 191–200.

Chemero, A. (2009). *Radical Embodied Cognitive Science*. Cambridge, MA: MIT Press.

Chen, Y., Chang, R. & Guo, J. (2021). Effects of data augmentation method Borderline-SMOTE on emotion recognition of EEG signals based on convolutional neural network. *IEEE Access* 9: 47491–502.

Chladenius, J. M. (1752). *Allgemeine Geschichtswissenschaft: worinnen der Grund zu einer neuen Einsicht in allen Arten der Gelahrtheit gelegt wird*. Friedrich Lanckischens Erben.

Christen, M., Bittlinger M., Walter, H., Brugger, P. & Müller, S. (2012). Dealing with side effects of deep brain stimulation: Lessons learned from stimulating the STN. *American Journal of Bioethics Neuroscience* 3(1): 37–43.

Christensen, E. (1999). Foroeldre i foengsel—en undersøgelse af børns og foroeldres erfaringer. Report no. 99/5. Copenhagen: Socialforskningsinstituttet.

Christensen, J. F., Di Costa, S., Beck, B. & Haggard, P. (2019). I just lost it! Fear and anger reduce the sense of agency: A study using intentional binding. *Experimental Brain Research* 237(5): 1205–12.

Christensen, W., Sutton, J. & McIlwain, D. J. 2016. Cognition in skilled action: Meshed control and the varieties of skill experience. *Mind & Language* 31(1): 37–66.

Christman J. (2009). *The Politics of Persons.* Cambridge: Cambridge University Press.

Christman J. (2004). Relational autonomy, liberal individualism, and the social constitution of selves. *Philosophical Studies* 117(1): 143–64.

Christoff, K., Cosmelli, D., Legrand, D. & Thompson, E. (2011) Specifying the self for cognitive neuroscience. *Trends in Cognitive Sciences* 15: 104–12.

Ciaunica, A., Charlton, J. & Farmer, H. (2021). When the window cracks: Transparency and the fractured self in depersonalisation. *Phenomenology and the Cognitive Sciences* 20(1): 1–19. https://doi.org/10.1007/s11097-020-09677-z

Ciaunica, A. & Fotopoulou, A. (2017). The touched self: Psychological and philosophical perspectives on proximal intersubjectivity and the self, in C. Durt, T. Fuchs, and C. Tewes (eds), *Embodiment, Enaction, and Culture: Investigating the Constitution of the Shared World* (173–92). Cambridge, MA: MIT Press.

Ciaunica, A., Hesp, C., Seth, A., Limanowski, J. & Friston, K. (2021). I overthink—therefore I am not: Altered sense of self in depersonalization. *PsyArXiv*, 23 Feb 2021 https://doi.org/10.31234/osf.io/k9d2n.

Cioffi, M. C., Banissy, M. J. & Moore, J. W. (2016). "Am I moving?" An illusion of agency and ownership in mirror-touch synaesthesia. *Cognition* 146: 426–30.

Clare, L., Rowlands, J., Bruce, E., Surr, C. & Downs, M. (2008). "I don't do like I used to do": A grounded theory approach to conceptualising awareness in people with moderate to severe dementia living in long-term care. *Social Science and Medicine* 66(11): 2366–77.

Clark, A. (2017). Busting out: Predictive brains, embodied minds, and the puzzle of the evidentiary veil. *Noûs* 51(4): 727–53.

Clark, A. (2015). Predicting peace: The end of the representation wars, in *Open mind.* Open MIND. Frankfurt am Main: MIND Group. file:///Users/sgllghr1/Downloads/The%20End%20of%20the%20Representation%20Wars.pdf

Clark, A. (2007). Soft selves and ecological control, in D. Ross, D. Spurrett, H. Kinkaid, and G. L. Stephens (eds), *Distributed Cognition and the Will: Individual Volition and Social Context* (101–22). Cambridge: MIT, A Bradford Book.

Clark, D. M. (1988). A cognitive model of panic attacks, in S. Rachman and J. D. Maser (eds), *Panic: Psychological Perspectives* (71–89). Mahwah, NJ: Lawrence Erlbaum Associates, Inc.

Clark, L. A., Cuthbert, B., Lewis-Fernández, R., Narrow, W. E. & Reed, G. M. (2017). Three approaches to understanding and classifying mental disorder: ICD-11, DSM-5, and the National Institute of Mental Health's Research Domain Criteria (RDoC). *Psychological Science in the Public Interest* 18(2): 72–145.

Clarke, E., DeNora, T. & Vuoskoski, J. (2015). Music, empathy and cultural understanding. *Physics of Life Reviews* 15: 61–88.

Cloud, D. H., Drucker, E., Browne, A., et al. (2015). Public health and solitary confinement in the United States. *American Journal of Public Health* 105:18–26.

Clowes, R. (2013). The cognitive integration of e-memory. *Review of Philosophy & Psychology* 4(1): 107–33.

Code, L. (2011). Self, subjectivity and the instituted social imaginary, in S. Gallagher (ed.), *The Oxford Handbook of the Self* (715–38). Oxford: Oxford University Press.

Cole, D. (1991). Artificial intelligence and personal identity. *Synthese* 88(3): 399–417.

Cole, J. (2007). The phenomenology of agency and intention in the face of paralysis and insentience. *Phenomenology and the Cognitive Sciences* 6(3): 309–25.

Cole, J., Crowle, S., Austwick, G. & Henderson Slater, D. (2009). Exploratory findings with virtual reality for phantom limb pain; from stump motion to agency and analgesia. *Disability and Rehabilitation* 31(10): 846–54.

Colombetti, G. 2014. *The Feeling Body: Affective Science meets the Enactive Mind.* Cambridge, MA: MIT Press.

Colombetti, G. & Roberts, T. (2015). Extending the extended mind: The case for extended affectivity. *Philosophical Studies* 172(5): 1243–63.

Colvert, E., Rutter, M., Kreppner, J., Beckett, C., Castle, J., Groothues, C., Hawkins, A., Stevens, S. & Sonuga-Barke, E. J. (2008). Do theory of mind and executive function deficits underlie the adverse outcomes associated with profound early deprivation? Findings from the English and Romanian adoptees study. *Journal of Abnormal Child Psychology* 36(7): 1057–68. doi: 10.1007/s10802-008-9232-x

Condillac, de, E. B. (1793). *Traité des sensations* (Vol. 3). chez les Librairies Associés.

Coninx, S. & Stilwell, P. (2023). Chronic pain, enactivism, and the challenges of integration. *Philsci-Archive.* http://philsci-archive.pitt.edu/20813/1/Coninx%26Stilwell_Chronic%20Pain%2C%20Enactivism%2C%20%26%20the%20Challenges%20of%20Integration.pdf

Constant, A., Badcock, P., Friston, K. & Kirmayer, L. J. (2022). Integrating evolutionary, cultural, and computational psychiatry: A multilevel systemic approach. *Frontiers in Psychiatry* 13:763380. doi: 10.3389/fpsyt.2022.763380

Constant, A., Clark, A. & Friston, K. J. (2021). Representation wars: Enacting an armistice through active inference. *Frontiers in Psychology* 11: 3798.

Conze, E. (1953). The way of wisdom. *The Wheel Publication,* 65/66.

Cook J. L., Blakemore S. J. & Press C. (2013). Atypical basic movement kinematics in autism spectrum conditions. *Brain* 136: 2816–24.

Cooper, K., Loades, M. E. & Russell, A. (2018). Adapting psychological therapies for autism. *Research in Autism Spectrum Disorders* 45: 43–50. https://doi.org/https://doi.org/10.1016/j.rasd.2017.11.002

Corlett, P. (2018). Delusions and prediction error, in L. Bortolotti (ed.), *Delusions in Context* (35–66). Cham: Palgrave/Springer Nature.

Cowan, H. R., Mittal, V. A. & McAdams, D. P. (2021). Narrative identity in the psychosis spectrum: A systematic review and developmental model. *Clinical Psychology Review* 88: 102067. https://doi.org/10.1016/j.cpr.2021.102067

Craik, F. I. M., Moroz, T. M., Moscovitch, M., Stuss, D. T., Winocur, G., Tulving, E. & Kapur, S. (1999). In search of the self: A positron emission tomography study. *Psychological Science* 10: 26–34.

Craver, C. F. 2007. *Explaining the Brain: Mechanisms and the Mosaic Unity of Neuroscience.* Oxford: Oxford University Press.

Craver, C. F. & Bechtel, W. 2007. Top-down causation without top-down causes. *Biology and Philosophy* 22: 547–63.

Craver, C. F. & Darden, L. (2013). *In Search of Mechanisms: Discoveries across the Life Sciences.* Chicago: University of Chicago Press.

Critchley, H. & Seth, A. (2012). Will studies of macaque insula reveal the neural mechanisms of self-awareness? *Neuron* 74: 423–6. doi: 10.1016/j.neuron.2012.04.012

Cullen, B., Eichel, K., Lindahl, J. R., Rahrig, H., Kini, N., Flahive, J. & Britton, W. B. (2021). The contributions of focused attention and open monitoring in mindfulness-based cognitive therapy for affective disturbances: A 3-armed randomized dismantling trial. *PLOS One* 16(1): e0244838.

Dahl C. J., Lutz, A. & Davidson, R. J. (2015). Reconstructing and deconstructing the self: Cognitive mechanisms in meditation practice. *Trends in Cognitive Sciences* 19(9): 515–23. https://doi.org/10.1016/j.tics.2015.07.001

Dainton, B. (2008). *The Phenomenal Self*. Oxford: Oxford University Press. doi: 10.1093/acprof:oso/9780199288847.001.0001

Dainton, B. (2016). I—the sense of self. *Aristotelian Society* 90: 113–43. doi: 10.1093/arisup/akw007

Dalai Lama (1966). *The Opening of the Wisdom-Eye: And the History of the Advancement of Buddhadharma in Tibet*. Wheaton, IL: Quest Books.

Dalgleish, T., Black, M., Johnston, D. & Bevan, A. (2020). Transdiagnostic approaches to mental health problems: Current status and future directions. *Journal of Consulting and Clinical Psychology* 88(3): 179–95. https://doi.org/10.1037/ccp0000482

Daly, A. & Gallagher, S. (2019) Towards a phenomenology of self-patterns in psychopathological diagnosis and therapy. *Psychopathology* 52: 33–49. doi.org/10.1159/000499315

Danion, J. M., Rizzo, L. & Bruant, A. (1999). Functional mechanisms underlying impaired recognition memory and conscious awareness in patients with schizophrenia. *Archives of General Psychiatry* 56(7): 639–44.

Damasio, A. (1999). *The Feeling of What Happens*. San Diego, CA: Harcourt.

Daprati, E., Franck, N., Georgieff, N., Proust, J., Pacherie, E., Dalery, J. & Jeannerod, M. (1997). Looking for the agent: An investigation into consciousness of action and self-consciousness in schizophrenic patients. *Cognition* 65: 71–86.

D'Argembeau, A., Ruby, P., Collette, F., Degueldre, C., Balteau, E., Luxen, A., Maquet, P. & Salmon, E. (2007). Distinct regions of the medial prefrontal cortex are associated with self-referential processing and perspective-taking. *Journal of Cognitive Neuroscience* 19: 935–44.

Davidson, J. (2003). *Phobic Geographies: The Phenomenology of Spatial Identity*. London: Ashgate Press.

Davidson, J. (2002). "Putting on a face": Sartre, Goffman, and agoraphobic anxiety in social space. *Environment and Planning* D 21(1): 107–22.

Davis, J. H. & Thompson, E. (2013). From the five aggregates to phenomenal consciousness: Towards a cross-cultural cognitive science, in S. M. Emmanuel (ed.), *A Companion to Buddhist Philosophy* (585–97). Malden, MA: Wiley & Blackwell.

Dawson, G., Hill, D., Spencer, A., Galpert, L. & Watson, L. (1990). Affective exchanges between young autistic children and their mothers. *Journal of Abnormal Child Psychology* 18(3): 335–45.

Deane, G., Miller, M. & Wilkinson, S. (2020). Losing ourselves: Active inference, depersonalization, and meditation. *Frontiers in Psychology* 11:539726. doi: 10.3389/fpsyg.2020.539726

de Boer, N. S., de Bruin, L. C., Geurts, J. J. G. & Glas, G. (2021) The network theory of psychiatric disorders: A critical assessment of the inclusion of environmental factors. *Frontiers in Psycholology* 12: 623970. doi: 10.3389/fpsyg.2021.623970

Decety, J. & Sommerville, J. A. (2003). Shared representations between self and other: A social cognitive neuroscience view. *Trends in Cognitive Sciences* 7: 527–33. doi: 10.1016/j.tics.2003.10.004

de Haan, S. (2020). *Enactive Psychiatry*. Cambridge: Cambridge University Press.

de Haan, S. (2010). Comment: The minimal self is a social self, in T. Fuchs, H. C. Sattel, and P. Henningsen (eds), *The Embodied Self* (12–17). Stuttgart: Schattauer.

de Haan, S. & Fuchs, T. (2010). The ghost in the machine: Disembodiment in schizophrenia–two case studies. *Psychopathology* 43(5): 327–33.

de Haan, S., Rietveld, E., Stokhof, M. & Denys, D. (2017). Becoming more oneself? Changes in personality following DBS treatment for psychiatric disorders: Experiences of OCD patients and general considerations. *PLOS One* 12(4): e0175748.

de Haan, S., Rietveld, E., Stokhof, M. & Denys, D. (2015). Effects of deep brain stimulation on the lived experience of obsessive-compulsive disorder patients: In-depth interviews with 18 patients. *PLOS One* 10(8): e0135524. doi:10.1371/journal.pone.0135524

de Haan, S., Rietveld, E., Stokhof, M. & Denys, D. (2013). The phenomenology of deep brain stimulation-induced changes in OCD: An enactive affordance-based model. *Frontiers in Human Neuroscience* 7: 653. doi:10.3389/fnhum.2013.00653

De Jaegher, H. (2013). Embodiment and sense-making in autism. *Frontiers in Integrative Neuroscience* 7: 15. doi: 10.3389/fnint.2013.00015

De Jaegher, H. & Di Paolo, E. (2007). Participatory sense-making. *Phenomenology and the Cognitive Sciences* 6(4): 485–507.

De Jaegher, H., Di Paolo, E. & Gallagher, S. (2010). Does social interaction constitute social cognition? *Trends in Cognitive Sciences* 14(10): 441–7.

de Koning, P. P., Figee, M., Van den Munckhof, P., Schuurman, R. & Denys, D. (2011). Current status of deep brain stimulation for obsessive-compulsive disorder: A clinical review of different targets. *Current Psychiatry Reports* 13(4): 274–82. doi:10.1007/s11920-011-0200-8; PMID21505875

Delafield-Butt, J. T. & Trevarthen, C. (2015). The ontogenesis of narrative: From moving to meaning. *Frontiers in Psycholology* 6: 1157. doi:10.3389/fpsyg.2015.01157

Della Sala, S., Marchetti, C. & Spinnler, H. (1994). The anarchic hand: A frontomesial sign, in F. Boller and J. Grafman (eds), *Handbook of Neuropsychology*, Vol. IX (233–55). Amsterdam: Elsevier.

Della Sala S., Marchetti, C. & Spinnler, H. (1991). Right-sided anarchic (alien) hand: A longitudinal study. *Neuropsychologia* 29(11): 1113–27.

de Marchena, A. & Eigsti, I. M. (2010). Conversational gestures in autism spectrum disorder: Asynchrony but not decreased frequency. *Autism Research* 3: 311–22. doi: 10.1002/aur.159

Dengsø, M. J. (2022). Wrong brains at the wrong time? Understanding ADHD through the diachronic constitution of minds. *Advances in Neurodevelopment Disorders* 6 (2): 184–195. https://doi.org/10.1007/s41252-022-00244-y

Dennett, D. C. (2003). Review of *Making Ourselves at Home in our Machines: The Illusion of Conscious Will* by Daniel Wegner. MIT Press 2002. *Journal of Mathematical Psychology* 47(1): 101–4.

Dennett, D. C. (1996). *Kinds of Minds: Towards an Understanding of Consciousness*. New York: Basic Books.

Dennett, D. C. (1991a). *Consciousness Explained*. Boston: Little, Brown and Co.

Dennett, D. C. (1991b). Real patterns. *The Journal of Philosophy* 88(1): 27–51.

Dennett, D. C. & Kinsbourne, M. (1992). Time and the observer: The where and when of consciousness in the brain. *Behavioral and Brain Sciences* 15(2): 183–201.

Denys, D., Mantione, M., Figee, M., van den Munckhof, P., Koerselman, F., Westenberg, H., Bosch, A. & Schuurman, R. (2010). Deep brain stimulation of the nucleus accumbens for treatment-refractory obsessive-compulsive disorder. *Archives of General Psychiatry* 67(10): 1061–8. doi:10.1001/archgenpsychiatry.2010.122; PMID20921122

De Pirro, S., Lush, P., Parkinson, J., Duka, T., Critchley, H. D. & Badiani, A. (2019). Effect of alcohol on the sense of agency in healthy humans. *Addiction Biology* 25 (4): e12796.

De Ridder, D., Vanneste, S., Gillett, G., Manning, P., Glue, P. & Langguth, B. (2016). Psychosurgery reduces uncertainty and increases free will? A review. *Neuromodulation* 19: 239–48. doi:10.1111/ner.12405; PMID26899938 de Vignemont, F. 2017. Agency and bodily ownership: The bodyguard hypothesis, in F. de Vignemont and A. Alsmith (eds), *The Subject's Matter* (217–37). Cambridge, MA: MIT Press.

de Vignemont, F. (2011). Embodiment, ownership and disownership. *Consciousness and Cognition* 20(1): 82–93.

de Vignemont, F. (2010). Embodiment, ownership and disownership. *Consciousness and Cognition* 20(1): 82–93.

de Vignemont, F. (2007). Habeas corpus: The sense of ownership of one's own body. *Mind & Language* 22: 427–49.

Dewey, J. (1988). *Human Nature and Conduct: The Middle Works, Vol. 14*. Carbondale and Edwardsville: Southern Illinois University Press.

Dewey, J. (1938). *Logic: The Theory of Inquiry*. NewYork: Holt, Rinehart, & Winston.

Dewey, J. (1937). The unity of the human being, in J. Boydston (ed.), *Later Works of John Dewey, Vol. 13* (323–37). Carbondale, IL: Southern Illinois University Press, 1991. [Originally, an Address to the American College of Physicians, St. Louis, MO, April 21, 1937].

Dewey, J. (1922). *Human Nature and Conduct: An Introduction to Social Psychology*. New York: Modern Library.

Dewey, J. A. & Knoblich, G. (2014). Do implicit and explicit measures of the sense of agency measure the same thing? *PLOS One* 9(10): e110118.

Di Cesare, G., Sparaci, L., Pelosi, A., Mazzone, L., Giovagnoli, G., Menghini, D., Ruffaldi, E. & Vicari S. (2017). Differences in action style recognition in children with autism spectrum disorders. *Frontiers in Psychology* 8: 1456. doi: 10.3389/fpsyg.2017.01456

Dickens, C. (1957). *American Notes and Pictures from Italy*. Oxford: Oxford University Press (Originally published 1842).

Difede, J., Cukor, J., Jayasinghe, N., Patt, I., Jedel, S., Spielman, L., Giosan, C. & Hoffman, H. G. (2007). Virtual reality exposure therapy for the treatment of posttraumatic stress disorder following September 11, 2001. *Journal of Clinical Psychiatry* 68(11): 1639.

Di Francesco, M., Marraffa, M. & Paternoster, A. (2016). *The Self and its Defenses: From Psychodynamics to Cognitive Science*. London: Palgrave Macmillan.

DiFrisco, J. (2014). Hylomorphism and the metabolic closure conception of life. *Acta Biotheoretica* 62(4): 499–525.

Dilthey, W. (1988). The understanding of other persons and their life-expressions, trans. K. Mueller-Vollmer in K. Mueller-Vollmer (ed.), *The Hermeneutics Reader* (152–64). New York: Continuum.

Dings, R. (2018). Understanding phenonenological differences in how affordances solicit action: An exploration. *Phenomenology and the Cognitive Sciences* 17(4): 681–99.

Dings, R. & de Bruin, L. (2022). What's special about "not feeling like oneself"? A deflationary account of self(-illness) ambiguity. *Philosophical Explorations* 25 (3): 269–289 doi: 10.1080/13869795.2022.2051592

Dings, R. & de Bruin, L. (2016). Situating the self: Understanding the effects of deep brain stimulation. *Phenomenology and the Cognitive Sciences* 15(2): 151–65.

Dings, R. & Newen, A. (2021). Constructing the past: The relevance of the narrative self in modulating episodic memory. *Review of Philosophy and Psychology* 14 (1): 87–112. https://doi.org/10.1007/s13164-021-00581-2

Di Paolo, E. A. (2021). Enactive becoming. *Phenomenology and the Cognitive Sciences* 20(5): 783–809.

Di Paolo, E. (2009). Extended life. *Topoi* 28(1): 9–21.

Di Paolo, E. A. (2005). Autopoiesis, adaptivity, teleology, agency. *Phenomenology and the Cognitive Sciences* 4(4): 429–52.

Di Paolo, E. A., Cuffari, E. C. & De Jaegher, H. (2018). *Linguistic Bodies: The Continuity between Life and Language*. Cambridge, MA: MIT Press.

Di Paolo, E., Thompson, E. & Beer, R. (2022). Laying down a forking path: Tensions between enaction and the free energy principle. *Philosophy and the Mind Sciences* 3 (2): 1–39. https://doi.org/10.33735/phimisci.2022.9187

Di Plinio, S., Arnò, S., Perrucci, M. G. & Ebisch, S. J. (2019). Environmental control and psychosis-relevant traits modulate the prospective sense of agency in non-clinical individuals. *Consciousness and Cognition* 73: 102776.

Dixon, M. L. & Gross, J. J. (2021). Dynamic network organization of the self: Implications for affective experience. *Current Opinion in Behavioral Sciences* 39: 1–9.

Dokic, J. (2003). The sense of ownership: An analogy between sensation and action, in J. Roessler and N. Eilan (eds), *Agency and Self-Awareness* (321–44). Oxford: Oxford University Press.

Dolan, R. J. & Fletcher, P. C. (1997). Dissociating prefrontal and hippocampal function in episodic memory encoding. *Nature* 388: 582–5.

Dolk, T., Hommel, B., Colzato, L. S., Schütz-Bosbach, S., Prinz, W. & Liepelt, R. (2014). The joint Simon effect: A review and theoretical integration. *Frontiers in Psychology* 5: 974.

Dolk, T., Hommel, B., Colzato, L. S., Schütz-Bosbach, S., Prinz, W. & Liepelt, R. (2011). How "social" is the social Simon effect? *Frontiers in Psychology* 2: 84.

Donald, M. (2006). An evolutionary rationale for the emergence of language from mimetic representation. Plenary paper presented at Language Culture and Mind Conference (July 17–20, 2006): Paris.

Dor-Ziderman, Y., Ataria, Y., Fulder, S., Goldstein, A. & Berkovich-Ohana, A. (2016). Self-specific processing in the meditating brain: A MEG neurophenomenology study. *Neuroscience of Consciousness* 2016(1): niw019.

Dor-Ziderman, Y., Berkovich-Ohana, A., Glicksohn, J. & Goldstein, A. (2013). Mindfulness-induced selflessness: A MEG neurophenomenological study. *Frontiers in Human Neuroscience* 7: 582.

Downey, A. (2020). It just doesn't feel right: OCD and the "scaling up" problem. *Phenomenology and the Cognitive Sciences* 19(4): 705–27.

Dreher, J. C., Banquet, J. P., Allilaire, J. F., Paillère-Martinot, M. L., Dubois, B. & Burnod, Y. (2001). Temporal order and spatial memory in schizophrenia: A parametric study. *Schizophrenia Research* 51(2–3): 137–47.

Dreon, R. (2022). *Human Landscapes Contributions to a Pragmatist Anthropology*. Albany: SUNY Press.

Dreyfus, G. (2011). Self and subjectivity: A middle way approach, in M. Siderits, E. Thompson, and D. Zahavi (eds), *Self, No Self? Perspectives from Analytical, Phenomenological, and Indian Traditions* (114–56). Oxford: Oxford University Press.

Duerler, P., Brem, S., Fraga-González, G., Neef, T., Allen, M., Zeidman, P., Stämpfli, P., Vollenweider, F. X. & Preller, K. H. (2022). Psilocybin induces aberrant prediction error processing of tactile mismatch responses—A simultaneous EEG–FMRI study. *Cerebral Cortex* 32(1): 186–96.

Dumas, G., de Guzman, G. C., Tognoli, E. & Kelso, J. A. S. (2014). The human dynamic clamp as a paradigm for social interaction. *Proceedings of the National Academy of Sciences* 111(35): E3726–34. https://doi.org/10.1073/pnas.1407486111

Dumas, G., Kelso, J. A. S. & Nadel, J. (2014). Tackling the social cognition paradox through multi-scale approaches. *Frontiers in Psychology* 5: 882.

Duncan, S. (2005). Spatiomotor imagery, affect, and time in discourse. Conference presentation for Deuxieme Congres de l'International Society for Gesture Studies (ISGS): Interacting bodies. (Lyons, June 15–18, 2005).

Dunne, J. D. (2015). Buddhist styles of mindfulness: a heuristic approach, in B. D. Ostafin, M. D. Robinson, and B. P. Meier (eds), *Handbook of Mindfulness and Self-Regulation* (251–70). New York: Springer.

Dunne, J. D. (2011). Toward an understanding of non-dual mindfulness. *Contemporary Buddhism* 12 (1): 71–88.

Eccles, J. C. (1994). *How the Self Controls its Brain*. Berlin: Springer-Verlag.

Eccles, J. C. (1989). *Evolution of the Brain, Creation of the Self*. London: Routledge.

Edey, R., Cook, J., Brewer, R., Johnson, M. H., Bird, G. & Press, C. (2016). Interaction takes two: Typical adults exhibit mind-blindness towards those with autism spectrum disorder. *Journal of Abnormal Psychology* 125: 879–85. doi: 10.1037/abn0000199

Ehring, T. & Watkins, E. R. (2008). Repetitive negative thinking as a transdiagnostic process. *International Journal of Cognitive Therapy* 1(3): 192–205.

Eich, S., Müller, O. & Schulze-Bonhage, A. (2019). Changes in self-perception in patients treated with neurostimulating devices. *Epilepsy & Behavior* 90: 25–30.

Elbau, I. G., Binder, E. B. & Spoormaker, V. I. (2019). Symptoms are not the solution but the problem: Why psychiatric research should focus on processes rather than symptoms. *Behavioral and Brain Sciences* 42, E7. doi:10.1017/S0140525X18001000

Emmelkamp, P. M., Krijn, M., Hulsbosch, A. M., De Vries, S., Schuemie, M. J. & van der Mast, C. A. (2002). Virtual reality treatment versus exposure in vivo: A comparative evaluation in acrophobia. *Behaviour Research and Therapy* 40(5): 509–16.

Engel, A. K., Friston, K., Kelso, J. A., König, P., Kovács, I., MacDonald III, A., Miller, E. K., Phillips, W. A., Silverstein, S. M., Tallon-Baudry, C. & Triesch, J. (2010). Coordination in behavior and cognition, in C. von der Malsburg, W. A. Phillips, and W. Singer (eds), *Dynamic Coordination in the Brain: From Neurons to Mind* (267–300). Cambridge, MA: MIT Press.

Engel, G. L. (1980). The clinical application of the biopsychosocial model. *American Journal of Psychiatry* 137(5): 535–44.

Engel, G. L. (1977). The need for a new medical model: A challenge for biomedicine. *Science* 196(4286): 129–36.

Eronen, M. I. (2021). The levels problem in psychopathology. *Psychological Medicine* 51(6): 927–33.

Eronen, M. I. (2015). Levels of organization: A deflationary account. *Biology & Philosophy* 30(1): 39–58.

Erskine, R. G. (2014). Nonverbal stories: The body in psychotherapy. *International Journal of Integrative Psychotherapy* 5(1): 21–33.

Ethics Commission. 2017. Ethics Commission Automated and Connected Driving, Report June 2017. Federal Ministry of Transport and Digital Infrastructure (Germany). https://bmdv.bund.de/SharedDocs/EN/publications/report-ethics-commission-automated-and-connected-driving.pdf?__blob=publicationFile

Evans, G. (1982). *The Varieties of Reference*. Oxford: Clarendon Press.

Fabbri-Destro M., Cattaneo L., Boria, S. & Rizzolatti, G. (2009). Planning actions in autism. *Experimental Brain Research* 192: 521–5.

Fabry, R. E. (2020). Into the dark room: a predictive processing account of major depressive disorder. *Phenomenology and the Cognitive Sciences* 19(4): 685–704.

Farb, N. A. S., Segal, Z. V., Mayberg, H., Bean, J., McKeon, D., et al. (2007). Attending to the present: Mindfulness meditation reveals distinct neural modes of self-reference. *Social, Cognitive and Affective Neuroscience* 2(4): 313–22.

Farias, M., Maraldi, E., Wallenkampf, K. C. & Lucchetti, G. (2020). Adverse events in meditation practices and meditation-based therapies: A systematic review. *Acta Psychiatrica Scandinavica* 142(5): 374–93. https://doi.org/10.1111/acps.13225

Farrer, C., Franck, N., Georgieff, N., Frith, C. D., Decety, J. & Jeannerod, M. (2003). Modulating the experience of agency: A positron emission tomography study. *NeuroImage* 18: 324–33.

Farrer, C. & Frith, C. D. (2002). Experiencing oneself vs. another person as being the cause of an action: The neural correlates of the experience of agency. *NeuroImage* 15: 596–603.

Feldman, C. F., Bruner, J., Renderer, B. & Spitzer, S. (1990). Narrative comprehension, in B. K. Britton and A. D. Pellegrini (eds), *Narrative Thought and Narrative Language* (1–78). Hillsdale, NJ: Lawrence Erlbaum Associates.

Fellous, J. M., Sapiro, G., Rossi, A., Mayberg, H. & Ferrante, M. (2019). Explainable artificial intelligence for neuroscience: Behavioral neurostimulation. *Frontiers in Neuroscience* 13: 1346.

Feyaerts, J., Henriksen, M. G., Vanheule, S., Myin-Germeys, I., & Sass, L. A. (2021). Delusions beyond beliefs: A critical overview of diagnostic, aetiological, and therapeutic schizophrenia research from a clinical-phenomenological perspective. *Lancet Psychiatry* 8: 237–49.

Feyaerts, J. & Kusters, W. (2022). On philosophy and schizophrenia: The case of thought insertion. Preprint: https://psyarxiv.com/jby3g/download?format=pdf

Fingelkurts, A. A. & Fingelkurts, A. A. (2018). Alterations in the three components of selfhood in persons with post-traumatic stress disorder symptoms: A pilot qEEG neuroimaging study. *The Open Neuroimaging Journal* 12: 42–54.

Fingelkurts, A. A. & Fingelkurts, A. A. 2017. Three-dimensional components of selfhood in treatment-naive patients with major depressive disorder: A resting-state qEEG imaging study. *Neuropsychologia* 99: 30–6.

Fingelkurts, A. A., Fingelkurts, A. A. & Kallio-Tamminen, T. (2021). Self, me and I in the repertoire of spontaneously occurring altered states of selfhood: Eight neurophenomenological case study reports. *Cognitive Neurodynamics* 16: 255–282 https://link.springer.com/article/10.1007/s11571-021-09719-5

First, M. B. (2005). Desire for amputation of a limb: Paraphilia, psychosis, or a new type of identity disorder. *Psychological Medicine* 35(6): 919–28.

Fitts, P. M. & Posner, M. I. (1967). *Human Performance*. Belmont, CA: Wadsworth.

Fitzpatrick, P., Diorio, R., Richardson, M. J. & Schmidt, R. C. (2013) Dynamical methods for evaluating the time-dependent unfolding of social coordination in children with autism. *Frontiers in Integrative Neuroscience* 7: 21. doi: 10.3389/fnint.2013.00021

Fitzpatrick, P., Frazier, J. A., Cochran, D. M., Mitchell, T., Coleman, C. & Schmidt, R. C. (2016) Impairments of social motor synchrony evident in autism spectrum disorder. *Frontiers in Psychology* 7: 1323. doi: 10.3389/fpsyg.2016.01323

Fitzpatrick, P., Romero, V., Amaral, J. L., Duncan, A., Barnard, H., Richardson, M. J. & Schmidt, R. C. (2017). Evaluating the importance of social motor synchronization and motor skill for understanding autism. *Autism Research* 10(10): 1687–99.

Fleming, K., Goldberg, T. E., Binks, S., Randolph, C., Gold, J. M. & Weinberger, D. R. (1997). Visuospatial working memory in patients with schizophrenia. *Biological Psychiatry* 41(1): 43–9.

Fletcher, P. C. & Frith, C. D. (2009). Perceiving is believing: A Bayesian approach to explaining the positive symptoms of schizophrenia. *Nature Reviews Neuroscience* 10: 48–58.

Flint, J. & Kendler, K. S. (2014). The genetics of major depression. *Neuron* 81(3): 484–503.

Floridi, L. (2011). The informational nature of personal identity. *Minds and Machines* 21(4): 549.

Fossati, P., Hevenor, S. J., Graham, S. J., Grady, C., Keightley, M. L., Craik, F. & Mayberg, H. (2003). In search of the emotional self: An fMRI study using positive and negative emotional words. *American Journal of Psychiatry* 160: 1938–45.

Fotia, F., Van Dam, L., Sykes, J. J., Ambrosini, E., Costantini, M. & Ferri, F. (2022). Body structural representation in schizotypy. *Schizophrenia Research* 239: 1–10.

Fotopoulou, A. (2012). Towards a psychodymamic neuroscience, in A. Fotopoulou, D. Pfaff, and M. A. Conway (eds), *From the Couch to the Lab: Trends in Psychodynamic Neuroscience* (25–48). Oxford: Oxford University Press.

Foxx, J. J. & Simpson, G. V. 2002. Flow of activation from V1 to frontal cortex in humans: A framework for defining "early" visual processing. *Experimental Brain Research* 142: 139–50.

Frank, M. J., Samanta, J., Moustafa, A. A., Sherman, S. J. (2007). Hold your horses: Impulsivity, deep brain stimulation, and medication in Parkinsonism. *Science* 318: 1309–12. PMID: 17962524

Frankfurt, H. G. (1988). *The Importance of What We Care about: Philosophical Essays*. Cambridge: Cambridge University Press.

Frankfurt, H. G. (1971). Freedom of the will and the concept of a person. *The Journal of Philosophy* 68(1): 5–20.

Freeman, D. (2008). Studying and treating schizophrenia using virtual reality: A new paradigm. *Schizophrenia Bulletin* 34(4): 605–10.

Freeman, D., Reeve, S., Robinson, A., Ehlers, A., Clark, D., Spanlang, B. & Slater, M. (2017). Virtual reality in the assessment, understanding, and treatment of mental health disorders. *Psychological Medicine* 47(14): 2393–400.

Freeman, T., Cameron, J. L. & McGhie, A. (2013). *Chronic Schizophrenia*. London: Routledge.

Fridland, E. (2017a). Skill and motor control: Intelligence all the way down. *Philosophical Studies* 174: 1539–60.

Fridland, E. (2017b). Automatically minded. *Synthese* 19(11): 4337–63.

Fridland, E. (2015). Skill, nonpropositional thought, and the cognitive penetrability of perception. *Journal for General Philosophy of Science* 46(1): 105–20.

Frijda, N. H. (1986). *The Emotions. Studies in Emotions and Social Interactions*. New York: Cambridge University Press.

Frisoli, A., Borelli, L., Montagner, A., Marcheschi, S., Procopio, C., Salsedo, F. . . . & Rossi, B. (2007). Arm rehabilitation with a robotic exoskeleleton in Virtual Reality, in *2007 IEEE 10th International Conference on Rehabilitation Robotics* (631–42). Piscataway, NJ: IEEE.

Frisoli, A., Salsedo, F., Bergamasco, M., Rossi, B. & Carboncini, M. C. (2009). A force-feedback exoskeleton for upper-limb rehabilitation in virtual reality. *Applied Bionics and Biomechanics* 6(2): 115–26.

Friston, K. (2011). Embodied inference: or "I think therefore I am, if I am what I think," in W. Tschacher and C. Bergomi (eds), *The Implications of Embodiment: Cognition and Communication* (89–125). Exeter: Imprint Academic.

Friston, K. (2010). The free-energy principle: a unified brain theory? *Nature Reviews Neuroscience* 11: 127–38.

Friston, K. J., Daunizeau, J., Kilner, J. & Kiebel, S. J. (2010). Action and behavior: A free-energy formulation. *Biological Cybernetics* 102(3): 227–60.

Frith, C. (2011). Explaining delusions of control: The comparator model 20 years on. *Consciousness and Cognition* 21: 52–4.

Frith, C. (2004). Comments on Shaun Gallagher: "Neurocognitive models of schizophrenia: A neurophenomenological critique." *Psychopathology* 37(1): 20–2.

Frith, C. (1992). *The Cognitive Neuropsychology of Schizophrenia*. New York: Psychology Press.

Frith, C. D., Blakemore, S. J. & Wolpert, D. M. (2000). Explaining the symptoms of schizophrenia: Abnormalities in the awareness of action. *Brain Research Reviews* 31(2–3): 357–63.

Frith, C. D., Friston, K. J., Herold, S., Silbersweig, D., Fletcher, P., Cahill, C., Dolan, R. J., Frackowiak, R. S. J. & Liddle, P. F. (1995). Regional brain activity in chronic schizophrenic patients during the performance of a verbal fluency task. *The British Journal of Psychiatry* 167(3): 343–9.

Frith, C. & Gallagher, S. (2002). Models of the pathological mind: An interview with Christopher Frith. *Journal of Consciousness Studies* 9(4): 57–80.

Frith, C. D. & Haggard, P. (2018). Volition and the brain—revisiting a classic experimental study. *Trends in Neurosciences* 41(7): 405–7.

Frith, C. D. & Metzinger, T. (2016). What's the use of consciousness, in A. K. Engel, K. J. Friston, and D. Kragic (eds), *The Pragmatic Turn: Toward Action-Oriented Views in Cognitive Science*. Strüngmann Forum Reports, vol. 18. Cambridge, MA: MIT Press.

Frith, U. & Happé, F. (1999). Theory of mind and self-consciousness: What is it like to be autistic? *Mind & Language* 14(1): 82–9.

Fuchs, T. (2020). The circularity of the embodied mind. *Frontiers in Psychology* 11: 1707.

Fuchs, T. (2017). Self across time: The diachronic unity of bodily existence. *Phenomenology and the Cognitive Sciences* 16(2): 291–315.

Fuchs, T. (2012). Are mental illnesses diseases of the brain, in S. Choudhury and J. Slaby, (eds). *Critical Neuroscience: A Handbook of the Social and Cultural Contexts of Neuroscience* (331–44). Oxford: John Wiley & Sons.

Fuchs, T. (2007). Fragmented selves: Temporality and identity in borderline personality disorder. *Psychopathology* 40(6): 379–87.

Fuchs, T. (2005). Corporealized and disembodied minds: A phenomenological view of the body in melancholia and schizophrenia. *Philosophy, Psychiatry, & Psychology* 12(2): 95–107.

Fuchs, T. (2001). Melancholia as a desynchronization: Towards a psychopathology of interpersonal time. *Psychopathology* 34(4): 179–86.

Fuchs, T. & De Jaegher, H. (2009). Enactive intersubjectivity: Participatory sense-making and mutual incorporation. *Phenomenology and the Cognitive Sciences* 8(4): 465–86.

Fuchs, T. & Schlimme, J. E. (2009). Embodiment and psychopathology: A phenomenological perspective. *Current Opinion in Psychiatry* 22(6): 570–5.

Fulceri, F., Tonacci, A., Lucaferro, A., Apicella, F., Narzisi, A., Vincenti, G., Muratori, F. & Contaldo, A. (2018). Interpersonal motor coordination during joint actions in children with and without autism spectrum disorder: The role of motor information. *Research in Developmental Disabilities* 80: 13–23.

Fulford, K. W. M. & Sartorius, N. (2009). A secret history of ICD and the hidden future of DSM, in M. Broome and L. Bortolotti (eds), *Psychiatry as Cognitive Neuroscience: Philosophical Perspectives* (29–48). Oxford: Oxford University Press.

Fuster, J. M. (1999). Synopsis of function and dysfunction of the frontal lobe. *Acta Psychiatrica Scandinavica* 99: 51–7.

Gadamer, H. G. (2018). *The Enigma of Health: The Art of Healing in a Scientific Age*. New York: John Wiley & Sons.

Gadamer, H. G. (2004). *Truth and Method*. Trans. J. Weinsheimer and D. G. Marshall. London: Bloomsbury.

Gallagher, S. (2023). *Embodied and Enactive Approaches to Cognition*. Cambridge: Cambridge University Press.

Gallagher, S. (2022). Integration and causality in enactive approaches to psychiatry. *Frontiers in Psychiatry* 13: 870122. doi: 10.3389/fpsyt.2022.870122

Gallagher, S. (2021a). *Performance/Art: The Venetian Lectures*. Milan: Mimesis International Edizioni.

Gallagher, S. (2021b). Deep brain stimulation, self and relational autonomy. *Neuroethics* 14(1): 31–43. doi: 10.1007/s12152-018-9355-x

Gallagher, S. (2020a). *Action and Interaction*. Oxford: Oxford University Press.

Gallagher, S. (2020b). Phenomenology of agency and the cognitive sciences, in C. Erhard and T. Keiling (eds), *The Routledge Handbook of the Phenomenology of Agency* (334–48). London: Routledge.

Gallagher, S. (2020c). Mindful performance, in A. Pennisi and A. Falzone (eds), *The Extended Theory of Cognitive Creativity—Interdisciplinary Approaches to Performativity* (43–58). Berlin: Springer.

Gallagher, S. (2020d). Phenomenology of agency and the cognitive sciences, in C. Erhard and T. Keiling (eds), *The Routledge Handbook of the Phenomenology of Agency* (334–48). London: Routledge.

Gallagher, S. (2018a). Rethinking nature: Phenomenology and a non-reductionist cognitive science. *Australasian Philosophical Review* 2(2): 125–37.

Gallagher, S. (2018b). New mechanisms and the enactivist concept of constitution, in M. P. Guta (ed.), *Consciousness and the Ontology of Properties* (207–20). London: Routlege. doi: 10.4324/9781315104706

Gallagher, S. (2017a). *Enactivist Interventions: Rethinking the Mind*. Oxford: Oxford University Press.

Gallagher, S. (2017b). Self-defense: Deflecting deflationary and eliminativist critiques of the sense of ownership. *Frontiers in Human Neuroscience* 8: 1612. https://doi.org/10.3389/fpsyg.2017.01612

Gallagher, S. (2015). Seeing without an I: Another look at immunity to error through misidentification, in D. Moyal-Sharrock, A. Coliva, and V. Munz (eds), *Mind, Language, and Action: Proceedings of the 36th International Wittgenstein Symposium* (549–68). Berlin: Walter de Gruyter.

Gallagher, S. (2014). The cruel and unusual phenomenology of solitary confinement. *Frontiers in Psychology* 5: 585.

Gallagher, S. (2013). A pattern theory of self. *Frontiers in Human Neuroscience* 7(443): 1–7. doi: 10.3389/fnhum.2013.00443

Gallagher, S. (2012a). Multiple aspects of agency. *New Ideas in Psychology* 30: 15–31.

Gallagher, S. (2012b). In defense of phenomenological approaches to social cognition: Interacting with the critics. *Review of Philosophy and Psychology* 3(2): 187–212.

Gallagher, S. (ed.) (2011). *Oxford Handbook of the Self*. Oxford: Oxford University Press.

Gallagher, S. (2009a). Delusional realities, in L. Bortolotti and M. Broome (eds), *Psychiatry as Cognitive Neuroscience* (245–66). Oxford: Oxford University Press.

Gallagher, S. (2009b). Deep and dynamic interaction: Response to Hanne De Jaegher. *Consciousness and Cognition* 18(2): 547–8.

Gallagher, S. (2008). Direct perception in the intersubjective context. *Consciousness and Cognition* 17: 535–43.

Gallagher, S. (2005). Dynamic models of body schematic processes, in H. De Preester and V. Knockaert (eds), *Body Image and Body Schema* (233–50). Amsterdam: John Benjamins Publishers.

Gallagher, S. (2004a). Neurocognitive models of schizophrenia: A neurophenomenological critique. *Psychopathology* 37: 8–19.

Gallagher, S. (2004b). Understanding interpersonal problems in autism: Interaction theory as an alternative to theory of mind. *Philosophy, Psychiatry, & Psychology* 11(3): 199–217.

Gallagher, S. (2003). Self-narrative in schizophrenia, in A. S. David and T. Kircher (eds), *The Self in Neuroscience and Psychiatry* (336–57). Cambridge: Cambridge University Press.

Gallagher, S. (2001). The practice of mind: Theory, simulation or primary interaction? *Journal of Consciousness Studies* 8(5–7): 83–108.

Gallagher, S. (2000a). Philosophical conceptions of the self: Implications for cognitive science. *Trends in Cognitive Science* 4: 14–12.

Gallagher, S. (2000b). Self-reference and schizophrenia: A cognitive model of immunity to error through misidentification, in D. Zahavi (ed.), *Exploring the Self: Philosophical and Psychopathological Perspectives on Self-experience* (203–39). Amsterdam & Philadelphia: John Benjamins.

Gallagher, S. (1998). *The Inordinance of Time*. Evanston: Northwestern University Press.

Gallagher, S. & Aguda, B. (2020). Anchoring know-how: Action, affordance and anticipation. *Journal of Consciousness Studies* 27(3–4): 3–37.

Gallagher, S. & Allen, M. (2018). Active inference, enactivism and the hermeneutics of social cognition. *Synthese* 195(6): 2627–48. doi:10.1007/s11229-016-1269-8

Gallagher, S. & Cole, J. (2011). Dissociation in self-narrative. *Consciousness and Cognition* 20(1): 149–55.

Gallagher, S. & Cole, J. (1995). Body schema and body image in a deafferented subject. *Journal of Mind and Behavior* 16: 369–90.

Gallagher, S. & Daly, A. (2018). Dynamical relations in the self-pattern. *Frontiers in Psychology* 9: 664. doi: 10.3389/fpsyg.2018.00664.

Gallagher, S. and Hutto, D. (2019). Narrative in embodied therapeutic practice: Getting the story straight. In H. Payne, J. Tantia, S. Koch, and T. Fuchs (eds.), *The Routledge International Handbook of Embodied Perspectives in Psychotherapy* (28-39). London: Routledge.

Gallagher, S. & Hutto, D. (2008). Understanding others through primary interaction and narrative practice, in J. Zlatev, T. Racine, C. Sinha, and E. Itkonen (eds), *The Shared Mind: Perspectives on Intersubjectivity* (17–38). Amsterdam: John Benjamins.

Gallagher, S., Hutto, D. & Hipólito, I. (2022) Predictive processing and some disillusions about illusions. *Review of Philosophy and Psychology* 13(4): 999–1017. https://doi.org/10.1007/s13164-021-00588-9

Gallagher, S. & Marcel, A. J. (1999). The self in contextualized action. *Journal of Consciousness Studies* 6(4): 4–30.

Gallagher, S. & Petracca, E. (2022). Trust as the glue of cognitive institutions. *Phenomenological Psychology*. Online. doi: 10.1080/09515089.2022.2134767

Gallagher, S., Raffone, A., Berkovich-Ohana, A., Barendregt, H. P., Bauer, P. R., Brown, K. W., Giommi, F., Nyklíček, I., Ostafin, B. D., Slagter, H., Trautwein, F.-M. & Vago, D. R. (2023). The self-pattern and Buddhist psychology. *Mindfulness* 1–9. https://doi.org/10.1007/s12671-023-02118-3

Gallagher, S. & Shear, J. (1999). *Models of the Self*. Exeter: Imprint Academic.

Gallagher, S. & Trigg, D. (2016). Agency and anxiety: Delusions of control and loss of control in schizophrenia and agoraphobia. *Frontiers in Neuroscience* 10: 459. doi: 10.3389/fnhum.2016.00459

Gallagher, S. & Varela, F. 2003. Redrawing the map and resetting the time: Phenomenology and the cognitive sciences. *Canadian Journal of Philosophy*, Supplementary Volume 29: 93–132.

Gallagher, S. and Varga, S. (2020). The meshed architecture of performance as a model of situated cognition. *Frontiers in Psychology* 11: 2140. doi: 10.3389/fpsyg.2020.02140

Gallagher, S. & Varga, S. (2015). Conceptual issues in autism spectrum disorders. *Current Opinion in Psychiatry* 28(2): 127–32. doi: 10.1097/YCO.0000000000000142

Gallagher, S. & Varga, S. (2014). Social constraints on the direct perception of emotions and intentions. *Topoi* 33(1): 185–99. doi: 10.1007/s11245-013-9203-x

Gallagher, S., Varga, S. & Sparaci, L. (2022). Disruptions of the meshed architecture in autism spectrum disorder. *Psychoanalytic Inquiry* 42(1): 76–95. doi.org/10.1080/07351690.2022.2007032

Gallagher, S. & Zahavi, D. (2021). *The Phenomenological Mind* (3rd edn). London: Routledge.

Gallagher, S. & Zahavi, D. (2020). Phenomenological approaches to self-consciousness. *The Stanford Encyclopedia of Philosophy*. https://plato.stanford.edu/archives/sum2021/entries/self-consciousness-phenomenological/

Gallese V., Rochat M. J. & Berchio C. (2013). The mirror mechanism and its potential role in autism spectrum disorder. *Developmental Medicine and Child Neurology* 55: 15–22.

García, E., Di Paolo, E. A. & De Jaegher, H. (2021). Embodiment in online psychotherapy: A qualitative study. *Psychology and Psychotherapy: Theory, Research and Practice* 95 (1): 191–211. https://doi.org/10.1111/papt.12359

García-Pérez, R. M., Lee, A. & Hobson, R. P. (2007). On intersubjective engagement in autism: A controlled study of nonverbal aspects of conversation. *Journal of Autism and Developmental Disorders* 37(7): 1310–22.

Garfield, J. (2021). Throwing out the Buddha with the offering water: Comments on Evan Thompson's *Why I Am Not a Buddhist*. *APA Newsletter: Asian and Asian American Philosophers and Philosophies* 20 (2): 21–6.

Gatens, M. (1996). *Bodies: Ethics, Power, and Corporeality*. New York, London: Routledge.

Gazzaniga, M. S. (1998). Brain and conscious experience. *Advances in Neurology* 77: 181–92.

Gazzaniga, M. S. (1995). Principles of human brain organization derived from split-brain studies. *Neuron* 14(2): 217–28.

Gazzaniga, M. S. & Gallagher, S. (1998). A neuronal Platonist: An interview with Michael Gazzaniga. *Journal of Consciousness Studies* 5: 706–17.

Genette, G. (1983). *Narrative Discourse: An Essay in Method*, trans. J. E. Lewin. Ithaca: Cornell University Press.

Gennaro, R. J. (2021). Inserted thoughts and the higher-order thought theory of consciousness, in *Psychiatry and Neuroscience Update* (61–71). Cham: Springer.

Gentsch, A., Schütz-Bosbach, S., Endrass, T. & Kathmann, N. (2012). Dysfunctional forward model mechanisms and aberrant sense of agency in obsessive-compulsive disorder. *Biological Psychiatry* 71(7): 652–9.

Georgie, Y. K., Schillaci, G. & Hafner, V. V. (2019). An interdisciplinary overview of developmental indices and behavioral measures of the minimal self, in *2019 Joint IEEE 9th International Conference on Development and Learning and Epigenetic Robotics (ICDL-EpiRob)* (129–36). Piscataway, NJ: IEEE.

Georgieff, N. & Jeannerod, M. (1998). Beyond consciousness of external events: A "who" system for consciousness of action and self-consciousness. *Consciousness and Cognition* 7: 465–77.

Gergen, K. (2011). The social construction of the self, in S. Gallagher (ed.), *The Oxford Handbook of the Self* (633–53). Oxford: Oxford University Press.

Gerrans, P. (2022). Alienation and identification in addiction. *Philosophical Psychology*. doi.org/10.1080/09515089.2022.2067034

Gerrans, P. (2020). Pain asymbolia as depersonalization for pain experience: An interoceptive active inference account. *Frontiers in Psychology* 11. 523710: 1–10 https://www.ncbi.nlm.nih.gov/pmc/articles/PMC7658103/

Gerrans, P. (2014). *The Measure of Madness: Philosophy of Mind, Cognitive Neuroscience, and Delusional Thought*. Cambridge, MA: MIT Press.

Gethin, R. (1998) *The Foundations of Buddhism*. Oxford: Oxford University Press.

Ghaemi, S. N. (2009). Nosologomania: DSM & Karl Jaspers' critique of Kraepelin. *Philosophy, Ethics, and Humanities in Medicine* 4: 10.

Gibson, J. J. (1977). The theory of affordances, in R. Shaw and J. Bransford (eds), *Perceiving, Acting, and Knowing* (67–82). Hillsdale, NJ: Erlbaum.

Gidley Larson, J. C. & Mostofsky, S. H. (2008). Evidence that the pattern of visuomotor sequence learning is altered in children with autism. *Autism Research* 1(6): 341–53.

Gilbert, F. (2015). A threat to autonomy? The intrusion of predictive brain implants. *Ajob Neuroscience* 6(4), 4–11.

Gilbert, F. 2013. Deep brain stimulation for treatment resistant depression: Postoperative feelings of self-estrangement, suicide attempt and impulsive-aggressive behaviours. *Neuroethics* 6(3): 473–81. doi: 10.1007/s12152-013-9178-8

Gilbert, F., Viaña, J. N. M. & Ineichen, C. (2021). Deflating the "DBS causes personality changes" bubble. *Neuroethics* 14(1): 1–17. https://doi.org/10.1007/s1215 2-018-9373-8

Gillett, C. (2013). Constitution, and multiple Constitution, in the sciences: Using the neuron to construct a starting framework. *Minds & Machines* 23: 309–37.

Gillihan S. J. & Farah M. J. 2005. Is self special? A critical review of evidence from experimental psychology and cognitive neuroscience. *Psychological Bulletin* 131(1): 76–97.

Giommi, F., Bauer, P. R., Berkovich-Ohana, A., Barendregt, H., Brown K. W., Gallagher, S., Nyklíček, I., Ostafin, B., Raffone, A., Slagter, H. A., Trautwein, F.-M. & Vago, D. (2023). The (in)flexible self: Psychopathology, mindfulness, and neuroscience. *International Journal of Clinical and Health Psychology* 23: 100381. doi.org/10.1016/j.ijchp.2023.100381

Giuliani, M., Martoni, R. M., Crespi, S. A., O'Neill, J., Erzegovesi, S., de'Sperati, C. & Grgic, R. G. (2021). Did I do that? Cognitive flexibility and self-agency in patients with obsessive compulsive disorder. *Psychiatry Research* 304: 114170.

Glannon, W. (2009). Stimulating brains, altering minds. *Journal of Medical Ethics* 35: 289–92. doi:10.1136/jme.2008.027789; PMID19407032

Goddard E. (2017). Deep brain stimulation through the "lens of agency": Clarifying threats to personal identity from neurological intervention. *Neuroethics* 10(3): 325–35. doi:10.1007/s12152-016-9297-0

Godfrin, K. A. & Van Heeringen, C. (2010). The effects of mindfulness-based cognitive therapy on recurrence of depressive episodes, mental health and quality of life: A randomized controlled study. *Behaviour Research and Therapy* 48(8): 738–46.

Goffman, E. (1961). *Asylums: Essays on the Social Situation of Mental Patients and Other Inmates.* Harmondsworth: Penguin.

Gold, I. & Hohwy, J. (2000). Rationality and schizophrenic delusion. *Mind & Language* 15(1): 146–67.

Goldberg, S. B., Riordan, K. M., Sun, S. & Davidson, R. J. (2022). The empirical status of mindfulness-based interventions: A systematic review of 44 meta-analyses of randomized controlled trials. *Perspectives on Psychological Science* 17(1): 108–30.

Goldberg, S. B., Tucker, R. P., Greene, P. A., Davidson, R. J., Wampold, B. E., Kearney, D. J. & Simpson, T. L. (2018). Mindfulness-based interventions for psychiatric disorders: A systematic review and meta-analysis. *Clinical Psychology Review* 59: 52–60.

Goldie, P. (2011). Grief: A narrative account. *Ratio* 24(2): 119–37.

Goldie, P. (2000). *The Emotions: A Philosophical Exploration.* Oxford: Oxford University Press.

Goldman-Rakic, P. S. (1994). Working memory dysfunction in schizophrenia, in S. P. Salloway, P. F. Malloy, and J. D. Duffy (eds), *The Frontal Lobes and Neuropsychiatric Illness* (71–81). Washington, DC: American Psychiatric Publishing.

Goldscheider, A. (1894). *Ueber den Schmerz in Physiologischer und Klinischer Hinsicht.* Berlin: Hirschwald.

Goldstein, K. & M. Scheerer. (1964). *Abstract and Concrete Behavior: An Experimental Study with Special Tests.* Evanston, IL: Northwestern University. Reprint of *Psychological Monographs* 53(2): 1941.

Goleman, D. (1977). *The Varieties of Meditative Experience*. New York: E. P. Dutton.

Gombrich, R. F. (2005). Recovering the Buddha's message. *Buddhism: Critical Concepts in Religious Studies* 1: 113–28.

Goodman, W. K. & Alterman, R. L. (2012). Deep brain stimulation for intractable psychiatric disorders. *Annual Review of Medicine* 63: 511–24. doi:10.1146/annurev-med-052209-100401; PMID22034866

Goodwin, C. (2017). *Co-operative Action*. Cambridge: Cambridge University Press.

Goodwin, C. (2000). Action and embodiment within situated human interaction. *Journal of Pragmatics* 32(10): 1489–522.

Gopnik, A. & Meltzoff, A. N. (1997). *Words, Thoughts, and Theories*. Cambridge, MA: MIT Press.

Graesser, A. C., Jeon, M., Yan, Y. & Cai, C. (2007). Discourse cohesion in text and tutorial dialogue. *Information Design Journal* 15: 199–213.

Graesser, A. C., McNamara, D. S., Louwerse, M. & Cai, Z. (2004). Coh-metrix: Analysis of text on cohesion and language. *Behavioral Research Methods, Instruments, and Computers* 36: 193–202.

Graham, G. & Stephens, G. L. (1994). Mind and mine, in G. Graham and G. L. Stephens (eds), *Philosophical Psychopathology* (91–109). Cambridge, MA: MIT Press.

Graham K. T., Martin-Iverson M. T., Holmes N. P., Jablensky A. & Waters F. (2014). Deficits in agency in schizophrenia, and additional deficits in body image, body schema, internal timing in passivity symptoms. *Frontiers in Psychiatry* 5:126. doi:10.3389/fpsyt.2014.00126

Granucci, A. F. (1969). "Nor cruel and unusual punishments inflicted": The original meaning. *California Law Review* 57(4): 839–65.

Grassian, S. (1983). Psychopathological effects of solitary confinement. *American Journal of Psychiatry* 140(11): 1450–4.

Greenberg, B., Malone, D., Friehs, G., et al. (2006). Three-year outcomes in deep brain stimulation for highly resistant obsessive–compulsive disorder. *Neuropsychopharmacology* 31: 2384–93. doi:10.1038/sj.npp.1301165

Greenspan, S. I. (2001). The affect diathesis hypothesis: The role of emotions in the core deficit in autism and in the development of intelligence and social skills. *Journal of Developmental and Learning Disorders* 5(1): 1–45.

Grenanderm, U. (1994). *General Pattern Theory*. Oxford: Oxford Science Publications.

Grossman, P., Niemann, L., Schmidt, S. & Walach, H. (2004). Mindfulness-based stress reduction and health benefits: A meta-analysis. *Journal of Psychosomatic Research* 57(1): 35–43.

Gruber, J. & Kring, A. M. (2008). Narrating emotional events in schizophrenia. *Journal of Abnormal Psychology* 117(3): 520–33.

Grünbaum, T. (2015). The feeling of agency hypothesis: a critique. *Synthese* 192(10), 3313–3337.

Grünbaum, T. (2010). Action and agency, in S. Gallagher and D. Schmicking (eds), *Handbook of Phenomenology and Cognitive Science* (337–54). Dordrecht: Springer.

Guajardo N. R. & Watson A. (2002). Narrative discourse and theory of mind development. *The Journal of Genetic Psychology* 163: 305–25.

Guenther, L. (2018). Unmaking and remaking the world in long-term solitary confinement. *Puncta: Journal of Critical Phenomenology* 1: 74–89. doi:10.31608/PJCP.v1i1.5

Guenther, L. (2013). *Solitary Confinement: Social Death and its Afterlives*. Minneapolis: University of Minnesota Press.

Guma, E., Plitman, E. & Chakravarty, M. M. (2019) The role of maternal immune activation in altering the neurodevelopmental trajectories of offspring: A translational review of neuroimaging studies with implications for autism spectrum disorder and schizophrenia. *Neuroscience and Biobehavioral Reviews* 104: 141–57.

Gupta, B. (1998). *The Disinterested Witness: A Fragment of Advaita Vedanta Phenomenology.* Evanston, IL: Northwestern University Press.

Gutchess, A. H., Kensinger, E. A., Yoon, C. & Schacter, D. L. (2007). Ageing and the self-reference effect in memory. *Memory* 15: 822–37.

Hacking, I. (1995). *Rewriting the Soul: Multiple Personality and the Sciences of Memory.* Princeton, NJ: Princeton University Press.

Hadwin, J., Baron-Cohen, S., Howlin, P. & Hill, K. (1997). Does teaching theory of mind have an effect on the ability to develop conversation in children with autism? *Journal of Autism and Developmental Disorders* 27(5): 519–37.

Haggard, P. (2005). Conscious intention and motor cognition. *Trends in Cognitive Sciences* 9(6), 290–295.

Haggard, P., Clark, S. & Kalogeras, J. (2002). Voluntary action and conscious awareness. *Nature Neuroscience* 5(4): 382–5.

Halliday, M. A. K. (1978). Meaning and the construction of reality in early childhood, in J. H. Pick Jr. & E. Saltzman (eds), *Psychological Modes of Perceiving and Processing Information* (67–98). Hillsdale, NJ: Erlbaum.

Halsema, A. (2011). The time of the self: A feminist reflection on Ricoeur's notion of narrative identity, in C. Schües, D. E. Olkowski, and H. A. Fielding (eds), *Time in Feminist Phenomenology* (111–31). Bloomington: Indiana University Press.

Hamilton, A. F. (2013). Reflecting on the mirror neuron system in autism: A systematic review of current theories. *Developmental Cognitive Neuroscience.* 3: 91–105.

Haney, C. (2003). Mental health issues in long-term solitary and "supermax" confinement. *Crime & Delinquency* 49(1): 124–56.

Happé, F. & Frith, U. (2020). Annual Research Review: Looking back to look forward—changes in the concept of autism and implications for future research. *Journal of Child Psychology and Psychiatry* 61(3): 218–32.

Happé, F. & Frith, U. (2014). Annual research review: Towards a developmental neuroscience of atypical social cognition. *Journal of Child Psychology and Psychiatry* 55(6): 553–77.

Harari, Y. N. (2017). Dataism is our new god. *New Perspectives Quarterly* 34(2), 36–43.

Harrison, A. & Tronick, E. (2022). Intersubjectivity: Conceptual considerations in meaning-making with a clinical illustration. *Frontiers in Psycholology* 12: 715873. doi:10.3389/fpsyg.2021.715873

Hartmann, E., Milofsky, E., Vaillant, G., Oldfield, M., Falke, R., & Ducey, C. (1984). Vulnerability to schizophrenia: Prediction of adult schizophrenia using childhood information. *Archives of General Psychiatry* 41(11), 1050–1056.

Harvey, A. G., Watkins, E. & Mansell, W. (2004). *Cognitive Behavioural Processes across Psychological Disorders: A Transdiagnostic Approach to Research and Treatment.* New York: Oxford University Press.

Harvey, P. (2013). *The Selfless Mind: Personality, Consciousness and Nirvana in Early Buddhism.* London: Routledge.

Harvey, P. (1995). Research article criteria for judging the unwholesomeness of actions in the texts of Theravaada Buddhism. *Journal of Buddhist Ethics* 2: 140–51.

Harvey, P. (1990). The transmission of truth in the Buddha's first sermon. *Buddhist Studies Review* 7(1–2): 19–24.

Hatfield, B. D. & S. E. Kerick (2007). The psychology of superior sport performance: A cognitive and affective neuroscience perspective, in G. Tenenbaum and R. C. Eklund (eds), *Handbook of Sport Psychology*, 3rd edn (84–109). Hoboken: Wiley.

Hastings, A., Browne, A., Kall, K., et al. (2015). *Keeping Vulnerable Populations Safe under PREA: Alternative Strategies to the Use of Segregation in Prisons and Jails*. New York: Vera Institute of Justice, National PREA Resource Center, March 2015

Haugeland, J. (1998). *Having Thought: Essays in the Metaphysics of Mind*. Cambridge, MA: Harvard University Press.

Hawking, S. (2013). Brain could exist outside body. *The Guardian*, September 21. https://www.theguardian.com/science/2013/sep/21/stephen-hawking-brain-outside-body

Hawley, K. (2014). Trust, distrust and commitment. *Noûs* 48(1): 1–20. https://doi.org/10.1111/nous.12000

Heatherton, T. F., Wyland, C. L., Macrae, C. N., Demos, K. E., Denny, B. T. & Kelley, W. M. (2006). Medial prefrontal activity differentiates self from close others. *Social Cognitive Affective Neuroscience* 1: 18–25.

Heckers, S. & Kendler, K. S. (2020). The evolution of Kraepelin's nosological principles. *World Psychiatry* 19(3): 381–8.

Heckers, S., Rauch, S., Goff, D., Savage, C., Schacter, D., Fischman, A. & Alpert, N. (1998). Impaired recruitment of the hippocampus during conscious recollection in schizophrenia. *Nature Neuroscience* 1(4): 318–23.

Heersmink, R. (2022). Preserving narrative identity for dementia patients: Embodiment, active environments, and distributed memory. *Neuroethics* 15(1): 1–16.

Heersmink, R. (2021). Varieties of artifacts: Embodied, perceptual, cognitive, and affective. *Topics in Cognitive Science* 13(4): 573–96. https://doi.org/10.1111/tops.12549

Heersmink, R. (2018). The narrative self, distributed memory, and evocative objects. *Philosophical Studies* 175(8): 1829–49.

Heersmink, R. (2017). Distributed selves: Personal identity and extended memory systems. *Synthese* 194(8): 3135–51.

Heidegger, M. (1988). *The Basic Problems of Phenomenology*, trans. A. Hofstadter. Bloomington: Indiana University Press.

Heidegger, M. (1962). *Being and Time*, trans. J. Macquarrie and E. Robinson. New York: Harper and Row.

Henderson, G. E. (2020). Autism and social interaction: A discursive psychological study. PhD Thesis, Victoria University of Wellington. https://openaccess.wgtn.ac.nz/ndownloader/files/28945308

Henriksen, M. G., Parnas, J. & Zahavi, D. (2019). Thought insertion and disturbed for-me-ness (minimal selfhood) in schizophrenia. *Consciousness and Cognition* 74: 102770.

Heyes, C. & Catmur, C. (2021). What happened to mirror neurons? *Perspectives on Psychological Science* 17(1): 153–168. https://doi.org/10.1177/1745691621990638

Higgins, J. (2018). Biosocial selfhood: Overcoming the "body-social problem" within the individuation of the human self. *Phenomenology and the Cognitive Sciences* 17(3): 433–54.

Hilton, C., Zhang, Y., White, M., et al. (2012). Motor impairment concordant and discordant for autism spectrum disorders. *Autism* 16: 430–41.

Hobson, P. (2004). *The Cradle of Thought: Exploring the Origins of Thinking*. London: Pan Macmillan.

Hobson, R. P. (1993). The emotional origins of social understanding. *Philosophical Psychology* 6: 227–49.

Hobson, R. P. (1990). On the origins of self and the case of autism. *Development and Psychopathology* 2: 163–81.

Hobson, R. P., & Lee, A. (1999). Imitation and identification in autism. *The Journal of Child Psychology and Psychiatry and Allied Disciplines* 40(4), 649–659.

Hobson, R. P. & Lee, A. (1998). Hello and goodbye: A study of social engagement in autism. *Journal of Autism and Developmental Disorders* 28: 117–27.

Høffding, S. (2019). *A Phenomenology of Musical Absorption.* Dordrecht: Springer.

Høffding, S. & Satne, G. (2019). Interactive expertise in solo and joint musical perform-ance. *Synthese* 198(1): 427–45.

Hohwy, J. (2013). *The Predictive Mind.* Oxford: Oxford University Press.

Hölken, A., Kugele, S., Newen, A. & Franklin, S. (2023). Modeling interactions between the embodied and the narrative self: Dynamics of the self-pattern within LIDA. *Cognitive Systems Research* 81: 25–36.

Holmes, J., Mareva, S., Bennett, M. P., Black, M. J. & Guy, J. (2021). Higher-order dimen-sions of psychopathology in a neurodevelopmental transdiagnostic sample. *Journal of Abnormal Psychology* 130(8): 909–22.

Hölzel, B. K., Lazar, S. W., Gard, T., Schuman-Olivier, Z., Vago, D. R. & Ott, U. (2011). How does mindfulness meditation work? Proposing mechanisms of action from a conceptual and neural perspective. *Perspectives on Psychological Science* 6(6): 537–59.

Hood, B. (2012). *The Self Illusion: How the Social Brain Creates Identity.* Oxford: Oxford University Press.

Houlders, J. W., Bortolotti, L. & Broome, M. R. (2021). Threats to epistemic agency in young people with unusual experiences and beliefs. *Synthese* 199: 7689–704. https://doi.org/10.1007/s11229-021-03133-4

Howe, M. L. (2000). *The Fate of Early Memories: Developmental Science and the Retention of Childhood Experiences.* Cambridge, MA: MIT Press.

Hughes, G., Desantis, A. & Waszak, F. (2013) Attenuation of auditory N1 results from identity-specific action-effect prediction. *European Journal of Neuroscience* 37: 1152–8.

Hume, D. (1739). *A Treatise of Human Nature.* Oxford: Clarendon Press, 1896.

Humphreys, P. (1996). Aspects of emergence. *Philosophical Topics* 24(1): 53–70.

Humpston, C. S. (2018). The paradoxical self: Awareness, solipsism and first-rank symp-toms in schizophrenia. *Philosophical Psychology* 31(2): 210–31. doi:10.1080/0951508 9.2017.1410877

Hunt, H. T. (2007). "Dark nights of the soul": Phenomenology and neurocognition of spiritual suffering in mysticism and psychosis. *Review of General Psychology* 11(3): 209–34.

Hur, J.-W., Kwon, J. S., Lee, T. Y. & Park, S. (2014). The crisis of minimal self-awareness in schizophrenia: A meta-analytic review. *Schizophrenic Research* 152: 58–64. doi:10.1016/j.schres.2013.08.042

Husserl, E. (2001). *Logical Investigations,* 2 vols, trans. J. N. Findlay. London: Routledge.

Husserl, E. (1973a). *Zur Phänomenologie der Intersubjektivität. Texte aus dem Nachlass, Erster Teil, 1905–1920,* ed. I. Kern. The Hague, Netherlands: Martinus Nijhoff.

Husserl, E. (1973b). *Zur Phänomenologie der Intersubjektivität II. Texte aus dem Nachlass. Zweiter Teil. 1921–1928,* ed. I. Kern. The Hague, Netherlands: Martinus Nijhoff.

Husserl, E. (1973c). *Zur Phänomenologie der Intersubjektivität III. Texte aus dem Nachlass. Dritter Teil. 1929–1935,* ed. I. Kern. The Hague, Netherlands: Martinus Nijhoff.

Husserl, E. (1968). *Phänomenologische Psychologie. Vorlesungen Sommersemester. 1925.* [*Phenomenological psychology. Lectures from the summer semester. 1925.*], ed. W. Biemel. The Hague, Netherlands: Martinus Nijhoff.

Husserl, E. (1959). *Erste Philosophie (1923/4). Zweiter Teil: Theorie der phänomenologischen Reduktion*. [*First philosophy (1923/24). Second part: theory of phenomenological reduction*.], ed. R. Boehm. The Hague, Netherlands: Martinus Nijhoff.

Hutto, D. D. (2008). *Folk Psychological Narratives: The Sociocultural Basis of Understanding Reasons*. Cambridge, MA: MIT Press.

Hutto, D. D. (2007). The narrative practice hypothesis: Origins and applications of folk psychology. *Narrative and Understanding Persons. Royal Institute of Philosophy Supplement* 82: 43–68.

Hutto, D. (2006). Narrative practice and understanding reasons: Reply to Gallagher, in R. Menary (ed.), *Radical Enactivism*. Amsterdam: John Benjamins.

Hutto, D. & Gallagher, S. (2017). Re-authoring narrative therapy: Opening the way for future developments. *Philosophy, Psychiatry, & Psychology* 24(2): 157–67.

Hutto, D. D. & Myin, E. (2017). *Evolving Enactivism*. Cambridge, MA: MIT Press.

Iacoboni, M. & Dapretto, M. (2006). The mirror neuron system and the consequences of its dysfunction. *Nature Reviews Neuroscience* 7(12): 942–51.

Ikegami, T. (2022). How can an android become human? Paper presented at the ECogS Interaction Matters Conference, November 9. OIST, Okinawa, Japan.

Ingold, T. (2004). Culture on the ground: The world perceived through the feet. *Journal of Material Culture* 9(3): 315–40.

Insel, T., and Cuthbert, B. N. (2015). Brain disorders? Precisely: precision medicine comes to psychiatry. *Science* 348: 499–500. doi: 10.1126/science.aab2358

Isenhower, R. W., Marsh, K. L., Richardson, M. J., Helt, M., Schmidt, R. C. & Fein, D. (2012). Rhythmic bimanual coordination is impaired in young children with autism spectrum disorder. *Research in Autism Spectrum Disorders* 6(1): 25–31.

Issartel, J., Marin, L. & Cadopi, M. (2007). Unintended interpersonal co-ordination: "Can we march to the beat of our own drum?" *Neuroscience Letters* 411(3): 174–9.

Iverson, J. M., Northrup, J. B., Leezenbaum, N. B., Parladé, M. V., Koterba, E. A. & West, K. L. (2018). Early gesture and vocabulary development in infant siblings of children with autism spectrum disorder. *Journal of Autism and Developmental Disorders* 48(1): 55–71.

Iverson, J. M. & Wozniak, R. H. (2016). Transitions to intentional and symbolic communication in typical development and in autism spectrum disorder, in D. Keen, H. Meadan, N. C. Brady, and J. W. Halle (eds), *Prelinguistic and Minimally Verbal Communicators on the Autism Spectrum* (51–72). Singapore: Springer.

Izard, C. E., Ackerman, B. P., Schoff, K. M., and Fine, S. E. (2000). Self-organization of discrete emotions, emotion patterns, and emotion-cognition relations, in S. E. Lewis and I. Granic (eds), *Emotion, Development, and Self-Organization: Dynamic Systems Approaches to Emotional Development* (15–36). New York: Cambridge University Press.

Izard, C. E., Bartlett, E. S. & Marshall, A. G. (1972). *Patterns of Emotions*. New York: Academic Press.

Jablensky A. (2016). Psychiatric classifications: Validity and utility. *World Psychiatry* 15: 26–31.

Jackson, M. (2002). *Justice behind the Walls: Human Rights in Canadian Prisons*. Toronto: Douglas & McIntyre.

James, W. (1904). Does consciousness exist? *The Journal of Philosophy, Psychology and Scientific Methods* 1(18): 477–91.

James W. (1890). *Principles of Psychology*. 2 vols. New York: Basic Books, 1950.

James, W. (1884). What is an emotion. *Mind* 9: 188–205.

Jarvis, G. E. & Kirmayer, L. J. (2021). Situating mental disorders in cultural frames, in *Oxford Research Encyclopedia of Psychology* (np). Oxford: Oxford University Press. https://doi.org/10.1093/acrefore/9780190236557.013.627

Jaspers K. 1997. *General Psychopathology*. 2 vols. Baltimore, MD: Johns Hopkins University Press.

Jaynes, J. 2019. *The Julian Jaynes Collection*, ed. Marcel Kuijsten. Henderson NV: The Julian Jaynes Society.

Jeannerod, M. (2009). The sense of agency and its disturbances in schizophrenia: a reappraisal. *Experimental Brain Research* 192: 527. doi:10.1007/s00221-008-1533-3

Jékely, G., Godfrey-Smith, P., and Keijzer, F. (2021). Reafference and the origin of the self in early nervous system evolution. *Philosophical Transactions of the Royal Society* B 376: 20190764. https://doi.org/10.1098/rstb.2019.0764

Jiang, F., Jiang, Y., Zhi, H., Dong, Y., Li, H., Ma, S.... & Wang, Y. (2017). Artificial intelligence in healthcare: Past, present and future. *Stroke and Vascular Neurology* 2(4): e000101. doi:10.1136/svn-2017-000101

Johansson, V., Garwicz, M., Kanje, M., Schouenborg, J., Tingström, A., & Görman, U. (2011). Authenticity, depression, and deep brain stimulation. *Frontiers in Integrative Neuroscience* 5, 21.

Johnson, S. C., Baxter, L. C., Wilder, L. S., Pipe, J. G., Heiserman, J. E., and Prigatano, G. P. (2002). Neural correlates of self-reflection. *Brain* 125: 1808–14.

Jonas, H. (1966). *The Phenomenon of Life: Toward a Philosophical Biology*. Evanston, IL: Northwestern University Press.

Jonides, J., Naveh-Benjamin, M. & Palmer, J. (1985). Assessing automaticity. *Acta Psychologica* 60(2–3): 157–71.

Jørgensen, C. R. (2006). Disturbed sense of identity in borderline personality disorder. *Journal of Personality Disorders* 20(6): 618–44.

Jørgensen, C. R., Berntsen, D., Bech, M., Kjølbye, M., Bennedsen, B. E. & Ramsgaard, S. B. (2012). Identity-related autobiographical memories and cultural life scripts in patients with borderline personality disorder. *Consciousness and Cognition* 21(2): 788–98. https://doi.org/10.1016/j.concog.2012.01.010

Josipovic, Z. & Miskovic, V. (2020). Nondual awareness and minimal phenomenal experience. *Frontiers in Psychology* 11: 2087. doi.org/10.3389/fpsyg.2020.02087

Junghaenel, D., Smyth, J. M. & Santner, L. (2008). Linguistic dimensions of psychopathology: A quantitative analysis. *Journal of Social & Clinical Psychology* 27(1): 36–55.

Kabat-Zinn, J. (2013). *Full catastrophe living: Using the wisdom of your body and mind to face stress, pain, and illness*. New York: Bantam.

Kalckert, A. & Ehrsson, H. H. (2012). Moving a rubber hand that feels like your own: A dissociation of ownership and agency. *Frontiers in Human Neuroscience* 6: 40.

Karmarkar, U. R. & Buonomano, D. V. (2007). Timing in the absence of clocks: Encoding time in neural network states. *Neuron* 53: 427–38.

Kasari, C., Sigman, M., Mundy, P. & Yirmiya, N. (1990). Affective sharing in the context of joint attention interactions of normal, autistic, and mentally retarded children. *Journal of Autism and Developmental Disorders* 20(1): 87–100.

Kashdan, T. B. & Rottenberg, J. (2010). Psychological flexibility as a fundamental aspect of health. *Clinical Psychology Review* 30(7): 865–78.

Kaufmann, L. 1987. Self-reference and recursive forms. *Journal of Social and Biological Structure* 10: 53–72.

Kaur, M., Srinivasan, S. M. & Bhat, A. N. (2018). Comparing motor performance, praxis, coordination, and interpersonal synchrony between children with and without autism spectrum disorder (ASD). *Research in Developmental Disabilities* 72: 79–95. https://doi.org/10.1016/j.ridd.2017.10.025

Keefe, R. S., Lees-Roitman, S. E. & Dupre, R. L. (1997). Performance of patients with schizophrenia on a pen and paper visuospatial working memory task with short delay. *Schizophrenia Research* 26(1): 9–14.

Keleman, S. (1989). *Patterns of Distress: Emotional Insults and Human Form*. Berkeley, CA: Center Press.

Kelley, W. M., Macrae, C. N., Wyland, C. L., Caglar, S., Inati, S. & Heatherton, T. F. (2002). Finding the self? An event-related fMRI study. *Journal of Cognitive Neuroscience* 14: 785–94.

Kelly, B. D. (2018). Love as delusion, delusions of love: Erotomania, narcissism and shame. *Medical Humanities* 44(1): 15–19. doi:10.1136/medhum-2017-011198

Kelly, B. D. (2017). Hearing voices: Lessons from the history of psychiatry in Ireland. *Irish Medical Journal* 110(3): 537–7.

Kelso, J. A. S. (2020). Matter, movement and mind—The order is important. The B. F. Skinner Lecture, Association for Behavior Analysis International (ABAI) May 12. https://www.youtube.com/watch?v=27HIJwn16Co

Kelso, J. A. S. (2014). *Coordination dynamics and cognition*, in K. Davids, R. Hristovski, D. Araújo, N. Balagué Serre, C. Button, and P. Passos (eds), *Routledge Research in Sport and Exercise Science: Complex Systems in Sport* (18–43). London: Routledge/Taylor & Francis Group.

Kelso, J. A. S. (2009). Coordination dynamics, in R. A. Meyers (ed.), *Encyclopedia of Complexity and Systems Science* (1537–64). Heidelberg: Springer.

Kelso, J. A. S. (1995). *Dynamic Patterns*. Cambridge, MA: MIT Press.

Kelso, J. A. S., de Guzman, G. C., Reveley, C. & Tognoli, E. (2009). Virtual partner interaction (VPI): Exploring novel behaviors via coordination dynamics. *PLOS One* 4(6): e5749. https://doi.org/10.1371/journal.pone.0005749

Kelso, J. A. S., Saltzman, E. L. & Tuller, B. (1986). The dynamical perspective on speech production: Data and theory. *Journal of Phonetics* 14(1): 29–59.

Kelso, J. A. S. & Tognoli, E. (2009). Toward a complementary neuroscience: Metastable coordination dynamics of the brain, in N. Murphy, G. F. R. Ellis, and T. O'Connor (eds), *Downward Causation and the Neurobiology of Free Will* (103–24). Berlin: Springer.

Kelso, J. A. S., Tuller, B. & Fowler, C. A. (1982). The functional specificity of articulatory control and coordination. *The Journal of the Acoustical Society of America* 72(S1): S103–3.

Kendler, K. S. (2008). Disorders of agency in psychiatric syndromes, in K. S. Kendler and J. Parnas (eds), *Philosophical Issues in Psychiatry* (312–26). Baltimore: Johns Hopkins University Press.

Kendon, A. (1990). *Conducting Interaction: Patterns of Behavior in Focused Encounters*. Cambridge: Cambridge University Press.

Kerby, P. (1993). *Narrative and the Self*. Bloomington, IN: Indiana University Press.

Kernberg, O. F. (1985). *Borderline Conditions and Pathological Narcissism*. Rowman & Littlefield.

Keromnes, G., Motillon, T., Coulon, N., Berthoz, A., Du Boisgueheneuc, F., Wehrmann, M., Martin, B., Thirioux, B., Bonnot, O., Ridereau, R., Bellissant, E., Drapier, D., Levoyer, D., Jaafari, N. & Tordjman, S. (2018). Self-other recognition impairments in individuals with schizophrenia: A new experimental paradigm using a double mirror. *NPJ Schizophrenia* 4(1): 24. https://doi.org/10.1038/s41537-018-0065-5

Kertész, I. (2004). *Fatelessness*, trans. T. Wilkinson. New York: Knopf.

Killingsworth, M. A., & Gilbert, D. T. (2010). A wandering mind is an unhappy mind. *Science* 330, 932–932. http://dx.doi.org/10.1126/science.1192439

Kinnaird, E., Stewart, C. & Tchanturia, K. (2019). Investigating alexithymia in autism: A systematic review and meta-analysis. *European Psychiatry* 55: 80–9.

Kinsbourne, M. & Helt, M. (2011). Entrainment, mimicry, and interpersonal synchrony, in D. Fein (ed.), *The Neuropsychology of Autism* (339–65). Oxford: Oxford University Press.

Kircher, T. T. J., Senior, C., Phillips, M. L., Benson, P. J., Bullmore, E. T., Brammer, M., Simmons, A., Williams, S. C. R., Bartels, M. & David, A. S. (2000). Towards a functional neuroanatomy of self processing: Effects of faces and words. *Cognitive Brain Research* 10: 133–44.

Kirchhoff, M. (2017). From mutual manipulation to cognitive extension: Challenges and implications. *Phenomenology and the Cognitive Sciences* 16: 862–78. doi:10.1007/s11097-016-9483-x

Kirchhoff, M. (2015). Extended cognition and the causal-constitutive fallacy: In search for a diachronic and dynamical conception of constitution. *Philosophy and Phenomenological Research* 90(2): 320–60.

Kirchoff, M. D. & Froese, T. (2017). Where there is life there is mind: In support of a strong life-mind continuity thesis. *Entropy* 19(4): 169.

Kirk, S. A., Gomory, T. & Cohen, D. (2017). *Mad Science: Psychiatric Coercion, Diagnosis, and Drugs*. London & New York: Routledge.

Kiverstein, J., Rietveld, E. & Denys, D. (2021). World wide open. *Aeon*. https://aeon.co/essays/how-deep-brain-stimulation-changes-a-persons-sense-of-confidence?utm_source=Aeon%20Newsletter&utm_campaign=0e3bca95b6-EMAIL_CAMPAIGN_2021_07_05_01_15&utm_medium=email&utm_term=0_411a82e59d-0e3bca95b6-69406197&fbclid=IwAR1Yp7o0Lm-9DjmqCZeZbpvU_4CzT4jzI0t_qHRfboK7YBVMIM-riqtavmnE

Klaming, L. & Haselager, P. (2013). Did my brain implant make me do it? Questions raised by DBS regarding psychological continuity, responsibility for action and mental competence. *Neuroethics* 6: 527–39. doi:10.1007/s12152-010-9093-1; PMID24273622

Klerman, G. L., Vaillant, G. E., Spitzer, R. L., Michels, R. (1984). A debate on DSMIII. *American Journal of Psychiatry* 141: 539–53.

Klin, A., Jones, W., Schultz, R. & Volkmar, F. (2003). The enactive mind, or from actions to cognition: Lessons from autism. *Philosophical Transactions of the Royal Society of London. Series B: Biological Sciences* 358(1430): 345–60.

Kljajevic, V. (2021). *Consensual Illusion: The Mind in Virtual Reality*. Berlin: Springer Nature.

Knapp, T. (1988). *Westphal's "Die Agoraphobie" with Commentary: The Beginnings of Agoraphobia*, trans. M. T. Schumacher. Lanham: University Press of America.

Kobak, K. A., Dottl, S. L., Greist, J. H., Jefferson, J. W., Burroughs, D., Mantle, J. M., Katzelnick, D. J., Norton, R., Henk, H. J. & Serlin, R. C. (1997). A computer-administered telephone interview to identify mental disorders. *JAMA* 278(11): 905–10.

Koffka, K. (2013). *Principles of Gestalt psychology*. London: Routledge.

Korsgaard, C. M. (1996). *The Sources of Normativity*. Cambridge: Cambridge University Press.

Kostrubiec, V., Huys, R., Jas, B. & Kruck, J. (2018). Age-dependent relationship between socio-adaptability and motor coordination in high functioning children with autism spectrum disorder. *Journal of Autism and Developmental Disorders* 48(1): 209–24.

Kotov, R., Krueger, R. F., Watson, D., Achenbach, T. M., Althoff, R. R., Bagby, R. M., Brown, T. A., Carpenter, W. T., Caspi, A., Clark, L. A., Eaton, N. R., Forbes, M. K., Forbush, K. T., Goldberg, D., Hasin, D., Hyman, S. E., Ivanova, M. Y., Lynam, D. R., Markon, K. . . . Zimmerman, M. (2017). The Hierarchical Taxonomy of Psychopathology

(HiTOP): A dimensional alternative to traditional nosologies. *Journal of Abnormal Psychology* 4(4): 454–77. https://doi.org/10.1037/abn0000258

Koutsouleris, N., Kahn, R. S., Chekroud, A. M., Leucht, S., Falkai, P., Wobrock, T., Derks, E. M., Fleischhacker, W. W. & Hasan, A. (2016). Multisite prediction of 4-week and 52-week treatment outcomes in patients with first-episode psychosis: A machine learning approach. *The Lancet Psychiatry* 3: 935–46.

Kozáková, E., Bakštein, E., Havlíček, O., Bečev, O., Knytl, P., Zaytseva, Y. & Španiel, F. (2020). Disrupted sense of agency as a state marker of first-episode schizophrenia: A large-scale follow-up study. *Frontiers in Psychiatry* 11: 570570. doi:10.3389/fpsyt.2020.570570

Krackow E. (2010). Narratives distinguish experienced from imagined childhood events. *American Journal of Psychology* 123(1): 71–80.

Kraemer F. (2013). Me, myself and my brain implant: Deep brain stimulation raises questions of personal authenticity and alienation. *Neuroethics* 6:483–97. doi:10.1007/s12152-011-9115-7

Kraepelin, E. (1910). *Psychiatrie. Ein Lehrbuch für Studierende und Ärzte. Achte, vollständig umgearbeitete Auflage, Vol. 2: Klinische Psychiatrie, Part 1.* Leipzig: Barth.

Kraepelin, E. (1893). *Psychiatrie. Ein kurzes Lehrbuch für Studirende und Aerzte*, 4th edn, completely revised. Leipzig: Abel.

Kraepelin, E. (1887). *Psychiatrie. Ein kurzes Lehrbuch für Studirende und Aerzte*, 2nd edn, completely revised. Leipzig: Abel, 1887.

Krauss, L. M. (1995). *The Physics of Star Trek.* New York: Basic Books.

Krickel, B. (2018). Saving the mutual manipulability account of constitutive relevance. *Studies in History and Philosophy of Science Part A* 68: 58–67.

Krickel, B. (2017). Making sense of interlevel causation in mechanisms from a metaphysical perspective. *Journal for General Philosophy of Science/Zeitschrift für Allgemeine Wissenschaftstheorie* 48(3): 453–68.

Kronsted, C., Tollefsen, D., Gallagher, S. & Windsor, L. (2023). An enactivist account of the dynamics of lying. *Adaptive Behavior.* Online. https://doi.org/10.1177/10597123231166421

Krueger, J. (2021). Enactivism, other minds, and mental disorders. *Synthese* 198(1): 365–89.

Krueger, J. (2011). The who and the how of experience, in M. Siderits, E. Thompson, and D. Zahavi (eds), *Self, No Self? Perspectives from Analytical, Phenomenological, and Indian Traditions* (27–55). Oxford: Oxford University Press.

Krueger, J. & Maiese, M. (2018). Mental institutions, habits of mind, and an extended approach to autism. *Thaumàzein|Rivista di Filosofia* 6: 10–41.

Krueger, J. & Michael, J. (2012). Gestural coupling and social cognition: Möbius Syndrome as a case study. *Frontiers in Human Neuroscience* 6: 81.

Krueger, J. & Szanto, T. (2016). Extended emotions. *Philosophy Compass* 11(12): 863–78.

Krugwasser, A. R., Stern, Y., Faivre, N., Harel, E. V. & Salomon, R. (2021). Impaired sense of agency and associated confidence in psychosis. *HAL, Nature Publishing Group.* hal-03318445. https://hal.archives-ouvertes.fr/hal-03318445/document

Kühn, S., Nenchev, I., Haggard, P., Brass, M., Gallinat, J., et al. (2011) Whodunnit? Electrophysiological correlates of agency judgements. *PLOS One* 6: e28657.

Kurzweil, R. (2005). *The Singularity Is Near: When Humans Transcend Biology.* New York: Viking.

Kyselo, M. (2016). The minimal self needs a social update. *Philosophical Psychology* 29(7): 1057–65.

Kyselo, M. (2014). The body social: An enactive approach to the self. *Frontiers in Psychology* 5: doi10. 3389/fpsyg.2014.00986

Laakasuo, M., Drosinou, M., Koverola, M., Kunnari, A., Halonen, J., Lehtonen, N. & Palomäki, J. (2018). What makes people approve or condemn mind upload technology? Untangling the effects of sexual disgust, purity and science fiction familiarity. *Palgrave Communications* 4(1): 1–14.

Ladyman, J., Ross, D., Collier, J., Spurrett, D., Spurrett, D. & Collier, J. G. (2007). *Every Thing Must Go: Metaphysics Naturalized*. Oxford: Oxford University Press.

Lafargue, G., Paillard, J., Lamarre, Y., and Sirigu, Y. (2003). Production and perception of grip force without proprioception: Is there a sense of effort in deafferented subjects? *European Journal of Neuroscience* 17(12): 2741–9.

Lafleur, A., Soulières, I. & d'Arc, B. F. (2020). Sense of agency: Sensorimotor signals and social context are differentially weighed at implicit and explicit levels. *Consciousness and Cognition* 84: 103004.

Lakin, J. & Chartrand, T. L. (2003). Using nonconscious behavioral mimicry to create affiliation and rapport. *Psychological Science* 14: 334–9.

Langland-Hassan, P. (2008). Fractured phenomenologies: Thought insertion, inner speech, and the puzzle of extraneity. *Mind & Language* 23(4): 369–401.

Larkin, F., Hobson, J. A., Hobson, R. P. & Tolmie, A. (2017). Collaborative competence in dialogue: Pragmatic language impairment as a window onto the psychopathology of autism. *Research in Autism Spectrum Disorders* 43: 27–39.

Lavenne-Collot, N., Maubant, E., Deroulez, S., Bronsard, G., Botbol, M. & Berthoz, A. (2022). Self/other recognition and distinction in adolescents with anorexia nervosa: A double mirror paradigm. *Research Square Preprint*. https://doi.org/10.21203/rs.3.rs-1943634/v2

Lavenne-Collot, N., Tersiguel M., Dissaux N., Degrez C., Bronsard G., Botbol M. & Berthoz A. (2023). Self/other distinction in adolescents with autism spectrum disorder (ASD) assessed with a double mirror paradigm. *PLOS One* 18(3): e0275018.

Layton, A. S. F. & Sherrington, C. S. (1917). Observations on the excitable cortex of the chimpanzee, orangutan and gorilla. *Quarterly Journal of Experimental Physiology* 11: 135–222.

Leach-Scully, J. (2012). Disability and the thinking body, in S. Gonzalez-Arnal, G. Jagger, and K. Lennon (eds), *Embodied Selves* (139–59). London: Palgrave Macmillan.

Leder, D. (2018) Coping with chronic pain, illness and incarceration: what patients and prisoners have to teach each other (and all of us). *Medical Humanities* 44(2): 113–119.

Leder, D. (1984). Toward a phenomenology of pain. *Review of Existential Psychology & Psychiatry* 19(2–3): 255–66.

LeDoux, J. 2002. *The Synaptic Self*. New York: Penguin Putnam.

Leentjens, A. F. G., Visser-vandewalle, V., Temel, Y. & Verhey, F. R. J. (2004). Manipuleerbare wilsbekwaamheid: een ethisch probleem bij elektrostimulatie van de nucleus subthalamicus voor ernstige ziekte van Parkinson. [Manipulation of mental competence: An ethical problem in case of electrical stimulation of the subthalamic nucleus for severe Parkinson's disease]. *Nederlands Tijdschrift Geneeskunde* 148(28): 1394–8. PMID15291423

Leezenbaum, N. B. & Iverson, J. M. (2019). Trajectories of posture development in infants with and without familial risk for autism spectrum disorder. *Journal of Autism and Developmental Disorders* 49(8): 3257–77.

Legault, M., Bourdon, J. N. & Poirier, P. (2019). Neurocognitive variety in neurotypical environments: The source of "deficit" in autism. *Journal of Behavioral and Brain Science* 9(6): 246.

Legrand D. & Ruby P. (2009). What is self specific? A theoretical investigation and a critical review of neuroimaging results. *Psychological Review* 116(1): 252–82.

Lenggenhager, B., Tadi, T., Metzinger, T. & Blanke, O. (2007). Video ergo sum: Manipulating bodily self-consciousness. *Science* 317: 1096–9.

Lenzo, E. & Gallagher, S. (2021). Intrinsic temporality in depression, in C. Tewes and G. Stanghellini (eds), *Time, Body and the Other: Phenomenological and Psychopathologial Approaches* (289–310). Cambridge: Cambridge University Press.

Leong, V. & Schilbach, L. (2019). The promise of two-person neuroscience for developmental psychiatry: Using interaction-based sociometrics to identify disorders of social interaction. *British Journal of Psychiatry* 215(5): 636–8. https://doi.org/10.1192/bjp.2019.73

Leuridan, B. (2012). Three problems for the mutual manipulability account of constitutive relevance in mechanisms. *British Journal for the Philosophy of Science* 63: 399–427.

Levi, P. (1993). *The Drowned and the Saved*, trans. R. Rosenthal. London: Abacus.

Levi, P. (1959). *If This Is a Man*, trans. S. Woolf. New York: The Orion Press.

Levin, A. R., Zeanah Jr, C. H., Fox, N. A. & Nelson, C. A. (2014). Motor outcomes in children exposed to early psychosocial deprivation. *The Journal of Pediatrics* 164(1): 123–9.

Lewis, M. D. & Todd, R. M. (2007). The self-regulating brain: Cortical-subcortical feedback and the development of intelligent action. *Cognitive Development* 22(4): 406–30.

Lewontin, R. (1982). *The Dialectical Biologist*. Cambridge, MA: MIT Press.

Li, W., Garland, E. L., McGovern, P., O'Brien, J. E., Tronnier, C. & Howard, M. O. (2017). Mindfulness-oriented recovery enhancement for internet gaming disorder in US adults: A stage I randomized controlled trial. *Psychology of Addictive Behaviors* 31(4): 393.

Liesner, M., Hinz, N.-A., and Kunde, W. (2021). How action shapes body ownership momentarily and throughout the lifespan. *Frontiers in Human Neuroscience* 15: 697810. doi: 10.3389/fnhum.2021.697810

Limanowski, J. & Blankenburg, F. (2013). Minimal self-models and the free energy principle. *Frontiers in Human Neuroscience* 7, 547: 1–12. https://doi.org/10.3389/fnhum.2013.00547

Lindahl, J. R. & Britton, W. (2019). "I have this feeling of not really being here": Buddhist meditation and changes in the sense of self. *Journal of Consciousness Studies* 26(7–8): 157–83.

Lindahl, J. R., Cooper, D. J., Fisher, N. E., Kirmayer, L. J. & Britton, W. B. (2020). Progress or pathology? Differential diagnosis and intervention criteria for meditation-related challenges: Perspectives from Buddhist meditation teachers and practitioners. *Frontiers in Psychology* 11: 1905.

Lindblom, J., & Ziemke, T. (2008). Interacting socially through embodied action. In F. Morganti, A. Carassa & G. Riva, *Enacting Intersubjectivity: A Cognitive and Social Perspective on the Study of Interactions* (49-63). Amsterdam: IOS Press.

Lindemann, H. (2014). Second nature and the tragedy of Alzheimer's, in L.-C. Hydén, H. Lindemann, and J. Brockmeier (eds), *Beyond Loss: Dementia, Memory and Identity* (11–23). Oxford: Oxford University Press.

Ling, Y. R. & Liu, L. H. (2008). Body narrative in Western modernist literature. *Journal of Southwest University (Social Sciences Edition)* 3: 034.

Linson, A. & Friston, K. (2019). Reframing PTSD for computational psychiatry with the active inference framework. *Cognitive Neuropsychiatry* 24(5): 347–68.

Lipsman, N. I. R. & Glannon, W. (2013). Brain, mind and machine: What are the implications of deep brain stimulation for perceptions of personal identity, agency and free will? *Bioethics* 27(9): 465–70. doi:10.1111/j.1467-8519.2012.01978.x; PMID22681593

Locke, J. (1690). *An Essay Concerning Human Understanding*, ed. P. H. Nidditch. Oxford: Clarendon, 1979.

López-Silva, P. (2021). Atribuciones de agencia mental y el desafío desde la psicopatología. *Kriterion: Revista de Filosofia* 61(147): 835–50.

López-Silva, P. (2019). Me and I are not friends, just aquaintances: On thought insertion and self-awareness. *Review of Philosophy and Psychology* 10(2): 319–35.

Lorimer, F. (1929). *The Growth of Reason: A Study of the Role of Verbal Activity in the Growth of the Structure of the Human Mind.* London & New York: Routledge.

Lothe, J. (2000). *Narrative in Fiction and Film.* Oxford: Oxford University Press.

Lou, H. C., Luber, B., Crupain, M., Keenan, J. P., Nowak, M., Kjaer, T. W., et al. (2004). Parietal cortex and representation of the mental self. *Proceedings of the National Academy of Sciences*, USA 101: 6827–32.

Ludwig, A. M. 1975. The psychiatrist as physician. *Journal of the American Medical Association* 234: 603.

Luhrmann, T. M. (2006). Subjectivity. *Anthropological Theory* 6(3): 345–61.

Lutz, A., Jha, A. P., Dunne, J. D. & Saron, C. D. (2015). Investigating the phenomenological matrix of mindfulness-related practices from a neurocognitive perspective. *American Psychologist* 70(7): 632–58.

Luxton, D. D. (2014). Artificial intelligence in psychological practice: Current and future applications and implications. *Professional Psychology: Research and Practice* 45(5): 332.

Lysaker, P. H., Clements, C. A., Plascak-Hallberg, C., Knipschure, S. J. & Wright, D. E. (2002). Insight and personal narratives of illness in schizophrenia. *Psychiatry* 65: 197–206.

Lysaker, P. H., Davis, L. W., Eckert, G. J., Strasburger, A. M., Hunter, N. L. & Buck, K. D. (2005). Changes in narrative structure and content in schizophrenia in long-term individual psychotherapy: A single case study. *Clinical Psychology and Psychotherapy* 12: 406–16.

Lysaker, P. H. & Lysaker, J. T. (2002). Narrative structure in psychosis: Schizophrenia and disruptions in the dialogical self. *Theory and Psychology* 12(2): 207–20.

Lysaker, P. H., Wickett, A. & Davis, L. (2005). Narrative qualities in schizophrenia: Associations with impairments in neurocognition and negative symptoms. *Journal of Nervous & Mental Disease* 193(4): 244–9.

MacKay, D. M. (1980). The interdependence of mind and brain. *Neuroscience* 5: 1389–91.

MacKay, D. M. (1979). Reply to Bunge. *Neuroscience* 4: 454.

MacKay, D. M. (1978). Selves and brains. *Neuroscience* 3: 599–606.

Mackinger, H. F., Pachinger, M. M., Leibetseder, M. M. & Fartacek, R. R. (2000). Autobiographical memories in women remitted from major depression. *Journal of Abnormal Psychology* 109(2): 331–4.

Mackenzie C. (2007). Bare personhood? Velleman on selfhood. *Philosophical Explorations* 10(3): 263–81.

Mackenzie, C. (2000). Imagining oneself otherwise, in C. Mackenzie and N. Stoljar (eds), *Relational Autonomy: Feminist Perspectives on Automony, Agency, and the Social Self* (124–50). Oxford: Oxford University Press.

Mackenzie, C. & Stoljar, N. (2000). Introduction: Autonomy refigured, in C. Mackenzie and N. Stoljar (eds), *Relational Autonomy: Feminist Perspectives on Automony, Agency, and the Social Self* (3–31). Oxford: Oxford University Press.

Mackenzie, M. (2011). Enacting the self: Buddhist and enactivist approaches to the emergence of the self, in M. Siderits, E. Thompson, and D. Zahavi (eds), *Self, No Self? Perspectives from Analytical, Phenomenological, and Indian traditions* (239–73). Oxford: Oxford University Press.

Macpherson, M. C., Marie, D., Schön, S. & Miles, L. K. (2020). Evaluating the interplay between subclinical levels of mental health symptoms and coordination dynamics. *British Journal of Psychology* 111(4): 782–804.

Madeira, L., Carmenates, S., Costa, C., et al. (2017). Rejoinder to commentary: Panic, self-disorder, and EASE research: Methodological considerations. *Psychopathology* 50: 228–30.

Madsen, J. K. (2017). Time during time: Multi-scalar temporal cognition, in S. J. Cowley, F. Vallée-Tourangeau, and F. Vallée-Tourangeau (eds), *Cognition beyond the Brain* (155–74). Cham: Springer International Publishing.

Magai, C., Cohen, C., Gomberg, D., Malatesta, C., and Culver, C. (1996). Emotional expression during mid- to late-stage dementia. *International Psychogeriatrics* 8(3): 383–95.

Maguire, E. A., Frith, C. D. & Morris, R. G. M. (1999). The functional neuroanatomy of comprehension and memory: The importance of prior knowledge. *Brain* 122(10): 1839–50.

Maiese, M. (2022). *Autonomy, Enactivism, and Mental Disorder: A Philosophical Account.* London: Routledge.

Maiese, M. (2021). An enactivist reconceptualization of the medical model. *Philosophical Psychology*, doi: 10.1080/09515089.2021.1940119

Maiese, M. (2018). Embodiment, sociality and the life-shaping thesis. *Phenomenology and the Cognitive Sciences* 18(2): 353–74.

Malafouris, L. (2013). *How Things Shape the Mind.* Cambridge, MA: MIT Press.

Malafouris, L. (2008). Between brains, bodies and things: Tectonoetic awareness and the extended self. *Philosophical Transactions of the Royal Society B* 363: 1993–2002.

Manning, M. (1994). *Undercurrents: A Life beneath the Surface.* San Francisco: HarperCollins.

Marcel, A. (2003). The sense of agency: Awareness and ownership of action, in J. Roessler and N. Eilan (eds), *Agency and Awarness* (48–93). Oxford: Oxford University Press.

Marcel, A. J. (1992). The personal level in cognitive rehabilitation, in N. Von Steinbüchel, E. Pöppel, and D. Cramon (eds), *Neuropsychological Rehabilitation.* Berlin: Springer.

Marcus, G. & Davis, E. (2019). *Rebooting AI: Building Artificial Intelligence We Can Trust.* New York: Pantheon.

Marmelat, V. & Delignières, D. (2012). Strong anticipation: Complexity matching in interpersonal coordination. *Experimental Brain Research* 222: 137–48. doi:10.1007/s00221-012-3202-9

Marotta, A., Bombieri, F., Zampini, M., Schena, F., Dallocchio, C., Fiorio, M. & Tinazzi, M. (2017). The moving rubber hand illusion reveals that explicit sense of agency for tapping movements is preserved in functional movement disorders. *Frontiers in Human Neuroscience* 11: 291.

Marsh, K. L., Isenhower, R. W., Richardson, M. J., Helt, M., Verbalis, A. D., Schmidt, R. C. & Fein, D. (2013) Autism and social disconnection in interpersonal rocking. *Frontiers of Integrative Neuroscience* 7:4. doi:10.3389/fnint.2013.00004

Martin, M. G. F. (1995). Bodily awareness: A sense of ownership, in J. L. Bermúdez, T. Marcel, and N. Eilan (eds), *The Body and the Self* (267–89). Cambridge, MA: MIT Press.

Martino, F., Menchetti, M., Pozzi, E. & Berardi, D. (2012). Predictors of dropout among personality disorders in a specialist outpatients psychosocial treatment: a preliminary study. *Psychiatry and Clinical Neurosciences* 66(3): 180–6. https://doi.org/10.1111/j.1440-1819.2012.02329.x

Mathews, D. J. (2011). Deep brain stimulation, personal identity and policy. *International Review of Psychiatry* 23(5): 486–92. doi:10.3109/09540261.2011.632624; PMID22200138

Maturana, H. & Varela, F. J. (1980). *Autopoiesis and Cognition: The Realization of the Living*. Dordrecht, The Netherlands: D. Reidel.

Maung, H. H. (2021). Causation and causal selection in the biopsychosocial model of health and disease. *European Journal of Analytic Philosophy* 17(2): M5–27.

Mauss, M. (1979). *Sociology and Psychology: Essays*. London: Routledge & Kegan Paul.

Mazefsky, C. A., Herrington, J., Siegel, M., Scarpa, A., Maddox, B. B., Scahill, L. & White, S. W. (2013). The role of emotion regulation in autism spectrum disorder. *Journal of the American Academy of Child & Adolescent Psychiatry* 52(7): 679–88.

McCulloch, W. S. 1965. *Embodiments of Mind*. Cambridge, MA: MIT Press.

McDougal, M. S., Lasswell, H. D. & Chen, L. (1980). *Human Rights and World Public Order: The Basic Policies of an International Law of Human Dignity*. New Haven: Yale University Press.

McGeer, V. (2001). Psycho-practice, psycho-theory and the contrastive case of autism: How practices of mind become second nature. *Journal of Consciousness Studies* 8(5–6): 109–32.

McIntyre, A. (1981). *After Virtue: A Study in Moral Theory*. Notre Dame: University of Notre Dame Press.

McLean, K. C., Syed, M., Pasupathi, M., Adler, J. M., Dunlop, W. L., Drustrup, D....& McCoy, T. P. (2020). The empirical structure of narrative identity: The initial Big Three. *Journal of Personality and Social Psychology* 119(4): 920.

McNamara, D. S., Louwerse, M. M., Cai, Z. & Graesser, A. C. (2005). Coh-Metrix Version 1.4. Software retrieved Feb 8, 2007, from http//:cohmetrix.memphis.edu.

McTaggart, J. M. E. (1908). The unreality of time. *Mind* 17 (New Series, no. 68): 457–74.

Mead, G. H. (1962). *Mind, Self and Society: From the Standpoint of a Social Behaviorist*. Chicago: University of Chicago Press.

Mead, G. H. (1913). The social self. *The Journal of Philosophy, Psychology and Scientific Methods* 10(14): 374–80.

Meincke, A. S. (2019). Autopoiesis, biological autonomy and the process view of life. *European Journal for Philosophy of Science* 9(1): 1–16.

Menary, R. (2008). Embodied narratives. *Journal of Consciousness Studies* 15(6): 63–84.

Mendoça, D. (2012). Pattern of sentiment: following a Deweyan suggestion. *Trans. C. S. Peirce Society* 48: 209–227. doi:10.2979/ trancharpeirsoc.48.2.209

Merleau-Ponty, M. (2012). *Phenomenology of Perception*, trans. D. A. Landes. London: Routledge.

Merleau-Ponty, M. (1963). *The Structure of Behavior*, trans. A. Fisher. Boston: Beacon.

Metzinger, T. (2020). Minimal phenomenal experience: Meditation, tonic alertness, and the phenomenology of "pure" consciousness. *Philosophy and the Mind Sciences* 1(1): 1–44.

Metzinger, T. (2014). How does the brain encode epistemic reliability? Perceptual presence, phenomenal transparency, and counterfactual richness. *Cognitive Neuroscience* 5(2): 122–4.

Metzinger, T. (2013). The myth of cognitive agency: Subpersonal thinking as a cyclically recurring loss of mental autonomy. *Frontiers in Psychology* 4: 1–19. doi:10.3389/fpsyg.2013.00931

Metzinger, T. (2009). *The Ego Tunnel: The Science of the Mind and the Myth of the Self*. New York: Basic Books.

Metzinger, T. (2004). *Being No One: The Self-Model Theory of Subjectivity*. Cambridge, MA: MIT Press.

Meyer, M. & Hunnius, S. (2021). Neural processing of self-produced and externally generated events in 3-month-old infants. *Journal of Experimental Child Psychology* 204: 105039.

Michalak, J., Mischnat, J. & Teismann, T. (2014). Sitting posture makes a difference—embodiment effects on depressive memory bias. *Clinical Psychology & Psychotherapy* 21(6): 519–24.

Michalak, J., Rohde, K. & Troje, N. F. (2015). How we walk affects what we remember: Gait modifications through biofeedback change negative affective memory bias. *Journal of Behavior Therapy and Experimental Psychiatry* 46: 121–5.

Miles, L. K., Nind, L. K. & Macrae, C. N. (2009). The rhythm of rapport: Interpersonal synchrony and social perception. *Journal of Experimental Social Psychology* 45: 585–9.

Milgram, P. & Kishino, F. (1994). A taxonomy of mixed reality visual displays. *IEICE Transactions on Information and Systems* 77(12): 1321–9.

Miller, G. R. & Stiff, J. B. (1993). *Deceptive Communication*. Washington DC: Sage Publications.

Miller, M. & Clark, A. (2018). Happily entangled: Prediction, emotion, and the embodied mind. *Synthese* 195(6): 2559–75.

Millière, R., Carhart-Harris, R. L., Roseman, L., Trautwein, F.-M. & Berkovich-Ohana, A. (2018). Psychedelics, meditation, and self-consciousness. *Frontiers in Psychology* 9. https://doi.org/10.3389/fpsyg.2018.01475

Millière, R. & Newen, A. (2022). Selfless memories. *Erkenntnis* 1–22. Online. https://doi.org/10.1007/s10670-022-00562-6

Milojevic, M. (2020). Extended mind, functionalism, and personal identity. *Synthese* 197: 2143–70.

Milton, A. & Pleydell-Pearce, C. W. (2016). The phase of pre-stimulus alpha oscillations influences the visual perception of stimulus timing. *Neuroimage* 133: 53–61. doi:10.1016/j.neuroimage.2016.02.065pmid:26924284

Milton, D. E. M. (2012). On the ontological status of autism: The "double empathy problem." *Disability & Society* 27: 883–7. doi: 10.1080/09687599.2012.710008

Minkowski, E. (1970). *Lived Time: Phenomenological and Psychological Studies*, trans. N. Metzel. Evanston, IL: Northwestern University Press.

Mitchell, S. D. (2009). *Unsimple Truths: Science, Complexity and Policy*. Chicago: University of Chicago Press.

Mlakar, J., Jensterle, J. & Frith, C. D. (1994). Central monitoring deficiency and schizophrenic symptoms. *Psychological Medicine* 24(3): 557–64.

Möller, T. J., Georgie, Y. K., Schillaci, G., Voss, M., Hafner, V. V. & Kaltwasser, L. (2021). Computational models of the "active self" and its disturbances in schizophrenia. *Consciousness and Cognition* 93: 103155.

Montero, B. G. (2015). Thinking in the zone: The expert mind in action. *The Southern Journal of Philosophy* 53(S1): 126–40.

Moran, R. (2004). Precis of authority and estrangement: An essay on self-knowledge. *Philosophy and Phenomenological Research* 69(2): 423–6.

Moore, G. E. (1903). The refutation of idealism. *Mind* 12(48): 433–53.

Moore, J. W. & Obhi, S. S. (2012). Intentional binding and the sense of agency: A review. *Consciousness and Cognition* 21(1): 546–61.

Moore, J. W., Schneider, S. A., Schwingenschuh, P., Moretto, G., Bhatia, K. P. & Haggard, P. (2010). Dopaminergic medication boosts action–effect binding in Parkinson's disease. *Neuropsychologia* 48(4): 1125–32.

Moore, J. W., Tang, T. C. W. & Cioffi, M. C. (2020). Schizotypy and the vicarious experience of agency. *Psychology of Consciousness: Theory, Research, and Practice* 8(1): 65–73. https://doi.org/10.1037/cns0000225

Moore, J. W., Wegner, D. M. & Haggard, P. (2009). Modulating the sense of agency with external cues. *Consciousness and Cognition* 18(4): 1056–64. http://doi.org/10.1016/j.concog.2009.05.004

Morgan, C., Hazlett, G. M., Wang, S., Richardson, G., Schnurr, P. & Southwick, S. (2001). Symptoms of dissociation in humans experiencing acute, uncontrollable stress: A prospective investigation. *American Journal of Psychiatry* 158: 1239–47.

Morishita, T., Fayad, S. M., Higuchi, M. A., Nestor, K. A. & Foote, K. D. (2014). Deep brain stimulation for treatment-resistant depression: Systematic review of clinical outcomes. *Neurotherapeutics* 11(3): 475–84. doi:10.1007/s13311-014-0282-1; PMID24867326

Morris, L. & Mansell, W. (2018). A systematic review of the relationship between rigidity/flexibility and transdiagnostic cognitive and behavioral processes that maintain psychopathology. *Journal of Experimental Psychopathology* 9(3): 1–40 doi:10.1177/2043808718779431

Morrison, K. E., DeBrabander, K. M., Jones, D. R., Ackerman, R. A. & Sasson, N. J. (2020). Social cognition, social skill, and social motivation minimally predict social interaction outcomes for autistic and non-autistic adults. *Frontiers in Psychology* 11: 591100. doi:10.3389/fpsyg.2020.591100

Moseley, G. L., Olthof, N., Venema, A., Don, S., Wijers, M., Gallace, A. & Spence C. (2008). Psychologically induced cooling of a specific body part caused by the illusory ownership of an artificial counterpart. *Proceedings of the National Academy of Sciences of the United States of America* 105: 13169–73.

Mrazek, M. D., Smallwood, J. & Schooler, J. W. (2012). Mindfulness and mind-wandering: Finding convergence through opposing constructs. *Emotion* 12(3): 442.

Müller, B. C., Kühn, S., van Baaren, R. B., Dotsch, R., Brass, M. & Dijksterhuis, A. (2011). Perspective taking eliminates differences in co-representation of out-group members' actions. *Experimental Brain Research* 211(3): 423–8.

Müller, O., Bittner, U. & Krug, H. (2010). Narrative Identität bei Therapie mit 'Hirnschrittmacher'. *Ethik in der Medizin* 22(4): 303–15.

Müller, S. & Christen, M. (2011). Deep brain stimulation in Parkinsonian patients—Ethical evaluation of cognitive, affective, and behavioral sequelae. *American Journal of Behavioral Neuroscience* 2(1): 3–13.

Mundale, J. & Gallagher, S. (2009). Delusional experience, in J. Bickle (ed.), *Oxford Handbook of Philosophy and Neuroscience* (513–21). Oxford: Oxford University Press.

Murphy, A. (2008). Feminism and race theory, in R. Diprose and J. Reynolds (eds), *Merleau-Ponty: Key Concepts* (197–206). London: Routledge.

Murphy, D. P. (2008). Levels of explanation in psychiatry, in K. S. Kendler and J. Parnas (eds), *Philosophical Issues in Psychiatry* (99–124). Baltimore: Johns Hopkins University Press.

Murray, L. & Trevarthen, C. (1985). Emotional regulation of interactions between two-month-olds and their mothers, in T. Field and N. A. Fox (eds.), *Social Perception in Infants* (177–97). New York: Ablex Publishing Corporation.

Nagaraj, B., Al-Turjman, F., Mascella, R. & Deng, Y. (eds) (2022). Artificial intelligence applications in mobile virtual reality technology. Special issue of *Wireless Communications and Mobile Computing*. https://www.hindawi.com/journals/wcmc/si/724104/page/1/

Ñāṇananda, B. (1997). *Concept and Reality in the Buddhist Thought*. Kandy: BPS.

Natorp, P. (1888). *Einleitung in die Psychologie nach kritischer Methode*. Freiburg i.b: Mohr.

Nave, O., Trautwein, F. M., Ataria, Y., Dor-Ziderman, Y., Schweitzer, Y., Fulder, S. & Berkovich-Ohana, A. (2021). Self-boundary dissolution in meditation: A phenomenological investigation. *Brain Sciences* 11(6): 819.

Neimeyer, R. A. (2016). Meaning reconstruction in the wake of loss: Evolution of a research program. *Behaviour Change* 33(2), 65–79.

Neimeyer, R. A. (2004). Fostering posttraumatic growth: A narrative elaboration. *Psychological Inquiry* 15(1): 53–9.

Neisser, U. (1991). Two perceptually given aspects of the self and their development. *Developmental Review* 11(3): 197–209.

Neisser, U. (1988). Five kinds of self-knowledge. *Philosophical Psychology* 1: 35–59.

Nekovarova, T., Fajnerova, I., Horacek, J. & Spaniel, F. (2014) Bridging disparate symptoms of schizophrenia: A triple network dysfunction theory. *Frontiers in Behavioral Neuroscience* 8: 171. doi: 10.3389/fnbeh.2014.00171

Nelson, B., Lavoie, S., Li, E., Sass, L. A., Koren, D., McGorry, P. D., Jack, B.N., Parnas, J., Polari, A., Allott, K. and Hartmann, J.A. & Whitford, T. J. (2020). The neurophenomenology of early psychosis: an integrative empirical study. *Consciousness and Cognition* 77, 102845.

Nelson, K. (2009). Narrative practices and folk psychology: A perspective from developmental psychology. *Journal of Consciousness Studies* 16(6–8): 69–93.

Nelson K. (2003). Narrative and the emergence of a consciousness of self, in G. D. Fireman, T. E. J. McVay, and O. Flanagan (eds), *Narrative and Consciousness* (17–36). Oxford: Oxford University Press.

Newen, A. (2018). The embodied self, the pattern theory of self, and the predictive mind. *Frontiers in Psychology* 9: 2270.

Newen, A., De Bruin, L. & Gallagher, S. (2018). *The Oxford Handbook of 4E Cognition*. Oxford: Oxford University Press.

Newen, A., Welpinghus, A. & Juckel, G. (2015). Emotion recognition as pattern recognition: The relevance of perception. *Mind & Language* 30(2): 187–208.

Nielsen, K. & Ward, T. (2020). Mental disorder as both natural and normative: Developing the normative dimension of the 3E conceptual framework for psychopathology. *Journal of Theoretical and Philosophical Psychology*, 40(2): 107–23.

Nijenhuis, E. R. & Van der Hart, O. (2011). Dissociation in trauma: A new definition and comparison with previous formulations. *Journal of Trauma & Dissociation* 12(4): 416–45.

Nijenhuis, E. R., Vanderlinden, J. & Spinhoven, P. (1998). Animal defensive reactions as a model for trauma-induced dissociative reactions. *Journal of Traumatic Stress* 11: 243–60.

Noël, X., Brevers, D. & Bechara, A. (2013). A neurocognitive approach to understanding the neurobiology of addiction. *Current Opinion in Neurobiology* 23(4): 632–8.

Northoff, G. & Bermpohl, F. (2004). Cortical midline structures and the self. *Trends in Cognitive Sciences* 8: 102–7.

Northoff, G., Heinzel, A., de Greck, M., Bennpohl, F., Dobrowolny, H., Panksepp, J. (2006). Self-referential processing in our brain: A meta-analysis of imaging studies on the self. *Neuroimage* 31: 440–57.

Northoff, G. & Panksepp, J. (2008). The trans-species concept of self and the subcortical–cortical midline system. *Trends in Cognitive Sciences* 12(7): 259–64.

Nyklíček, I., Hoogwegt, F. & Westgeest, T. (2015). Psychological distress across twelve months in patients with rheumatoid arthritis: The role of disease activity, disability, and mindfulness. *Journal of Psychosomatic Research* 78(2): 162–7.

Oakley, B. F., Jones, E. J., Crawley, D., Charman, T., Buitelaar, J., Tillmann, J., Murphy, D. G. & Loth, E. (2022). Alexithymia in autism: Cross-sectional and longitudinal associations with social-communication difficulties, anxiety and depression symptoms. *Psychological Medicine* 52(8): 1458–70. doi:10.1017/S0033291720003244

Øberg, G. K, Norman, B. & Gallagher, S. (2015). Embodied clinical reasoning in neurological physical therapy. *Physical Therapy: Theory and Practice* 31(4): 244–52. http://dx.doi.org/10.3109/09593985.2014.1002873

Oberman, L. M. & Ramachandran, V. S. (2007). The simulating social mind: The role of the mirror neuron system and simulation in the social and communicative deficits of autism spectrum disorders. *Psychological Bulletin* 133(2): 310–27.

O'Brien, S. (2004). *The Family Silver: A Memoir of Depression and Inheritance.* Chicago: University of Chicago Press.

Okun, M. S., Gallo, B. V., Mandybur, G., et al. (2012). Subthalamic deep brain stimulation with a constant-current device in Parkinson's disease: An open-label randomised controlled trial. *The Lancet Neurology* 11(2): 140–9. doi:10.1016/S1474-4422(11)70308-8; PMID22239915

Okun, M. S., Mann, G., Foote, K. D., et al. (2007). Deep brain stimulation in the internal capsule and nucleus accumbens region: Responses observed during active and sham programming. *Journal of Neurology, Neurosurgery & Psychiatry* 78(3): 310–14. doi:10.1136/jnnp.2006.095315; PMID17012341

Ola, L. & Gullon-Scott, F. (2020). Facial emotion recognition in autistic adult females correlates with alexithymia, not autism. *Autism* 24(8): 2021–34.

Ooms, P., Mantione, M., Figee, M., et al. (2014) Deep brain stimulation for obsessive-compulsive disorders: Long-term analysis of quality of life. *Journal of Neurology, Neurosurgery, and Psychiatry* 85: 153–8. doi: 10.1136/jnnp-2012-302550. PMID23715912

Opel, N., Redlich, R., Zwanzger, P., Grotegerd, D., Arolt, V., Heindel, W., Konrad, C., Kugel, H. & Dannlowski, U. (2014). Hippocampal atrophy in major depression: A function of childhood maltreatment rather than diagnosis? *Neuropsychopharmacology* 39: 2723–31.

Oppenheim, P. & Putnam, H. (1958). Unity of science as a working hypothesis. *Minnesota Studies in the Philosophy of Science* 2: 3–36.

Oren, E., Friedmann, N., & Dar, R. (2016). Things happen: Individuals with high obsessive-compulsive tendencies omit agency in their spoken language. *Consciousness and Cognition* 42, 125–34. doi: 10.1016/j.concog.2016.03.012

Otis, L. (1984). Adverse effects of transcendental meditation, in D. Shapiro and R. Walsh (eds), *Meditation: Classic and Contemporary Perspectives* (201–8). New York: Aldine.

Oullier, O., de Guzman, G. C., Jantzen, K. J., Lagarde, J. & Kelso, J. A. S. (2008). Social coordination dynamics: Measuring human bonding. *Social Neuroscience* 3(2): 178–92. doi:10.1080/17470910701563392

Pacherie, E. (2008). The phenomenology of action: A conceptual framework. *Cognition* 107 (1): 179–217.

Pacherie, E. (2007a). The sense of control and the sense of agency. *Psyche* 13(1): Online. https://journalpsyche.org/files/0xab10.pdf

Pacherie, E. (2007b). The anarchic hand syndrome and utilization behavior: A window onto agentive self-awareness. *Functional Neurology* 22(4): 211–17.

Pacherie, E. (2006). Towards a dynamic theory of intentions, in S. Pockett, W. P. Banks and S. Gallagher (eds), *Does Consciousness Cause Behavior? An Investigation of the Nature of Volition* (145–67). Cambridge, MA: MIT Press.

Pacherie, E., Green, M. & Bayne, T. (2006). Phenomenology and delusions: Who put the "alien"in alien control? *Consciousness and Cognition* 15(3): 566–77.

Pacherie, E., and Mylopoulos, M. (2021). Beyond automaticity: The psychological complexity of skill. *Topoi* 40(3): 649–62.

Palermos, S. O. 2014. Loops, constitution, and cognitive extension. *Cognitive Systems Research* 27: 25–41.

Papineau, D. (2013). In the zone. *Royal Institute of Philosophy* Supplement 73: 175–96.

Park, H. D. & Blanke, O. (2019). Coupling inner and outer body for self-consciousness. *Trends in Cognitive Sciences* 23(5): 377–88.

Park, J. & Kitayama, S. (2014). Interdependent selves show face-induced facilitation of error processing: Cultural neuroscience of self-threat. *Social Cognitive and Affective Neuroscience* 9(2): 201–8.

Parker, S. W. & Nelson, C. A. (2005). The impact of early institutional rearing on the ability to discriminate facial expressions of emotion: An event-related potential study. *Child Development* 76(1): 54–72.

Parnas, J. (2012). The core Gestalt of schizophrenia. *World Psychiatry* 11(2): 67–9.

Parnas, J., Bovet, P. & Innocenti, G. M. (1996). Schizophrenic trait features, binding, and cortico-cortical connectivity: A neurodevelopmental pathogenetic hypothesis. *Neurology, Psychiatry and Brain Research* 4(4): 185–96.

Parnas, J. & Gallagher, S. (2015). Phenomenology and the interpretation of psychopathological experience, in L. Kirmayer, R. Lemelson, and C. Cummings (eds), *Revisioning Psychiatry Integrating Biological, Clinical and Cultural Perspectives* (65–80). Cambridge: Cambridge University Press.

Parnas, J. & Henriksen, M. G. (2016). Mysticism and schizophrenia: A phenomenological exploration of the structure of consciousness in the schizophrenia spectrum disorders. *Consciousness and Cognition* 43: 75–88.

Parnas, J. & Henriksen, M. G. (2014). Disordered self in the schizophrenia spectrum: A clinical and research perspective. *Harvard Review of Psychiatry* 22(5): 251.

Parnas, J., Møller, P., Kircher, T., Thalbitzer, J., Jansson, L., Handest, P., Zahavi, D. (2005). EASE: Examination of Anomalous Self-Experience. *Psychopathology* 38: 236–58.

Parnas, J. & Zandersen, M. (2018). Self and schizophrenia: Current status and diagnostic implications. *World Psychiatry* 17(2): 220–1. https://doi.org/10.1002/wps.20528

Parvizi, J. (2009). Corticocentric myopia: Old bias in new cognitive sciences. *Trends in Cognitive Sciences* 13(8): 354–9.

Paskaleva, A. (2011). A phenomenological assessment of depression narratives. Master's thesis, University of Osnabrück. *Publications of the Institute of Cognitive Science* 3.

Pasqualini, I., Blefari, M. L., Tadi, T., Serino, A. & Blanke, O. (2018). The architectonic experience of body and space in augmented interiors. *Frontiers in Psychology* 9, 375: 1–15.

Paulus, M. P., Feinstein, J. S. & Khalsa, S. S. (2019). An active inference approach to interoceptive psychopathology. *Annual Review of Clinical Psychology* 15: 97–122.

Paxton, A. & Dale, R. (2013). Argument disrupts interpersonal synchrony. *Quarterly Journal of Experimental Psychology* 66(11): 2092–102.

Pedrini, P. (2015). Rescuing the "loss-of-agency" account of thought insertion. *Philosophy, Psychiatry, & Psychology* 22(3): 221–33.

Pellegrino, E. D. (2008). Letter of transmittal to the President of the United States, in President's Council on Bioethics (eds), *Human Dignity and Bioethics: Essays Commissioned by the President's Council on Bioethics*. Washington, DC. US Government Printing Office.

Pennebaker, J. W., Mehl, M. R. & Niederhoffer, K. G. (2003). Psychological aspects of natural language use: Our words, our selves. *Annual Review of Psychology* 54: 547–77.

Peper, C. E., van der Wal, S. J. & Begeer, S. (2016) Autism in action: Reduced bodily connectedness during social interactions? *Frontiers in Psychology* 7:1862. doi:10.3389/fpsyg.2016.01862

Pereira, A. F., Smith, L. B. & Yu, C. (2014). A bottom-up view of toddler word learning. *Psychonomic Bulletin & Review* 21(1): 178–85.

Petitmengin, C. (2014). Researching the microdynamics of intuitive experience, in *Handbook of Research Methods on Intuition* (188–98). Cheltenham: Edward Elgar Publishing. doi.org/10.4337/9781782545996.00024

Petitmengin, C. (2006). Describing one's subjective experience in the second person: An interview method for the science of consciousness. *Phenomenology and the Cognitive Sciences* 5(3): 229–69.

Philippi, C. L., Feinstein, J. S., Khalsa, S. S., Damasio, A., Tranel, D., Landini, G., Williford, K. & Rudrauf, D. (2012). Preserved self-awareness following extensive bilateral brain damage to the insula, anterior cingulate, and medial prefrontal cortices. *PLOS One* 7(8): e38413. https://doi.org/10.1371/journal.pone.0038413

Phillips, J. (2013). Technology and psychiatry, in K. W. M. Fulford, M. Davies, R. Gipps, G. Graham, J. Sadler, G. Stanghellini, and T. Thornton (eds), *The Oxford Handbook of Philosophy and Psychiatry* (176–16). Oxford: Oxford University Press.

Phillips, J. (2003). Schizophrenia and the narrative self, in A. S. David and T. Kircher (eds), *The Self in Neuroscience and Psychiatry* (319–35). Cambridge: Cambridge University Press.

Piredda, G. (2020). What is an affective artifact? A further development in situated affectivity. *Phenomenology and the Cognitive Sciences* 19: 549–67.

Platek, S. M., Myers, T. E., Critton, S. R. & Gallup, G. G. (2003). A left-hand advantage for self-description: The impact of schizotypal personality traits. *Schizophrenia Research* 65: 147–51.

Plessner, H. (1970). *Laughing and Crying: A Study of the Limits of Human Behavior.* Evanston, IL: Northwestern University Press.

Pöppel, E. (1994). Temporal mechanisms in perception. *International Review of Neurobiology* 37: 185–202.

Popper, K. R. & Eccles, J. C. (1977). *The Self and its Brain: An Argument for Interactionism.* New York: Springer-Verlag.

Preston, C. & Newport, R. (2014). Noisy visual feedback training impairs detection of self-generated movement error: Implications for anosognosia for hemiplegia. *Frontiers of Human Neuroscience* 8: 456. doi:10.3389/fnhum.2014.00456

Prikken, M., van der Weiden, A., Renes, R. A., Koevoets, M. G., Heering, H. D., Kahn R. S., et al. (2017). Abnormal agency experiences in schizophrenia patients: Examining the role of psychotic symptoms and familial risk. *Psychiatry Research* 250: 270–6. doi:10.1016/j.psychres.2016.10.077

Prinz, J. (2004). *Gut Reactions. A Perceptual Theory of Emotion.* NewYork: Oxford University Press.

Proust, J. (2009). Is there a sense of agency for thoughts? In L. O'Brien and M. Soteriou (eds), *Mental Actions* (253–79). Oxford: Oxford University Press.

Provenza, N. R., Paulk, A. C., Peled, N., Restrepo, M. I., Cash, S. S., Dougherty, D. D., Eskandar, E. N., Borton, D. A. & Widge, A. S. (2019). Decoding task engagement from distributed network electrophysiology in humans. *Journal of Neural Engineering* 16(5), 056015.

Pugh, J. (2020). Clarifying the normative significance of "personality changes" following deep brain stimulation. *Science and Engineering Ethics* 26(3): 1655–80.

Qin, P. & Northoff, G. (2011). How is our self related to midline regions and the default-mode network? *Neuroimage* 57(3): 1221–33.

Raballo, A. (2012). Self-disorders and the experiential core of schizophrenia spectrum vulnerability. *Psychiatria Danubina* 24(Suppl 3): S303–10.

Raballo, A., Monducci, E., Ferrara, M., Fiori Nastro, P., Dario, C. & Group, R. (2018). Developmental vulnerability to psychosis: Selective aggregation of basic self-disturbance in early onset schizophrenia. *Schizophrenia Research* 201: 367–72.

Rabjam, S. (2007). *The Great Medicine That Conquers Clinging to the Notion of Reality: Steps in Meditation on the Enlightened Mind.* Boulder, CO: Shambhala Publications.

Radden, J. (2009). *Moody Minds Distempered: Essays on Melancholy and Depression.* Oxford: Oxford University Press.

Radin, M. J. (1978). The jurisprudence of death: Evolving standards for the cruel and unusual punishments clause. *University of Pennsylvania Law Review* 126: 989–1064.

Raffard, S., D'Argembeau, A., Lardi, C., Bayard, S., Boulenger, J. P. & Van der Linden, M. (2010). Narrative identity in schizophrenia. *Consciousness and Cognition* 19(1): 328–40.

Raffone, A., & Barendregt, H. P. (2020). Global workspace models of consciousness in a broader perspective. In J. Mogensen, and M.S. Overgaard (eds.), *Beyond the Neural Correlates of Consciousness* (104-130). London: Psychology Press & Routledge.

Rainteau, N., Salesse, R. N., Macgregor, A., Macioce, V., Raffard, S. & Capdevielle, D. (2020). Why you can't be in sync with schizophrenia patients. *Schizophrenia Research* 216: 504–6.

Ramírez-Vizcaya, S. & Froese, T. (2019). The enactive approach to habits: New concepts for the cognitive science of bad habits and addiction. *Frontiers in Psychology* 10: 301.

Ramseyer, F. & Tschacher, W. (2011). Nonverbal synchrony in psychotherapy: Coordinated body movement reflects relationship quality and outcome. *Journal of Consulting and Clinical Psychology* 79(3): 284.

Ramstead, M. J., Veissière, S. P. & Kirmayer, L. J. (2016). Cultural affordances: Scaffolding local worlds through shared intentionality and regimes of attention. *Frontiers in Psychology* 7: 1090.

Ratcliffe, M. (2017). Selfhood, schizophrenia, and the interpersonal regulation of experience, in C. Durt, T. Fuchs, and C. Tewes (eds), *Embodiment, Enaction, and Culture: Investigating the Constitution of the Shared World* (149–72). Cambridge, MA: MIT Press.

Ratcliffe, M. (2014). *Experiences of Depression: A Study in Phenomenology.* Oxford: Oxford University Press.

Ratcliffe, M. (2012a). The phenomenology of existential feeling, in J. Fingerhut and S. Marienberg (eds), *Feelings of Being Alive* (23–54). Berlin: De Gruyter.

Ratcliffe, M. (2008). *Feelings of Being: Phenomenology, Psychiatry and the Sense of Reality.* Oxford: Oxford University Press.

Ratcliffe, M. (2006). *Rethinking Commonsense Psychology.* London: Palgrave Macmillan.

Ratcliffe, M. & Bortolan, A. (2020). Emotion regulation in a disordered world, in C. Tewes and G. Stanghellini (eds), *Time and Body: Phenomenological and Psychopathological Approaches* (177–200). Cambridge: Cambridge University Press.,

Reddy, V. (2008). *How Infants Know Minds.* Cambridge, MA: Harvard University Press.

Reed, J. & Ones, D. S. (2006). The effect of acute aerobic exercise on positive activated affect: A meta-analysis. *Psychology of Sport and Exercise* 7(5): 477–514.

Ricoeur, P. (1992). *Oneself as Another*, trans. K. Blamey. Chicago: University of Chicago Press.

Rietveld, E. (2008). Situated normativity: The normative aspect of embodied cognition in unreflective action. *Mind* 117(468): 973–1001. https://doi.org/10.1093/mind/fzn050

Rietveld, E. & Kiverstein, J. (2014). A rich landscape of affordances. *Ecological Psychology* 26(4): 325–52.

Riva, G., Bacchetta, M., Baruffi, M., Rinaldi, S. & Molinari, E. (1999). Virtual reality based experiential cognitive treatment of anorexia nervosa. *Journal of Behavior Therapy and Experimental Psychiatry* 30(3): 221–30.

Robinson, T. & Berridge, K. (2000). The psychology and neurobiology of addiction: An incentive-sensitization view. *Addiction* 95(8s2): 91–117.

Robinson, T. & Berridge, K. (1993). The neural basis of drug craving: An incentive-sensitization theory of addiction. *Brain Research Review* 18(3): 247–91.

Rochat, P. (2011). What is it like to be a newborn? in S. Gallagher (ed.), *The Oxford Handbook of the Self* (57–79). Oxford: Oxford University Press.

Rochat, P. (2001). *The Infant's World*. Cambridge, MA: Harvard University Press.

Roche, T. D. (2014). Happiness and external goods, in R. Polansky (ed.), *The Cambridge Companion to Aristotle's* Nicomachean Ethics (34–63). Cambridge: Cambridge University Press.

Roefs, A., Fried, E. I., Kindt, M., Martijn, C., Elzinga, B., Evers, A. W.... & Jansen, A. (2022). A new science of mental disorders: Using personalised, transdiagnostic, dynamical systems to understand, model, diagnose, and treat psychopathology. *Behaviour Research and Therapy* 153: 104096.

Roese, N. J., Epstude, K., Fessel, F., Morrison, M., Smallman, R., Summerville, A., Galinsky A. D. & Segerstrom S. (2009). Repetitive regret, depression, and anxiety: Findings from a nationally representative survey. *Journal of Social and Clinical Psychology* 28: 671–88.

Röhricht, F., Gallagher, S., Geuter, U. & Hutto, D. D. (2014). Embodied cognition and body psychotherapy: The construction of new therapeutic environments. *Sensoria: A Journal of Mind, Brain & Culture* 10(1): 11–20. http://dx.doi.org/10.7790/sa.v10i1.389

Röhricht F. & Priebe S. (2006). Effect of body-oriented psychological therapy on negative symptoms in schizophrenia: A randomized controlled trial. *Psychological Medicine* 36: 669–78.

Ronconi, L. & Melcher, D. (2017). The role of oscillatory phase in determining the temporal organization of perception: Evidence from sensory entrainment. *Journal of Neuroscience* 37(44): 10636–44.

Rosen, R. (1970). *Dynamical System Theory in Biology*. New York: Wiley-Interscience.

Rothbaum, B. O. & Hodges, L. F. (1999). The use of virtual reality exposure in the treatment of anxiety disorders. *Behavior Modification* 23(4): 507–25.

Rothbaum, B. O., Hodges, L. F., Kooper, R., Opdyke, D., Williford, J. S., & North, M. (1995). Virtual reality graded exposure in the treatment of acrophobia: A case report. *Behavior Therapy* 26(3), 547–554.

Ruby, P., Collette, F., D'Argembeau, A., Peters, F., Degueldre, C., Balteau, E., Luxen, A., Maquet, P., & Salmon, E. (2009). Perspective taking to assess self-personality: What's modified in Alzheimer's disease? *Neurobiology of Aging* 30: 1637–51.

Rueve, M. E. & Welton, R. S. (2008). Violence and mental illness. *Psychiatry* 5(5): 34–48.

Rus-Calafell, M., Garety, P., Sason, E., Craig, T. J. K. & Valmaggia, L. R. (2018). Virtual reality in the assessment and treatment of psychosis: A systematic review of its utility, acceptability and effectiveness. *Psychological Medicine* 48(3): 362–91.

Rutter, M., Andersen-Wood, L., Beckett, C., Bredenkamp, D., Casde, J. Groothues, C., Kreppner, J., Keaveriey, L., Lord, C., O'Connor T. G. & the English and Romanian Adoptees Study Team (1999). Quasi-autistic patterns following severe early global privation. *Journal of Child Psychology and Psychiatry* 40: 537–49.

Rutter, M., Kreppner, J., Croft, C., Murin, M., Colvert, E., Beckett, C. . . . & Sonuga-Barke, E. (2007). Early adolescent outcomes of institutionally deprived and non-deprived adoptees, III: Quasi-autism. *Journal of Child Psychology and Psychiatry* 48(12): 1200–7.

Ryan, K., Agrawal, P. & Franklin, S. (2020). The pattern theory of self in artificial general intelligence: A theoretical framework for modeling self in biologically inspired cognitive architectures. *Cognitive Systems Research* 62: 44–56.

Ryan, K. & Gallagher, S. (2020). Between ecological psychology and enactivism: Is there resonance? *Frontiers in Psychology* 11: 1147. https://doi.org/10.3389/fpsyg.2020.01147

Ryle, G. (1949). *The Concept of Mind*. London: Hutchinson's.

Salice, A., Høffding, S. & Gallagher, S. (2017). Putting plural self-awareness into practice: The phenomenology of expert musicianship. *Topoi* 38(1): 197–209. doi:10.1007/s11245-017-9451-2

Saltzman, E. L. & Munhall, K. G. (1989). A dynamical approach to gestural patterning in speech production. *Ecological Psychology* 1(4): 333–82.

Sandsten, K. E., Zahavi, D. & Parnas, J. (2022). Disorder of selfhood in schizophrenia: A symptom or a gestalt? *Psychopathology* 55(5): 273–281

Sartre, J.-P. 1956. *Being and Nothingness: An Essay on Phenomenological Ontology*, trans. H. E. Barnes. London: Routledge.

Sass, L. A. (2014). Self-disturbance and schizophrenia: Structure, specificity, pathogenesis. *Schizophrenia Research* 152(1): 5–11.

Sass, L. A. (2000). Schizophrenia, self-experience, and the so-called negative symptoms, in D. Zahavi (ed.), *Exploring the Self: Philosophical and Psychopathological Perspectives on Self-experience* (149–82). Amsterdam & Philadelphia: John Benjamins.

Sass, L. (1999). Schizophrenia, self-consciousness, and the modern mind, in S. Gallagher and J. Shear (eds), *Models of the Self* (319–41). Exeter: Imprint Academic

Sass, L. A. (1998). Schizophrenia, self-consciousness, and the modern mind. *Journal of Consciousness Studies* 5(5–6): 543–65.

Sass, L. (1995). *The Paradoxes of Delusion: Wittgenstein, Schreber, and the Schizophrenic Mind*. Ithaca: Cornell University Press.

Sass, L. A. (1992). Heidegger, schizophrenia and the ontological difference. *Philosophical Psychology* 5(2): 109–32.

Sass, L., Borda, J. P., Madeira, L., Pienkos, E. & Nelson, B. (2018). Varieties of self disorder: A bio-pheno-social model of schizophrenia. *Schizophrenia Bulletin* 44(4): 720–7.

Sass, L. A. & Parnas, J. (2003). Schizophrenia, consciousness, and the self. *Schizophrenia Bulletin* 29(3): 427–44.

Sass, L., Parnas, J. & Zahavi, D. (2011). Phenomenological psychopathology and schizophrenia: Contemporary approaches and misunderstandings. *Philosophy, Psychiatry, & Psychology* 18(1): 1–23.

Sass, L. & Pienkos, E. (2013). Varieties of self-experience: A comparative phenomenology of melancholia, mania, and schizophrenia, part I. *Journal of Consciousness Studies* 20(7–8): 103–30.

Sass L., Pienkos E., Nelson B. & Medford N. (2013). Anomalous self-experience in depersonalization and schizophrenia: A comparative investigation. *Consciousness and Cognition* 22: 430–41.

Sass, L., Pienkos, E., Skodlar, B., Stanghellini, B., Fuchs, T., Parnas, J. & Jones, N. (2017). EAWE: Examination of Anomalous World Experience. *Psychopathology* 50(1): 10–54.

Sass, L. & Ratcliffe, M. (2017). Atmosphere: On the phenomenology of "atmospheric" alterations in Schizophrenia—Overall sense of reality, familiarity, vitality, meaning, or relevance (Ancillary Article to EAWE Domain 5). *Psychopathology* 50(1): 90–7.

Sato, A. & Yasuda, A. (2005). Illusion of sense of self-agency: Discrepancy between the predicted and actual sensory consequences of actions modulates the sense of self-agency, but not the sense of self-ownership. *Cognition* 94: 241–55.

Sayadaw, M. (2016). *Manual of Insight*. New York: Simon and Schuster.

Scaer, R. C. (2014). *Body Bears the Burden, Vol. 3*. New York: Routledge.

Schaffner, K. F. (1993). *Discovery and Explanation in Biology and Medicine*. Chicago: University of Chicago Press.

Schechtman, M. (2015). The size of the self: Minimalist selves and narrative self-constitution, in A. Speight (ed.), *Narrative, Philosophy and Life* (33–47). Dordrecht: Springer.

Schechtman, M. (2011). The narrative self, in S. Gallagher (ed.), *The Oxford Handbook of the Self* (394–417). Oxford: Oxford University Press.

Schechtman, M. (2010). Philosophical reflections on narrative and deep brain stimulation. *The Journal of Clinical Ethics* 21(2): 133–9. PMID20866019

Schechtman, M. (2007). Stories, lives, and basic survival: A refinement and defense of the narrative view. *Royal Institute of Philosophy Supplements* 60: 155–78.

Schechtman, M. (1996). *The Constitution of Selves*. Ithaca, NY: Cornell University Press.

Schermer, M. (2011). Ethical issues in deep brain stimulation. *Frontiers in Integrative Neuroscience* 5: 17.

Schermer M. (2009). Changes in the self: The need for conceptual research next to empirical research. *The American Journal of Bioethics* 9(5): 45–7. doi.org/10.1080/15265160902788744; PMID19396686

Schloesser, D. S., Kello, C. T. & Marmelat, V. (2019). Complexity matching and coordination in individual and dyadic performance. *Human Movement Science* 66: 258–72.

Schlosser, M., Sparby, T., Vörös, S., Jones, R. & Marchant, N. L. (2019). Unpleasant meditation-related experiences in regular meditators: Prevalence, predictors, and conceptual considerations. *PLOS One* 14: e0216643.

Schmidt, P. (2021). Nobody? Disturbed self-experience in borderline personality disorder and five kinds of instabilities, in C. Tewes and S. G. Stanghellini (ed.), *Time, Body and the Other: Phenomenological and Psychopathologial Approaches* (206–29). Cambridge: Cambridge University Press.

Schmidt, P. & Fuchs, T. (2021). The unbearable dispersal of being: Narrativity and personal identity in borderline personality disorder. *Phenomenology and the Cognitive Sciences* 20(2): 321–40.

Schmidt, R. E. & Van der Linden, M. (2013). Feeling too regretful to fall asleep: Experimental activation of regret delays sleep onset. *Cognitive Therapy and Research* 37: 872–80.

Schmitz, L., Vesper, C., Sebanz, N. & Knoblich, G. (2017). Co-representation of others' task constraints in joint action. *Journal of Experimental Psychology: Human Perception and Performance* 43(8): 1480.

Schneider, S. (2019). *Artificial You: AI and the Future of Your Mind*. Princeton: Princeton University Press.

Schneider, S. (2009). Mindscan: Transcending and enhancing the human brain, in S. Schneider (ed.), *Science Fiction and Philosophy* (241–55). Oxford: Blackwell Publishing.

Schneider, S. & Mandik, P. (2018). How philosophy of mind can shape the future. *Philosophy of Mind in the 20th and 21th Century*. Abingdon: Routledge.

Schoenberg, P. L. & Vago, D. R. (2019). Mapping meditative states and stages with electrophysiology: Concepts, classifications, and methods. *Current Opinion in Psychology* 28: 211–17.

Scholz, S. (2000). *Body Narratives: Writing the Nation and Fashioning the Subject in Early Modern England*. London: Palgrave Macmillan.

Schultz, P. W. & Searleman, A. (2002). Rigidity of thought and behavior: 100 years of research. *Genetic, Social, and General Psychology Monographs* 128(2): 165.

Schüpbach, M., Gargiulo, M., Welter, M. L., Mallet, C., Béhar, C. & Houeto, J. L. (2006). Neurosurgery in Parkinson disease: A distressed mind in a repaired body? *Neurology* 66: 1811–16. doi:10.1212/01.wnl.0000234880.51322.16; PMID16801642

Searle, J. (1983). *Intentionality: An Essay in the Philosophy of Mind*. Cambridge: Cambridge University Press.

Sebanz N., Bekkering H. & Knoblich G. (2006). Joint action: Bodies and minds moving together. *Trends in Cognitive Sciences* 10: 70–6.

Sebanz, N., Knoblich, G. & Prinz, W. (2003). Representing others' actions: Just like one's own? *Cognition* 88: B11–21.

Séchehaye, M. (1968). *Autobiography of a Schizophrenic Girl*, trans. by G. Rubin-Rabson, New York: Plume.

Seeger, M. (2015). Authorship of thoughts in thought insertion: What is it for a thought to be one's own? *Philosophical Psychology* 28(6): 837–55.

Segal, Z. V., Williams, J. M. G., Teasdale, J. D. (2013). *Mindfulness-Based Cognitive Therapy for Depression*. New York: Guilford.

Seth, A. K. (2013). Interoceptive inference, emotion, and the embodied self. *Trends in Cognitive Sciences* 17(11): 565–73.

Seth, A. K. & Friston, K. J. (2016). Active interoceptive inference and the emotional brain. *Philosophical Transactions of the Royal Society B: Biological Sciences* 371(1708): 20160007.

Seth, A. K., Suzuki, K. & Critchley, H. D. (2011). An interoceptive predictive coding model of conscious presence. *Frontiers in Psychology* 2: 395. doi:10.3389/fpsyg.2011.00395

Shalev, S. (2009). *Supermax: Controlling Risk through Solitary Confinement*. Portland, OR: Willan.

Shapiro D. H. (1992). Adverse effects of meditation: A preliminary investigation of long-term meditators. *International Journal of Psychosomatics* 39: 62–7.

Shawn, A. (2008). *Wish I Could be There: Notes from a Phobic Life*. New York: Penguin.

Shiffrin, R. M. & Schneider, W. (1977). Controlled and automatic human information processing: I & II. Perceptual learning, automatic attending and a general theory. *Psychological Review* 84(1&2).

Shockley, K., Richardson, D. C. & Dale, R. (2009). Conversation and coordinative structures. *Topics Cognitive Science* 1: 305–19.

Shoemaker, S. (2011). On what we are, in S. Gallagher (ed.), *The Oxford Handbook of the Self* (352–71). Oxford: Oxford University Press.

Shoemaker, S. (1968). Self-reference and self-awareness. *Journal of Philosophy* 65; reprinted in Shoemaker, *Identity, Cause, and Mind*, Cambridge: Cambridge University Press, 1984.

Sierra, M., Baker, D., Medford, N. & David, A. S. (2005). Unpacking the depersonalization syndrome: An exploratory factor analysis on the Cambridge Depersonalization Scale. *Psychological Medicine* 35: 1523–32.

Sierra, M. & Berrios, G. E. (2001). The phenomenological stability of depersonalization: Comparing the old with the new. *The Journal of Nervous and Mental Disease* 189(9): 629–36.

Sierra, M. & Berrios, G. (2000). The Cambridge Depersonalization Scale: A new instrument for the measurement of depersonalization. *Psychiatry Research* 93(2): 153–64.

Sierra, M. & David, A. S. (2011). Depersonalization: A selective impairment of self-awareness. *Consciousness and Cognition* 20: 99–108.

Sigman, M. D., Kasari, C., Kwon, J. H. & Yirmiya, N. (1992). Responses to the negative emotions of others by autistic, mentally retarded, and normal children. *Child Development* 63(4): 796–807.

Simanowski, R., Brodmer, M. & Chase, J. (2019). On the ethics of algorithmic intelligence. *Social Research: An International Quarterly* 86(2): 423–47.

Simeon, D. & Abugel, J. (2006). *Feeling Unreal: Depersonalization Disorder and the Loss of the Self.* Oxford: Oxford University Press.

Simeon, D., Kozin, D. S., Segal, K., Lerch, B., Dujour, R. & Giesbrecht, T. (2008). Deconstructing depersonalization: Further evidence for symptom-clusters. *Psychiatry Research* 157: 303–6.

Simon, J. R. (1969). Reactions toward the source of stimulation. *Journal of Experimental Psychology* 81(1): 174.

Simondon, G. (2005). L'Individuation à la Lumière des Notions de Forme et d'Information. Grenoble: Millon.

Simondon, G. (1958). *Individuation in Light of Notions of Form and Information.* Minneapolis, MN: University of Minnesota Press.

Sinclair, D. C. (1955). Cutaneous sensation and the doctrine of specific energy. *Brain* 78: 584–614. doi:10.1093/brain/78.4.584

Singh, J., Knight, R. T., Rosenlicht, N., Kotun, J. M., Beckley, D. J. & Woods, D. L. (1992). Abnormal premovement brain potentials in schizophrenia. *Schizophrenia Research* 8(1): 31–41.

Sivathasan, S., Fernandes, T. P., Burack, J. A. & Quintin, E. M. (2020). Emotion processing and autism spectrum disorder: A review of the relative contributions of alexithymia and verbal IQ. *Research in Autism Spectrum Disorders* 77: 101608.

Slaby, J., Paskaleva, A. & Stephan, A. (2013). Enactive emotion and impaired agency in depression. *Journal of Consciousness Studies* 20(7–8): 33–55.

Slaby, J. & Stephan, A. (2008). Affective intentionality and self-consciousness. *Consciousness and Cognition* 17(2): 506–13.

Slatman J. (2005). The sense of life: Husserl and Merleau-Ponty touching and being touched. *Chiasmi International* 7: 305–325.

Slors, M., Francken, J. C. & Strijbos, D. (2019). Intentional content in psychopathologies requires an expanded interpretivism. *Behavioral and Brain Sciences* 42: 1–3 doi:10.1017/S0140525X18001176

Słowiński, P., Zhai, C., Alderisio, F., Salesse, R., Gueugnon, M., Marin, L., et al. (2016). Dynamic similarity promotes interpersonal coordination in joint action. *Journal of the Royal Society Interface* 13: 20151093. doi:10.1098/rsif.2015.1093

Smigielski, L., Kometer, M., Scheidegger, M., Stress, C., Preller, K. H., Koenig, T. & Vollenweider, F. X. (2020). P300-mediated modulations in self–other processing under psychedelic psilocybin are related to connectedness and changed meaning: A window into the self–other overlap. *Human Brain Mapping* 41(17): 4982–96.

Smith, P. S. (2006). The effects of solitary confinement on prison inmates: A brief history and review of the literature. *Crime and Justice* 34(1): 441–528.

Smith, P. (1988). Wit and chutzpah: Review of *The Intentional Stance* and Jerry A. Fodor's *Psychosemantics. Times Higher Education Supplement* (August 7), p. 22.

Snoek, A., Kennett, J. & Fry, C. (2012). Beyond dualism: A plea for an extended taxonomy of agency impairment in addiction. *AJOB Neuroscience* 3(2): 56–7.

Sofsky, W. (1996). *The Order of Terror*, trans. W. Templer. Princeton: Princeton University Press.

Soliman, T. M. & Glenberg, A. M. (2014). The embodiment of culture, in L. Shapiro (ed.), *The Routledge Handbook of Embodied Cognition* (207–20). London: Routledge.

Solomon, A. (2001). *The Noonday Demon: An Atlas of Depression.* New York: Scribner.

Soto-Andrade, J., Jaramillo, S., Gutiérrez, C. & Letelier, J. C. (2011). Ouroboros avatars: A mathematical exploration of self-reference and metabolic closure, in *Advances in Artificial Life ECAL 2011: Proceedings of the Eleventh European Conference on the Synthesis and Simulation of Living systems* (763–70). Cambridge, MA: MIT Press.

Sousa, P. & Swiney, L. (2013). Thought insertion: Abnormal sense of thought agency or thought endorsement? *Phenomenology and the Cognitive Sciences* 12(4): 637–54.

Spaniel, F., Tintera, J., Rydlo, J., Ibrahim, I., Kasparek, T., Horacek, J.... & Hajek, T. (2016). Altered neural correlate of the self-agency experience in first-episode schizophrenia-spectrum patients: An fMRI study. *Schizophrenia Bulletin* 42(4): 916–25.

Sparaci, L., Formica, D., Lasorsa, F. R., Mazzone, L., Valeri, G. & Vicari, S. (2015). Untrivial pursuit: Measuring motor procedures learning in children with autism. *Autism Research* 8(4): 398–411.

Sparaci, L., Northrup, J. B., Capirci, O. & Iverson, J. M. (2018). From using tools to using language in infant siblings of children with autism. *Journal of Autism and Developmental Disorders* 48(7): 2319–34.

Sparaci, L., Stefanini, S., D'Elia, L., Vicari, S. & Rizzolatti, G. (2014). What and why understanding in autism spectrum disorders and Williams Syndrome: Similarities and differences. *Autism Research* 7: 421–32.

Sparks, G. G., Pellechia, M., and Irvine, C. (1999). The repressive coping style and fright reactions to mass media. *Communication Research* 26: 176–92. doi:10.1177/009365099026002004

Spencer-Brown, G. (1969). *Laws of Form.* London: Allen & Unwin.

Stanghellini, G. (2017). Abnormal time experiences in major depression: An empirical qualitative study. *Psychopathology* 50(2): 125–40.

Stanley, J. (2011). *Know How.* Oxford: Oxford University Press.

Stein, D. J. (2012). Dimensional or categorical: Different classifications and measures of anxiety and depression. *Medicographia* 34: 270–5.

Stenzel, A., Chinellato, E., Bou, M. A. T., Del Pobil, Á. P., Lappe, M. & Liepelt, R. (2012). When humanoid robots become human-like interaction partners: Corepresentation of robotic actions. *Journal of Experimental Psychology: Human Perception and Performance* 38(5): 1073.

Stephens, G. L. & Graham, G. 2000. *When Self-Consciousness Breaks: Alien Voices and Inserted Thoughts.* Cambridge, MA: MIT Press.

Sterelny, K. (2010). Minds: extended or scaffolded? *Phenomenology and the Cognitive Sciences* 9(4), 465–481.

Stern, D. N. (2010). *Forms of Vitality.* Oxford: Oxford University Press.

Sterzer, P., Adams, R. A., Fletcher, P., Frith, C., Lawrie, S. M., Muckli, L., Petrovic, P., Uhlhaas, P., Voss, M. & Corlett, P. R. (2018). The predictive coding account of psychosis. *Biological Psychiatry* 84(9): 634–43.

Stirman, S. W. & Pennebaker, J. W. (2001). Word use in the poetry of suicidal and non-suicidal poets. *Psychosomatic Medicine* 63(4): 517–22.

Stone, O. & Zahavi, D. (2022). Bare attention, dereification, and meta-awareness in mindfulness: A phenomenological critique, in *Routledge Handbook on the Philosophy of Meditation* (341–53). London: Routledge.

Strawson, G. (2004). Against narrativity. *Ratio* 17(4): 428–542.

Strawson, G. (1999). The self and the SESMET. *Journal of Consciousness Studies* 6: 99–135.

Strawson, G. (1997). The self. *Journal of Consciousness Studies* 4(5–6): 405–28.

Strawson, P. F. (1994). The first person—and others, in Q Cassam (ed.), *Self-knowledge* (210–15). Oxford: Oxford University Press.

Sterzer, P., Adams, R. A., Fletcher, P., Frith, C., Lawrie, S. M., Muckli, L., Petrovic, P., Uhlhaas, P., Voss, M. & Corlett, P. R. (2018). The predictive coding account of psychosis. *Biological Psychiatry* 84(9): 634–43.

Stuss, D. T., Gallup, G. G., Jr. & Alexander, M. P. (2001). The frontal lobes are necessary for "theory of mind." *Brain* 124: 279–86.

Stuss, D. T., Picton, T. W., Alexander, M. P. (2001) Consciousness, self-awareness and the frontal lobes, in S. Salloway, P. Malloy, and J. Duffy (eds), *The Frontal Lobes and Neuropsychiatric Illness* (101–9). Washington, DC: American Psychiatric Press.

Styron, W. (1990). *Darkness Visible: A Memoir of Madness*. New York: Random House.

Sutton, J. (2009). The feel of the world: Exograms, habits, and the confusion of types of memory, in A. Kania (ed.), *Philosophers on Memento* (65–86). London: Routledge.

Sutton, J., McIlwain, D., Christensen, W. & Geeves, A. (2011). Applying intelligence to the reflexes: Embodied skills and habits between Dreyfus and Descartes. *Journal of the British Society for Phenomenology* 42(1): 78–103.

Suzuki, K., Garfinkel, S., Critchley, H. & Seth, A. K. (2013). Multisensory integration across interoceptive and exteroceptive domains modulates self-experience in the rubber-hand illusion. *Neuropsychologia* 51(13): 2909–17.

Swanson, J. W. (2021). Introduction: Violence and mental illness. *Harvard Review of Psychiatry* 29(1): 1–5.

Syme, K. L. & Hagen, E. H. (2020). Mental health is biological health: Why tackling "diseases of the mind" is an imperative for biological anthropology in the 21st century. *American Journal of Physical Anthropology* 171: 87–117.

Synofzik, M. (2013). Functional neurosurgery and deep brain stimulation, in A. Chatterjee and M. J. Farah (eds), *Neuroethics in Practice* (189–208). Oxford: Oxford University Press.

Synofzik, M. & Schlaepfer, T. E. (2008). Stimulating personality: Ethical criteria for deep brain stimulation in psychiatric patients and for enhancement purposes. *Biotechnological Journal* 3: 1511–20.

Synofzik, M., Thier, P., Leube, D. T., Schlotterbeck, P. & Lindner, A. (2010). Misattributions of agency in schizophrenia are based on imprecise predictions about the sensory consequences of one's actions. *Brain* 133(1): 262–71. http://doi.org/10.1093/brain/awp291

Synofzik, M., Vosgerau, G., and Newen, A. (2008). Beyond the comparator model: A multifactorial two-step account of agency. *Consciousness and Cognition* 17(1): 219–39.

Szalai, J. (2021). The potential use of artificial intelligence in the therapy of borderline personality disorder. *Journal of Evaluation in Clinical Practice* 27(3): 491–6.

Tabb, K. & Schaffner, K. F. (2017). Causal pathways, random walks and tortuous paths: Moving from the descriptive to the etiological in psychiatry, in K. S. Kendler and J. Parnas (eds), *Philosophical Issues in Psychiatry IV: Psychiatric Nosology* (342–60). Oxford: Oxford University Press.

Tager-Flusberg, H. & Anderson, M. (1991). The development of contingent discourse ability in autistic children. *Journal of Child Psychology and Psychiatry* 32: 1123–34.

Takahama, S., Kumada, T. & Saiki, J. 2005. Perception of other's action influences performance in Simon task [Abstract]. *Journal of Vision* 5(8): 396, 396a.

Taylor, C. (1989). *Sources of the Self: The Making of the Modern Identity*. Cambridge, MA: Harvard University Press.

Thom, R. (1975). *Structural Stability and Morphogenesis: An Outline of a General Theory of Models*. Reading, MA: W. A. Benjamin.

Thompson, E. (2020). *Why I Am Not a Buddhist*. New Haven: Yale University Press.

Thompson, E. (2010). Self-no-self? Memory and reflexive awareness, in M. Siderits, E. Thompson, & D. Zahavi (eds), *Self, No Self? Perspectives from Analytical, Phenomenological, and Indian Traditions* (157–75). Oxford: Oxford University Press.

Thompson, E. (2007). *Mind in Life: Biology, Phenomenology, and the Sciences of Mind.* Cambridge, MA: Harvard University Press.

Thompson, E. & Stapleton, M. (2009). Making sense of sense-making: Reflections on enactive and extended mind theories. *Topoi* 28: 23–30.

Teitelbaum, P., Teitelbaum, O., Nye, J., Fryman, J., and Maurer, R. G. (1998). Movement analysis in infancy may be useful for early diagnosis of autism. *Proceedings of the National Academy of Science of the United State of America* 95(23): 13982–7.

Tewes, C. (2021). Embodied selfhood and personal identity in dementia, in C. Tewes and G. Stanghellini (eds), *Time and Body: Phenomenological and Psychopathological Approaches* (367–89). Cambridge: Cambridge University Press.

Tisserand, A., Philippi, N., Botzung, A., & Blanc, F. (2023). Me, Myself and My Insula: An Oasis in the Forefront of Self-Consciousness. *Biology* 12(4), 599.

Tognoli, E. & Kelso, J. A. S. (2015). The coordination dynamics of social neuromarkers. *Frontiers in Human Neuroscience* 9: 563.

Tognoli, E. & Kelso, J. A. S. (2014). The metastable brain. *Neuron* 81: 35–48. https://doi.org/10.1016/j.neuron.2013.12.022

Tognoli, E., Zhang, M., Fuchs, A., Beetle, C. & Kelso, J. A. S. (2020). Coordination dynamics: A foundation for understanding social behavior. *Frontiers in Human Neuroscience* 14, 317: 1–15. doi: 10.3389/fnhum.2020.00317

Tognoli E., Zhang M., Kelso J. A. S. (2018) On the nature of coordination in nature, in J. Delgado-García, X. Pan, R. Sánchez-Campusano, and R. Wang (eds), *Advances in Cognitive Neurodynamics (VI).* Singapore: Springer.

Tollefsen, D. & Gallagher, S. (2017). We-narratives and the stability and depth of shared agency. *Philosophy of the Social Sciences* 47(2): 95–110.

Torous, J. (2017). Digital psychiatry. *IEEE Spectrum* 54(7): 45–50.

Torous, J., Bucci, S., Bell, I. H., Kessing, L. V., Faurholt-Jepsen, M., Whelan, P. . . . & Firth, J. (2021). The growing field of digital psychiatry: Current evidence and the future of apps, social media, chatbots, and virtual reality. *World Psychiatry* 20(3): 318–35.

Torres, E. B. (2013). A typical signatures of motor variability found in an individual with ASD. *Neurocase* 19: 150–65.

Torres, E. B., Brincker, M., Isenhower, R. W., Yanovich, P., Stigler, K. A., Nurnberger, J. I., Metaxas, D. N. & José, J. V. (2013). Autism: The micro-movement perspective. *Frontiers in Integrative Neuroscience* 7, 32: 1–26.

Travis, F. & Shear, J. (2010). Focused attention, open monitoring and automatic self-transcending: Categories to organize meditations from Vedic, Buddhist and Chinese traditions. *Consciousness and Cognition* 19(4): 1110–18.

Trevarthen, C. (1979) Communication and cooperation in early infancy: A description of primary intersubjectivity, in M. Bullowa (ed.), *Before Speech* (321–47). Cambridge: Cambridge University Press.

Trevarthen, C., and Daniel, S. (2005). Disorganized rhythm and synchrony: Early signs of autism and Rett syndrome. *Brain and Development Journal* 27: S25–34. doi:10.1016/j.braindev.2005.03.016

Trevarthen, C. & Delafield-Butt, J. T. (2013). Biology of shared meaning and language development: Regulating the life of narratives, in M. Legerstee, D. Haley, and M. Bornstein (eds), *The Infant Mind: Origins of the Social Brain* (167–99). New York: Guilford Press.

Trevarthen, C. & Hubley, P. (1978). Secondary intersubjectivity: Confidence, confiding and acts of meaning in the first year, in A. Lock (ed.), *Action, Gesture and Symbol: The Emergence of Language* (183–229). London: Academic Press.

Trigg, D. (2016). *Topophobia: A Phenomenology of Anxiety.* London: Bloomsbury Publishing.

Trigg, D. (2014). *The Thing: A Phenomenology of Horror.* Washington: Zero Books.

Trigg, D. (2013). The body of the other: Intercorporeality and the phenomenology of agoraphobia. *Continental Philosophy Review* 46(3): 413–29.

Tronick, E., Als, H., Adamson, L., Wise, S. & Brazelton, T. B. (1978). The infants' response to entrapment between contradictory messages in face-to-face interactions. *Journal of the American Academy of Child Psychiatry* 17: 1–13.

Tsakiris, M., Bosbach, S., and Gallagher, S. (2007). On agency and body-ownership: Phenomenological and neuroscientific reflections. *Consciousness and Cognition* 16(3): 645–60.

Tsakiris, M. & Haggard, P. (2005). Experimenting with the acting self. *Cognitive Neuropsychology* 22(3/4): 387–407.

Tsakiris, M., & Haggard, P. (2003). Awareness of somatic events associated with a voluntary action. *Experimental Brain Research* 149, 439–446.

Tsakiris, M., Longo, M. R. & Haggard, P. (2010). Having a body versus moving your body: Neural signatures of agency and body-ownership. *Neuropsychologia* 48(9): 2740–9.

Turgon, R., Ruffault, A., Juneau, C., Blatier, C. & Shankland, R. (2019). Eating disorder treatment: A systematic review and meta-analysis of the efficacy of mindfulness-based programs. *Mindfulness* 10(11): 2225–44.

Turk, D. J., Heatherton, T. F., Macrae, C. N., Kelley, W. M. & Gazzaniga, M. S. (2003). Out of contact, out of mind: The distributed nature of the self. *Annals of the New York Academy of Science* 1001: 65–78.

Ugelvik, T., Boyle, R. E., Jewkes, Y. & Nyvoll, P. S. (2022). Disrupting "healthy prisons": Exploring the conceptual and experiential overlap between illness and imprisonment. *The Howard Journal of Crime and Justice* 62(2): 204–219. https://doi.org/10.1111/hojo.12498

Værnes, T. G., Røssberg, J. I. & Møller, P. (2018). Anomalous self-experiences: Markers of schizophrenia vulnerability or symptoms of depersonalization disorder? A phenomenological investigation of two cases. *Psychopathology* 51: 198–209.

Vago, D. R. & Silbersweig, D. A. (2012). Self-awareness, self-regulation, and self-transcendence (S-ART): A framework for understanding the neurobiological mechanisms of mindfulness. *Frontiers in Human Neuroscience* 6, 296: 1–30. doi: 10.3389/fnhum.2012.00296

Vallar, G. & Ronchi, R. (2009). Somatoparaphrenia: A body delusion. A review of the neuropsychological literature. *Experimental Brain Research* 192(3): 533–51.

Van Dam, N. T., van Vugt, M. K., Vago, D. R., Schmalzl, L., Saron, C. D., Olendzki, A., Meissner, T., Lazar, S. W., Kerr, C. E., Gorchov, J. & Fox, K. C. (2018). Mind the hype: A critical evaluation and prescriptive agenda for research on mindfulness and meditation. *Perspectives on Psychological Science* 13(1): 36–61.

Van Duppen, Z. 2017. The intersubjective dimension of Schizophrenia. *Philosophy, Psychiatry, & Psychology* 24(4): 399–418.

Van der Hart, O., Nijenhuis, E. R. S. & Steele, K. (2006). *The Haunted Self: Structural Dissociation and the Treatment of Chronic Traumatization.* New York/London: W. W. Norton & Co.

Van der Hart, O., Nijenhuis, E., Steele, K. & Brown, D. (2004). Trauma-related dissociation: Conceptual clarity lost and found. *Australian and New Zealand Journal of Psychiatry* 38: 906–14.

Van der Kolk, B. A., Brown, P. & Van der Hart, O. (1989). Pierre Janet on post-traumatic stress. *Journal of Traumatic Stress* 2(4): 365–78. https://doi.org/10.1002/jts.2490020403

van Dis, E. A., Bollen, J., Zuidema, W., van Rooij, R. & Bockting, C. L. (2023). ChatGPT: Five priorities for research. *Nature* 614(7947): 224–6.

Varela, F. J. (1999). The specious present: A neurophenomenology of time consciousness, in J. Petitot, F. J. Varela, B. Pachoud, and J.-M. Roy (eds), *Naturalizing Phenomenology: Issues in Contemporary Phenomenology and Cognitive Science* (266–314). Stanford: Stanford University Press.

Varela, F. (1997). Patterns of life: Intertwining identity and cognition. *Brain and Cognition* 34: 72–87.

Varela, F. (1991). Organism: A meshwork of selfless selves, in A. I. Tauber (ed.), *Organism and the Origins of Self*. Boston studies in the philosophy of science, Vol. 129 (79–108). Dordrecht: Kluwer Academic.

Varela, F. (1975). A calculus for self-reference. *International Journal for General Systems* 2: 5–24.

Varela, F. & Goguen, J. A. (1978). The arithmetic of closure. *Journal of Cybernetics* 8(3–4): 291–324.

Varela, F., Thompson, E. & Rosch, E. (1991). *The Embodied Mind: Cognitive Science and Human Experience*. Cambridge, MA: MIT Press.

Varga, S. (2019). *Scaffolded Minds: Integration and Disintegration*. Cambridge, MA: MIT Press.

Varga, S. (2015). *Naturalism, Interpretation, and Mental Disorder*. Oxford: Oxford University Press.

Varga, S. (2012). Depersonalization and the sense of realness. *Philosophy, Psychiatry, & Psychology* 19(2): 103–13.

Vass, Á., Csukly, G. & Farkas, K. (2022). Transdiagnostic conceptualization of schizophrenia and autism spectrum disorder: An integrative framework of minimal self disturbance. psyarxiv.com. Preprint doi:10.31234/osf.io/vfuzh

Velleman, J. D. (2007). *Self to Self: Selected Essays*. New York: Cambridge University Press.

Velleman, J. D. (2005). Self as narrator, in J. Christman and J. Anderson (eds), *Autonomy and the Challenges to Liberalism: New Essays* (56–76). New York: Cambridge University Press.

Verplanken, B. & Sui, J. (2019). Habit and identity: Behavioral, cognitive, affective, and motivational facets of an integrated self. *Frontiers in Psychology* 10, 1504: 1–11. doi.org/10.3389/fpsyg.2019.01504.

Vidler, A. (2002). *Warped Space: Art, Architecture, and Anxiety in Modern Culture*. Cambridge, MA: MIT Press.

Vogeley, K. & Gallagher, S. (2011). The self in the brain, in S. Gallagher (ed.), *The Oxford Handbook of the Self* (111–36). Oxford: Oxford University Press.

Vogeley, K., May, M., Ritzl, A., Falkai, P., Zilles, K., & Fink, G. R. (2004). Neural correlates of first-person perspective as one constituent of human self-consciousness. *Journal of Cognitive Neuroscience* 16: 817–27. doi:10.1162/089892904970799

Von Bertalanffy, L. (1950). An outline of general system theory. *The British Journal for the Philosophy of Science* 1(2), 134–165.

Voss, M., Moore, J., Hauser, M., Gallinat, J., Heinz, A. & Haggard, P. (2010). Altered awareness of action in schizophrenia: A specific deficit in predicting action consequences. *Brain* 133(10): 3104–12. http://doi.org/10.1093/brain/awq152

Vrij, A. (2001). *Detecting Lies and Deceit: The Psychology of Lying and Implications for Professional Practice*. Chichester: Wiley & Sons.

Vrij, A. & Heaven, S. (1999). Vocal and verbal indicators of deception as a function of lie complexity. *Psychology, Crime, and Law* 5: 203–15.

Vu, M. A. T., Adalı, T., Ba, D., Buzsáki, G., Carlson, D., Heller, K. . . . & Dzirasa, K. (2018). A shared vision for machine learning in neuroscience. *Journal of Neuroscience* 38(7): 1601–7.

Wabnitz, P., Gast, U. & Catani, C. (2013). Differences in trauma history and psychopathology between PTSD patients with and without co-occurring dissociative disorders. *European Journal of Psychotraumatology* 4(1). doi:10.3402/ejpt.v4i0.21452

Walker C. (2014). Karl Jaspers on the disease entity: Kantian ideas and Weberian ideal types. *History of Psychiatry* 25: 317–34.

Wallace, D. F. (1998). The depressed person. *Harper's Magazine* 296: 57–64. January 1998.

Wallis, P. & Edmonds, B. (2021). An enactivist account of mind reading in natural language understanding. *arXiv preprint arXiv:2111.06179*. https://doi.org/10.48550/arXiv.2111.06179

Weiler, M., Northoff, G., Damasceno, B. P. & Balthazar, M. L. F. (2016). Self, cortical midline structures and the resting state: Implications for Alzheimer's disease. *Neuroscience & Biobehavioral Reviews* 68: 245–55.

Weiss, G. (1999). *Body Images: Embodiment as Intercorporeality*. New York: Routledge.

Wek, S. R. & Husal, W. S. (1989). Distributed and massed practice effects on motor performance and learning of autistic children. *Perceptual and Motor Skills* 68: 107–13.

Werner-Seidler, A. & Moulds, M. L. (2011). Autobiographical memory characteristics in depression vulnerability: Formerly depressed individuals recall less vivid positive memoricitedes. *Cognition & Emotion* 25: 1087–103.

West, K. L., Leezenbaum, N. B., Northrup, J. B. & Iverson, J. M. (2019). The relation between walking and language in infant siblings of children with autism spectrum disorder. *Child Development* 90(3): e356–72.

Westerbeck, J. & Mutsaers, K. (2008). Depression narratives: How the self became a problem. *Literature and Medicine* 27(1): 25–53.

Wexler, B. E., Stevens, A. A., Bowers, A. A., Sernyak, M. J. & Goldman-Rakic, P. S. (1998). Word and tone working memory deficits in schizophrenia. *Archives of General Psychiatry* 55(12): 1093–6.

Whyatt, C. & Craig, C. (2013). Sensory–motor problems in autism. *Frontiers Integrative Neuroscience* 7: 51.

Wielgosz, J., Goldberg, S. B., Kral, T. R., Dunne, J. D. & Davidson, R. J. (2019). Mindfulness meditation and psychopathology. *Annual Review of Clinical Psychology* 15: 285–316.

Wiens, T. K. & Walker, L. J. (2015). The chronic disease concept of addiction: Helpful or harmful? *Addiction Research & Theory* 23(4): 309–21.

Wiers, C. E., Gladwin, T. E., Ludwig, V. U., Gröpper, S., Stuke, H., Gawron, C. K....Bermpohl, F. (2017). Comparing three cognitive biases for alcohol cues in alcohol dependence. *Alcohol and Alcoholism* 52(2): 242–8.

Wiese, W. & Metzinger, T. (2017). Vanilla PP for philosophers: A primer on predictive processing, in *Philosophy and Predictive Processing*. Frankfurt am Main: MIND Group.

Wilkes, C., Kydd, R., Sagar, M. & Broadbent, E. (2017). Upright posture improves affect and fatigue in people with depressive symptoms. *Journal of Behavior Therapy and Experimental Psychiatry* 54: 143–9.

Williams, T. F. & Simms, L. J. (2020). The conceptual foundations of descriptive psychopathology, in A. Wright and M. Hallquist (eds), *The Cambridge Handbook of Research Methods in Clinical Psychology* (33–44). Cambridge: Cambridge University Press. https://doi.org/10.1017/9781316995808.006

Wimpory, D. C., Hobson, R. P., Williams, J. M. G. & Nash, S. (2000). Are infants with autism socially engaged? A study of recent retrospective parental reports. *Journal of Autism and Developmental Disorders* 30(6): 525–36.

Wimsatt, W. C. (2007). The ontology of complex systems: Levels of organization, perspectives, and causal thickets, in W. C. Wimsatt (ed.), *Re-engineering Philosophy for Limited Beings:*

Piecewise Approximations to Reality (193–240). Cambridge, MA: Harvard University Press; originally published in the *Canadian Journal of Philosophy* (1994) S20: 207–274.

Witt, K., Kuhn J., Timmermann, L., Zurowski, M. & Woopen, C. (2013). Deep brain stimulation and the search for identity. *Neuroethics* 6: 499–511. doi:10.1007/s12152-011-9100-1; PMID24273620

Wittgenstein, L. (1953). *Philosophical Investigations.* Oxford: Blackwell.

Wittgenstein, L. (1958). *The Blue and Brown Books.* Oxford: Blackwell.

Wolpert, L. (1999). *Malignant Sadness: The Anatomy of Depression.* New York: Free Press.

Woodward, J. (2020). Levels: What are they and what are they good for? In K. S. Kendler, J. Parnas, and P. Zachar (eds), *Levels of Analysis in Psychopathology: Cross-Disciplinary Perspectives* (424–49). Cambridge: Cambridge University Press.

Woodward, J. (2014). Cause and explanation in psychiatry: an interventionist perspective. In K. S. Kendler and J. Parnas (eds.), *Philosophical Issues in Psychiatry: Explanation, Phenomenology and Nosology* (209-272). Baltimore: John Hopkins University Press).

Woodward, J. (2003). *Making Things Happen: A Theory of Causal Explanation.* Oxford: Oxford University Press.

Wurtzel, E. (1995). *Prozac Nation: Young and Depressed in America.* New York: Riverhead.

Wutz, A., Weisz, N., Braun, C. & Melcher, D. (2014) Temporal windows in visual processing: "Prestimulus brain state" and "poststimulus phase reset" segregate visual transients on different temporal scales. *Journal of Neuroscience* 34: 1554–65. doi:10.1523/JNEUROSCI.3187-13.2014; PMID24453342

Yaden, D. B., Haidt, J., Hood Jr, R. W., Vago, D. R. & Newberg, A. B. (2017). The varieties of self-transcendent experience. *Review of General Psychology* 21(2): 143–60.

Yamaguchi, S., Shiozawa, T., Matsunaga, A., Bernick, P., Sawada, U., Taneda, A., Osumi, T. & Fujii, C. (2020). Development and psychometric properties of a new brief scale for subjective personal agency (SPA-5) in people with schizophrenia. *Epidemiology and Psychiatric Sciences* 29(e111): 1–8. https://doi.org/10.1017/S2045796020000256

Young, I. M. (1980). Throwing like a girl: A phenomenology of feminine body comportment, motility and spatiality. *Human Studies* 3(2): 137–56.

Yu, C. & Smith, L. B. (2012). Embodied attention and word learning by toddlers. *Cognition* 125(2): 244–62.

Yu, K. H., Beam, A. L. & Kohane, I. S. (2018). Artificial intelligence in healthcare. *Nature Biomedical Engineering* 2(10): 719–31.

Yuk, V., Anagnostou, E. & Taylor, M. J. (2020). Altered connectivity during a false-belief task in adults with autism spectrum disorder. *Biological Psychiatry: Cognitive Neuroscience and Neuroimaging* 5(9): 901–12.

Zachar, P. (2008). Real kinds but no true taxonomy: An essay in psychiatric systematics, in K. S. Kendler and J. Parnas (eds), *Philosophical Issues in Psychiatry* (327–54). Baltimore: Johns Hopkins University Press.

Zachar, P. (2002). The practical kinds model as a pragmatist theory of classification. *Philosophy, Psychiatry, & Psychology* 9(3): 219–27.

Zahavi, D. (2017). Thin, thinner, thinnest: Defining the minimal self, in C. Durt, T. Fuchs, and C. Tewes (eds), *Embodiment, Enaction, and Culture: Investigating the Constitution of the Shared World* (193-9). Cambridge, MA: MIT Press.

Zahavi, D. (2011). Unity of consciousness and the problem of self, in S. Gallagher (ed.), The *Oxford Handbook of the Self.* Oxford: Oxford University Press.

Zahavi, D. (2005). *Subjectivity and Selfhood: Investigating the First-Person Perspective.* Cambridge, MA: MIT Press.

Zahavi, D. & Loidolt, S. (2022). Critical phenomenology and psychiatry. *Continental Philosophy Review* 55(1): 55–75.

Zapata-Fonseca, L., Dotov, D., Fossion, R. & Froese, T. (2016). Time-series analysis of embodied interaction: Movement variability and complexity matching as dyadic properties. *Frontiers in Psycholology* 7: 1940. doi:10.3389/fpsyg.2016.01940

Zapata-Fonseca, L., Dotov, D., Fossion, R., Froese, T., Schilbach, L., Vogeley, K. & Timmermans, B. (2019). Multi-scale coordination of distinctive movement patterns during embodied interaction between adults with high-functioning autism and neurotypicals. *Frontiers in Psychology* 9: 2760.

Zawadzki, P. (2021). Dimensions of the threat to the self posed by deep brain stimulation: Personal identity, authenticity, and autonomy. *Diametros* 18(69): 71–98. doi:10.33392/diam.1592

Zhang, M., Kalies, W. D., Kelso, J. S. & Tognoli, E. (2020). Topological portraits of multi-scale coordination dynamics. *Journal of Neuroscience Methods* 339(1): 108672.

Zhao, Z., Salesse, R. N., Marin, L., Gueugnon, M. & Bardy, B. G. (2017). Likability's effect on interpersonal motor coordination: Exploring natural gaze direction. *Frontiers in Psychology* 8: 1864.

Index

cognitive (*cont.*)
  terms 136, 184
  theories 65
  therapy 213–14, 224
  views 2, 172–3
  workload 138
coherence 6, 27–8, 47, 60, 62, 105, 110, 118,
    126–7, 132–3, 145, 151–2, 164–5, 167,
    179, 212–13
coherency 61, 63–4, 94, 97, 125, 220–1, 255–6
coherent
  aggregate 219
  experience 28
  global pattern 60n.13
  integration 40–1, 127
  meaning 146–7
  narrative 146
  organization 91
  patterns 116–17, 163
  phenomenon 37
  self 217, 232–3
  self-narrative 136
  self-pattern 100
  sense of body 112
  sense of self 149
  sequences 210
  story 16–17, 133–4
  world 244–5
Cole, D. 206n.3
Cole, J. 56–7, 105, 155, 158n.2, 195, 214
College of Physicians 1, 256
Colombetti, G. 15, 30–1, 71–2
Colvert, E. 248
communication 72, 77, 79, 81, 83–7, 89–90,
    89n.12, 110–11, 133, 135, 141–2, 209–10,
    212–13, 248
communicative
  actions 82, 189, 211–12
  behavior 83
  delays 84
  environment 84
  interactions 81, 87, 189, 212
  intertwinement 21n.4
  practices 87, 247
  processes 65–6
  style 84
comorbidity 1–2, 9–10, 9n.6, 180
comparator 43, 111n.12, 172–3
  mechanisms 159–60, 170–1
  models 42, 116, 159n.3, 160
  processes 150t, 159n.3
complex systems 16, 53, 62, 78–9
composition 42, 44, 139–40
  constituent 48

constitution 47–8, 54
  relations 47–8, 50
computation 110–11
  models of the mind 2
  predictive models 110–11
  processes 2n.2
  psychiatry 200–1
  theory of mind 16n.1
computer 170, 205–6, 211–12
  connections 206
  interface 209
  program 207
  science 61n.15
  screen 160, 205
  systems 211
computer-assisted interview program 209n.4
computer-based communication 212, 215
computer-based technologies 212
computer-generated avatar 89, 215
concentration camps 240n.1, 241–2
conceptual
  articulation 169–70
  distinction 25
  fuziness 24
  proliferation 222
  self 5
  self-consciousness 171–2
  sense of self 123–4, 224–5
  thought 32
  understanding 19t, 21, 123
Condillac, É. 26–7
Coninx, S. 46
conscious
  component 14
  content 98–9
  control 70
  experiences 54–5, 204, 222
  mental states 159
  monitoring 69
  perceptual clues 73n.7
  self 93
  self-model 99
  thinking 125, 156, 170–1
consciousness 4, 17, 19t, 20–1, 26–7, 55n.11,
    94–5, 133, 138, 147, 159n.3, 168–9, 202,
    204–5, 207, 212–13, 219–20, 222,
    225–6, 230–6
Constant, A. 2–3, 84–5, 110–11, 114n.16, 200–1
constraints 15, 19t, 21–3, 42–3, 60n.14, 70–2,
    112, 167–9, 187, 189–90, 208–9, 255–6
continuity 2n.1, 16–17, 16n.1, 19t, 21, 32, 63–4,
    94, 112, 118–19, 125, 141–2, 151, 207, 230
Conze, E. 221
Cook, J. L. 83–4